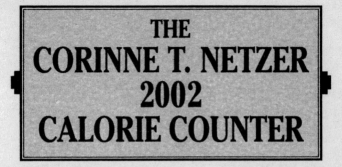

# THE
# CORINNE T. NETZER
# 2002
# CALORIE COUNTER

## Corinne T. Netzer

A Dell Book

13036306

Published by
Dell Publishing
a division of
Random House, Inc.
1540 Broadway
New York, New York 10036

Cover photo by Stockbyte

Dell books may be purchased for business or promotional use or for special sales. For information please write to: Special Markets Department, Random House, Inc., 1540 Broadway, New York, NY 10036.

Dell® is a registered trademark of Random House, Inc., and the colophon is a trademark of Random House, Inc.

ISBN: 0-440-23676-2

Printed in the United States of America

Published simultaneously in Canada

September 2001

10  9  8  7  6  5  4  3  2  1

OPM

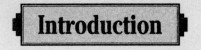

# Introduction

*The Corinne T. Netzer Calorie Counter* has been compiled with a twofold purpose: to keep you up to date with many of the changes made by the food industry, and to provide a handy source that you can carry in purse or pocket.

To keep this book concise yet comprehensive, I have grouped together listings of the same manufacturer whenever possible. Many brand-name yogurts, for example, are listed as "all fruit flavors." Therefore, instead of three pages filled with individual flavors of yogurt, all with identical calorie counts, I have been able to use the extra space for many other products. And for many basic foods and beverages (such as oil, milk, cream, and alcoholic beverages), I have used generic listings, rather than include numerous brands with the same or similar caloric values.

Finally, in the process of updating this edition, it was necessary to eliminate many previous listings and brands to accommodate new products and different brands. If you do not find a specific brand-name food that was listed in a previous edition of this book, this does not necessarily mean that the food product is no longer available. Also, since food producers are constantly revising and improving products, the calorie counts of your favorite foods may have changed even if the description of the product hasn't. Be sure to check for updated entries.

This book contains data from individual producers and manufacturers and from the United States government. It contains the most current information available as we go to press.

Good luck—and good eating.

*C.T.N.*

# Abbreviations

| | |
|---|---|
| approx. | approximately |
| cont. | container |
| diam. | diameter |
| fl. | fluid |
| lb. | pound |
| oz. | ounce |
| pc. | piece |
| pkg. | package |
| pkt. | packet |
| tbsp. | tablespoon |
| tsp. | teaspoon |
| w/ | with |

# Symbols

| | |
|---|---|
| " | inch |
| * | prepared according to basic package directions |
| < | less than |

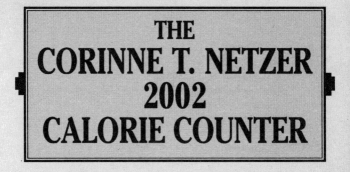

# THE
# CORINNE T. NETZER
# 2002
# CALORIE COUNTER

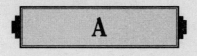

## A

**FOOD AND MEASURE**                             **CALORIES**

**Acerola juice,** fresh, 8 fl. oz. .....................................56
**Acorn squash,** fresh:
raw, 4"-diam., 15.2 oz. ...........................................172
baked, cubed, 1 cup ...............................................115
**Adzuki bean,** dry (*Arrowhead Mills*), ¼ cup ....................160
**Alfredo sauce, in jars,** ¼ cup:
(*Classico* Alfredo Di Roma) .....................................110
cheese, see "Cheese sauce, cooking"
garlic, roasted (*Classico* Di Sorrento) ......................110
sun-dried tomato (*Classico* Di Capri) ........................110
**Alfredo sauce, refrigerated,** ¼ cup:
(*Contadina Buitoni/Contadina Buitoni* Light) .................180
(*Di Giorno*) ..........................................................180
(*Di Giorno Light Varieties*) ......................................140
mushroom (*Contadina Buitoni* ) ...............................100
**Allspice,** 1 tsp. .........................................................5
**Almond,** shelled, except as noted:
(*Beer Nuts* Choice), 1 oz. ........................................170
natural, whole (*Dole*), ¼ cup, 1.23 oz. .......................170
natural, sliced (*Dole*), ⅓ cup, 1.1 oz. ........................170
blanched, whole (*Dole*), ¼ cup, 1.23 oz. ....................180
sliced (*Planters*), ⅓ cup ..........................................200
slivered (*Planters*), 2-oz. pkg. .................................340
dry roasted, whole kernels, ¼ cup ...............................206
honey roasted, whole kernels, 1 oz. .............................168
oil roasted, 1 oz., 22 kernels .....................................172
oil roasted, whole kernels, ¼ cup ................................238
smoked (*Planters*), 1 oz. ..........................................170
**Almond butter** (*Arrowhead Mills*), 2 tbsp. .....................210
**Amaranth leaf,** boiled, drained, 1 cup ..........................28
**Anchovy,** canned in olive oil, drained (*Duet*), 6 pcs. .........25
**Anchovy paste** (*Reese's*), 1 tbsp. ...............................30
**Andouille sausage,** cooked (*Aidell's*), 3.5-oz. link ...........220

**Angel hair pasta,** plain:

dry, see "Pasta"

refrigerated (*Contadina Buitoni*), 1¼ cups ...............................230

refrigerated (*Di Giorno*), 2 oz. .................................................160

**Angel hair pasta entree,** frozen, Alfredo (*Lean Cuisine
Everyday Favorites*), 10-oz. pkg...........................................240

**Angel hair pasta mix,** about 1 cup\*:

w/herbs or Parmesan cheese (*Pasta Roni*) .............................320

w/lemon and butter (*Pasta Roni*)............................................360

**Anise seed,** 1 tsp. .......................................................................7

**Apple,** fresh:

raw (*Dole Cameo*), 1 medium, 5.4 oz. ......................................80

raw (*Frieda's* Lady Apple), 5 oz. ..............................................80

raw, w/peel, sliced, 1 cup .........................................................65

raw, peeled, 1 medium, 2¾" diam., 5.3 oz. ................................72

raw, peeled, sliced, 1 cup .........................................................63

boiled, peeled, sliced, 1 cup .....................................................91

**Apple, canned:**

cinnamon (*Del Monte Fruitrageous* Cup), 4 oz. ........................80

spiced (*Del Monte Fruit Pleasures*), ½ cup..............................70

**Apple, dried,** sulfured, uncooked, 1 cup .................................209

**Apple, escalloped,** frozen (*Stouffer's*), ½ of 12-oz. pkg. ......180

**Apple, frozen,** sliced, unheated, 1 cup .....................................83

**Apple butter,** 1 tbsp.:

(*Lucky Leaf/Musselman's*) .......................................................30

all varieties (*Smucker's*) ..........................................................45

**Apple drink blend,** cranberry or grape (*Mott's*), 8 fl. oz. .......120

**Apple fritter,** frozen (*Mrs. Paul's*), 2 pcs. ...........................240

**Apple juice,** 8 fl. oz.:

(*Apple Time/Lincoln/Speas Farm*)...........................................120

(*Juicy Juice*) .........................................................................120

(*Lucky Leaf* Old Fashioned/Cider/Premium Select)..................120

(*Minute Maid*) .......................................................................110

(*Mott's* 16/64 oz.) .................................................................120

(*Musselman's/Musselman's* Premium/*Musselman's* Natural)..120

(*Musselman's* Premium Natural) ............................................130

unsweetened (*Mott's* Natural) ................................................110

sparkling cider (*Lucky Leaf/Musselman's*)...............................150

**Apple juice blend,** cranberry (*Mott's*), 11.5-fl.-oz. can............180

**Apple nectar** (*Libby's*), 11.5-fl.-oz. can ....................................200
**Applesauce,** canned:
natural/unsweetened:
    (*Apple Time* Original/*Lucky Leaf* Old Fashioned), 4 oz. ..........50
    (*Mott's*), 3.9-oz. cont. ....................................50
    cinnamon (*Apple Time* Original/*Lucky Leaf* ), 4-oz. cup........50
    cinnamon (*Lucky Leaf/Musselman's* Natural), 4 oz...............50
sweetened:
    (*Lucky Leaf/Lucky Leaf* Premium), 4 oz. ....................90
    (*Lucky Leaf/Musselman's*), 4-oz. cup........................80
    (*Mott's* Original), 4-oz. cont. .............................90
    (*Musselman's/Musselman's* Premium), 4 oz.....................90
    chunky (*Lucky Leaf* ), 4 oz. ...............................90
    chunky (*Musselman's* Homestyle), 4 oz. ...................100
    cinnamon (*Lucky Leaf* ), 4-oz. cup .........................80
    cinnamon (*Lucky Leaf/Lucky Leaf* Deluxe), 4 oz. .............100
    cinnamon (*Mott's*), 4-oz. cont. ...........................100
    cinnamon (*Musselman's*), 4-oz. cup ........................80
    cinnamon (*Musselman's* Deluxe), 4-oz. cup..................90
**Applesauce fruit blend,** 4-oz. cont.:
all flavors, except mango peach (*Mott's Fruitsations*).................90
berry, mixed (*Mott's*) ..............................................90
mango peach (*Mott's Fruitsations*)..................................100
strawberry (*Mott's*) ................................................80
**Apricot,** fresh:
(*Dole*), 3 medium, 4 oz...............................................60
pitted, halves, 1 cup ................................................74
pitted, sliced, 1 cup ................................................79
**Apricot, canned,** ½ cup, except as noted:
(*Del Monte* Lite)....................................................60
in juice, halves, w/skin, 1 cup .....................................117
in extra light syrup, halves, w/skin, 1 cup..........................121
in light syrup, halves (*Del Monte Orchard Select*)....................90
in light syrup, almond flavor (*Del Monte*) ..........................90
in heavy syrup, halves, w/out skin (*S&W*) ...........................120
in heavy syrup, halves, w/skin (*Del Monte*) .........................100
**Apricot, dried,** sulfured, halves, uncooked, 1 cup .................309
**Apricot nectar** (*Libby's*), 8 fl. oz. ............................150
**Apricot syrup** (*Smucker's*), ¼ cup ...............................210

**Arby's,** 1 serving:
breakfast items:

| | |
|---|---|
| bacon, 2 strips | 90 |
| biscuit w/margarine | 270 |
| croissant | 260 |
| eggs, scrambled | 70 |
| French *Toastix,* plain, 6 pcs. | 370 |
| ham | 50 |
| maple syrup, 1.5 oz. | 220 |
| sausage patty | 200 |

chicken sandwiches:

| | |
|---|---|
| chicken bacon 'n Swiss | 610 |
| chicken breast fillet | 560 |
| chicken Cordon Bleu | 650 |
| grilled chicken deluxe | 420 |
| roast chicken club | 540 |

roast beef sandwiches:

| | |
|---|---|
| *Arby's* melt w/cheddar or *Arby-Q* | 380 |
| beef 'n cheddar | 510 |
| *Big Montana* | 720 |
| giant roast beef | 550 |
| junior roast beef | 340 |
| regular roast beef | 400 |
| super roast beef | 530 |

sub sandwiches:

| | |
|---|---|
| French dip | 490 |
| hot ham 'n Swiss | 570 |
| Italian | 800 |
| Philly beef 'n Swiss | 780 |
| roast beef | 770 |
| turkey | 670 |

light menu:

| | |
|---|---|
| garden salad, w/crouton pkt. and 2 saltines | 110 |
| grilled chicken | 190 |
| grilled chicken salad | 230 |
| roast chicken deluxe | 260 |
| roast chicken salad | 200 |
| roast turkey deluxe | 230 |
| side salad, w/crouton pkt. and 2 saltines | 90 |

chicken finger snack .................................................610
chicken finger meal.................................................880
side items:
    curly fries, cheddar ...........................................450
    curly fries, large ..............................................600
    curly fries, medium .........................................380
    curly fries, small.............................................320
    homestyle fries, large......................................630
    homestyle fries, medium ................................420
    homestyle fries, small ....................................340
    *Jalapeno Bites*.............................................330
    mozzarella sticks ...........................................470
    onion petals.................................................410
    potato, baked, w/butter and sour cream.............500
    potato, baked, broccoli 'n cheddar....................550
    potato, baked, deluxe ....................................610
    potato cakes, 2 pcs. .....................................220
condiments:
    *Arby's Sauce,* pkt. ........................................15
    BBQ dipping sauce .........................................40
    beef stock au jus ...........................................10
    bleu cheese dressing ....................................390
    *Bronco Berry Sauce* .....................................90
    buttermilk ranch dressing ..............................210
    buttermilk ranch dressing, reduced calorie .........50
    German mustard, pkt. .......................................5
    honey French dressing....................................350
    honey mustard ..............................................130
    *Horsey Sauce,* pkt. .......................................60
    Italian dressing, reduced calorie .....................20
    ketchup, pkt.................................................10
    mayonnaise, pkt. ...........................................86
    mayonnaise, light, pkt. ...................................20
    marinara sauce..............................................35
    *Tangy Southwest Sauce*................................250
    Thousand Island dressing...............................350
desserts and shakes:
    apple turnover, iced........................................360
    cherry turnover, iced .....................................350

*Arby's* **desserts and shakes (*cont.*)**

shake, chocolate, 10.3 oz. .....................................390

shake, Jamocha, strawberry or vanilla, 10.3 oz. .......380

**Arrowhead,** boiled, drained, 1 medium, .4 oz. corm ...............10

**Artichoke,** French or globe, fresh:

raw (*Dole*), 1 medium, 4.5 oz. .............................60

raw, 1 large, 5.7 oz. ...........................................76

boiled, drained, 1 medium, 4.2 oz. ........................60

boiled, drained, hearts, ½ cup..............................42

**Artichoke, canned,** hearts (*Reese*), 2 pcs., w/liquid ...........50

**Artichoke, frozen,** hearts (*Birds Eye Deluxe*), ½ cup.............40

**Artichoke, Jerusalem,** see "Jerusalem artichoke"

**Artichoke, pickled,** in jars (*Braswell's*), 3 pcs., 1 oz. ...............15

**Artichoke dip** (*Victoria*), 2 tbsp..................................30

**Artichoke salad,** in jars (*Reese's*), ⅓ cup .....................150

**Arugula,** fresh, raw, ½ cup .........................................3

**Asparagus,** fresh:

raw (*Dole*), 5 spears, 3.3 oz. ................................25

raw (*Frieda's*), ⅔ cup, 3 oz. ...............................20

boiled, drained, 4 spears, ½" diam. base..................14

boiled, drained, ½ cup.......................................22

**Asparagus, canned:**

all styles (*Del Monte*), ½ cup .............................20

spears, extra large (*Le Sueur*), ½ cup ...................20

spears, extra long (*Green Giant*), 4.5 oz., approx. 5 spears .......20

cut spears (*Green Giant*), ½ cup...........................20

white, spears (*Haddon House*), 6 pcs., approx. 4.6 oz...............15

**Asparagus, frozen:**

(*Birds Eye* Stir Fry), 2 cups ...............................90

(*Freshlike*), 7 spears.........................................20

boiled, drained, 1 cup .......................................50

spears (*Birds Eye* Deluxe), 8 spears......................20

spears (*Seabrook Farms*), ⅓ cup..........................20

cuts (*Birds Eye* Deluxe), ½ cup............................25

cuts (*Green Giant*), ⅔ cup..................................20

cuts (*Freshlike* Select), ¾ cup.............................20

**Asparagus, pickled,** in jars (*Hogue Farms*), 3 spears ...............10

**Asparagus bean,** see "Winged bean"

**Atemoya** (*Frieda's*), 3-oz. fruit....................................80

**Au jus gravy,** in jars, ¼ cup:

(*Franco-American*).........................................................................10

(*Heinz* Home Style Bistro) ..............................................15

**Au jus gravy mix** (*Knorr*), 1 tsp. or ¼ cup*...........................10

**Aubergine,** see "Eggplant"

**Australian blue squash** (*Frieda's*), ¾ cup, 3 oz...........................30

**Avocado,** fresh

(*Frieda's Cocktail*), 1.4-oz. fruit..............................................60

all varieties, cubed, 1 cup......................................................242

California, trimmed, 1 fruit, peeled and seeded, 6 oz................306

California, pureed, 1 cup .........................................................407

Florida, trimmed, 1 fruit, peeled and seeded, 10.75 oz............340

Florida, pureed, 1 cup.............................................................258

**Avocado dip** (*Kraft*), 2 tbsp. ......................................................60

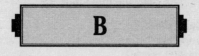

# B

**FOOD AND MEASURE**                **CALORIES**

**Bacon,** cooked, 2 slices, except as noted:
(*Hormel* Fully Cooked), 2½ slices ...............................................70
(*Oscar Mayer*) .....................................................................70
(*Oscar Mayer* Ready to Serve), 3 slices ....................................70
(*Plumrose* Premium) .............................................................80
thick sliced (*Oscar Mayer* Hearty), 1 slice................................60
**Bacon, Canadian style** (*Hormel*), 2 slices, 2 oz. ......................70
**"Bacon," vegetarian** (*Lightlife* Fakin' Bacon), 3 slices .............80
**Bacon bits,** 1 tbsp.:
bits (*Hormel* Real) ................................................................30
chips, crispy (*Hormel* Real).....................................................45
pieces (*Hormel* Real) ............................................................25
**"Bacon" bits, imitation** (*Bac*Os*), 1½ tbsp. .............................30
**Bacon dip,** 2 tbsp.:
horseradish (*Kraft/Kraft* Premium)...........................................60
onion (*Breakstone's/Kraft* Premium) ........................................60
**Bagel,** 1 pc., except as noted:
plain (*Awrey's*), 4 oz. ...........................................................270
plain (*Thomas'* New York Style) ..............................................280
plain or cinnamon raisin (*Awrey's*), 2.6 oz.................................190
plain or cinnamon raisin (*Awrey's*), 2 oz...................................150
blueberry or cinnamon raisin (*Awrey's*), 4 oz. ...........................280
blueberry or cinnamon swirl (*Thomas'* New York Style) ...........300
cinnamon raisin swirl (*Thomas'* New York Style) .....................290
**Bagel, frozen,** 2.8-oz. pc.:
all varieties, except cinnamon raisin (*Sara Lee*) .....................210
cinnamon raisin (*Sara Lee*)....................................................220
**Baked beans** (see also specific bean listings), ½ cup:
(*Allens*) ..............................................................................150
(*B&M* Original 8 oz.)..............................................................180
(*Campbell's* Old Fashioned/New England Style)......................180
(*Greene's Farm*) ...................................................................150
(*Van Camp's* Original/Southern Style) .....................................145

bacon and onion (*B&M*) ............................................................190
maple sugar (*S&W* Fat Free) ..................................................150
w/pork (*Van Camp's* Large) ...................................................100
w/pork (*Van Camp's* Small) ...................................................110
w/pork (*Van Camp's* Southwestern) .......................................125
w/pork (*Wagon Master/Trappey's*) .........................................110
w/pork, tomato sauce (*Campbell's*) ........................................130
vegetarian (*B&M*) ..................................................................150
**Baking mix** (see also "Biscuit mix"), all-purpose:
(*Bisquick* Original), ⅓ cup ....................................................160
(*Bisquick* Reduced Fat), ⅓ cup .............................................140
(*Bisquick* Sweet), ⅓ cup ......................................................170
(*"Jiffy"*), ¼ cup ....................................................................130
**Baking powder** (*Calumet*), ¼ tsp. ............................................0
**Baking soda,** 1 tsp. ....................................................................0
**Balsam pear,** fresh (*Frieda's* Bitter Melon), 1 cup, 3 oz. ....15
**Bamboo shoots,** fresh, boiled, drained, ½" slices, 1 cup ..........14
**Bamboo shoots, canned,** drained, sliced, 1 cup ......................25
**Banana** (see also "Plantain"), fresh:
(*Frieda's* Burro/Ice Cream/Nino), 3-oz. banana .....................80
(*Frieda's* Red), 5-oz. banana ...............................................130
8¾" banana ............................................................................105
sliced, 1 cup ..........................................................................138
**Banana, dried** (*Frieda's*), 1.2-oz. pc. .................................130
**Banana milk** (*Nesquik*), 1 cup...........................................200
**Banana nectar** (*Libby's*), 11.5-fl.-oz. can .........................190
**Banana squash** (*Frieda's*), ¾ cup, 3 oz. .............................30
**Barbecue dip,** sweet and spicy (*Kraft*), 2 tbsp. .....................60
**Barbecue pocket,** frozen (*Hot Pockets*), 4.5-oz. pc. .............340
**Barbecue sauce,** 2 tbsp.:
(*D. L. Jardine's* 5-Star) ........................................................40
(*Kraft* Char-Grill) .................................................................60
(*Kraft* Extra Rich Original/*Kraft Thick 'N Spicy* Original) .............50
(*Kraft* Original) ....................................................................40
all varieties (*Muir Glen* Organic) ..........................................40
brown sugar or hickory bacon (*Kraft Thick 'n Spicy*) ................60
hickory smoke (*Kraft Thick 'n Spicy*) ....................................50
hickory smoke, mesquite smoke, or hot (*Kraft*) ......................40
honey, roasted garlic, or Kansas City (*Kraft*) ..........................50

**Barbecue sauce (*cont.*)**

honey, honey mustard, or Kansas City (*Kraft Thick 'n Spicy*) ....60
honey hickory, honey mustard, or teriyaki (*Kraft*).....................60
hot (*D. L. Jardine's* Killer)...............................................................35
Korean style (*Sun Luck*) ................................................................45
mesquite smoke (*Kraft Thick 'n Spicy*)...........................................50
mesquite or Texas pecan (*D. L. Jardine's*) ...................................35
mustard (*D. L. Jardine's* Chik'n-Lik'n) ............................................40
molasses (*Kraft*)...............................................................................70
onion bits or hickory w/onion bits (*Kraft*) .....................................45
**Barbecue seasoning,** hickory (*Wyler's Shakers*), 1 tsp.............10
**Barley,** pearled:
dry (*Arrowhead Mills*), ¼ cup ....................................................170
cooked, 1 cup ..............................................................................193
**Barley flour or meal** (*Arrowhead Mills*), ¼ cup .........................93
**Basil,** fresh:
1 oz. ..................................................................................................8
5 medium leaves.............................................................................<1
**Basil, dried,** ground, 1 tsp. ............................................................4
**Bass** (see also "Sea bass"), meat only:
freshwater, raw, 4 oz......................................................................129
freshwater, baked, broiled, or microwaved, 4 oz......................166
striped, raw, 4 oz. ...........................................................................110
striped, baked, broiled, or microwaved, 4 oz. ...........................141
**Batter mix** (*Hodgson Mill Don's Chuck Wagon*), ¼ cup ..........100
**Bay leaf, dried,** crumbled, 1 tsp......................................................2
**Bean dip,** 2 tbsp.:
(*Fritos/Fritos Hot*) .............................................................................40
black bean (*Taco Bell Home Originals* Fat Free).........................30
**Bean dish,** see specific bean listings
**Bean salad:**
(*Cedarlane* Caribbean), ½ cup.....................................................160
(*Green Giant*), ½ cup .......................................................................70
4 (*Hanover*), ⅓ cup...........................................................................60
**Bean sauce,** brown, spicy (*House of Tsang*), 1 tsp. ..................15
**Bean sprouts** (see also specific listings), fresh
    (*Chang Farms*), 1 cup...............................................................30
**Bean,** see specific listings
**Beans and franks,** canned (*Hormel*), 7.5-oz. can...................290

**Beans and rice,** see "Rice dish, mix"
**Bearnaise sauce mix,** dry (*Knorr* Classic), 1 tsp. ......................10
**Beef,** meat only, choice grade, trimmed to ¼" fat,
   except as noted, 4 oz.:
brisket, whole, braised, lean w/fat ...............................................437
brisket, whole, braised, lean only ...............................................274
chuck, arm pot roast, braised, lean w/fat ...................................395
chuck, arm pot roast, braised, lean only ....................................255
chuck, blade roast, braised, lean w/fat .......................................412
chuck, blade roast, braised, lean only .........................................298
flank steak, trimmed to 0" fat, broiled, lean w/fat .....................256
flank steak, trimmed to 0" fat, broiled, lean only ......................235
ground, lean, broiled, medium ....................................................308
ground, lean, broiled, well done ..................................................318
ground, lean, pan-fried, medium .................................................312
ground, lean, pan-fried, well done ...............................................314
ground, regular, broiled, medium ................................................328
ground, regular, broiled, well done ..............................................331
ground, regular, pan-fried, medium ............................................347
ground, regular, pan-fried, well done ..........................................324
porterhouse steak, broiled, lean w/fat ........................................346
porterhouse steak, broiled, lean only .........................................247
rib, whole (ribs 6–12), roasted, lean w/fat .................................426
rib, whole (ribs 6–12), roasted, lean only ..................................276
rib, large end (ribs 6–9), roasted, lean w/fat .............................434
rib, large end (ribs 6–9), roasted, lean only ..............................284
rib, small end (ribs 10–12), roasted, lean w/fat ........................376
rib, small end (ribs 10–12), roasted, lean only .........................264
round, bottom, braised, lean w/fat ..............................................322
round, bottom, braised, lean only ...............................................249
round, eye of, roasted, lean w/fat ...............................................273
round, eye of, roasted, lean only .................................................198
round, full cut, broiled, lean w/fat ...............................................272
round, full cut, broiled, lean only .................................................217
round, tip, roasted, lean w/fat .....................................................280
round, tip, roasted, lean only .......................................................213
round, top, broiled, lean w/fat .....................................................254
round, top, broiled, lean only .......................................................214
round, top, pan fried, lean w/fat ..................................................314

**Beef (*cont.*)**

round, top, pan fried, lean only ...............................................257
shank, crosscuts, simmered, lean w/fat.................................298
shank, crosscuts, simmered, lean only ...................................228
short ribs, braised, lean w/fat.................................................534
short ribs, braised, lean only .................................................335
sirloin, top, broiled, lean w/fat...............................................305
sirloin, top, broiled, lean only ................................................229
sirloin, top, pan fried, lean w/fat............................................370
sirloin, top, pan fried, lean only .............................................270
T-bone steak, broiled, lean w/fat............................................338
T-bone steak, broiled, lean only.............................................243
tenderloin, broiled, lean w/fat................................................345
tenderloin, broiled, lean only .................................................252
tenderloin, roasted, lean w/fat...............................................384
tenderloin, roasted, lean only ................................................262
top loin, broiled, lean w/fat....................................................338
top loin, broiled, lean only.....................................................243

**Beef, corned** (see also "Beef lunch meat"):

brisket, cooked, 4 oz.............................................................285
canned (*Hormel*), 2 oz. .......................................................120

**Beef, dried:**

cured, 5 slices, ¾ oz...............................................................35
sliced, in jars (*Hormel*), 10 slices, 1 oz. ................................60
sliced, refrigerated (*Hormel Pillow Pack*), 10 slices, 1 oz. .........45

**Beef, refrigerated:**

roast, w/au jus (*Hormel Always Tender*), 5 oz..........................200
sirloin fillet, peppercorn (*Hormel Always Tender*), 4 oz. ..........160
sirloin fillet, teriyaki flavor (*Hormel Always Tender*), 4 oz. .......170
steak strips, grilled (*Louis Rich Carving Board*), 3 oz. .............110
tips, w/gravy (*Hormel Always Tender*), ½ cup .........................150

**Beef dinner,** frozen, 1 pkg.:

chicken fried steak (*Banquet Extra Helping*), 16 oz..................820
mesquite, barbecue sauce (*Healthy Choice* Meal), 11 oz..........320
oven roasted (*Healthy Choice* Meal), 10.15 oz...........................280
patty, char-broiled (*Healthy Choice* Meal), 11 oz. ....................300
pot roast (*Swanson Hungry-Man*), 16 oz. ...............................350
pot roast, Yankee (*Banquet Extra Helping*), 14.5 oz. ...............410
pot roast, Yankee (*Swanson*), 11.5 oz....................................250

Salisbury steak (*Banquet Extra Helping*), 16.5 oz.....................740
Salisbury steak (*Healthy Choice* Meal), 11.5 oz. ......................330
Salisbury steak (*Swanson Hungry-Man*), 16.25 oz. .................640
Stroganoff (*Healthy Choice* Meal), 11 oz. ...............................320
tips, portobello (*Healthy Choice* Meal), 11.25 oz. ....................270
tips, sirloin (*Swanson Hungry-Man*), 15.75 oz. ........................440
**Beef entree, canned or packaged** (see also "Beef hash"):
pot roast (*Dinty Moore American Classics*), 1 bowl.................200
roast, and gravy (*Hormel*), ½ cup .............................................150
roast, w/potato (*Dinty Moore American Classics*), 1 bowl .......240
Salisbury steak (*Dinty Moore American Classics*), 1 bowl.......320
stew (*Castleberry's* Original), 1 cup .........................................340
stew (*Chef Boyardee* Microwave Bowl), 1 bowl........................160
stew (*Dinty Moore*), 7.5-oz. can................................................190
stew (*Dinty Moore*), 1 cup.........................................................180
stew (*Dinty Moore* Microwave), 1 cup .......................................160
stew (*Dinty Moore American Classics*), 1 bowl........................250
stew (*Hormel* Microcup Meals), 1 cup.......................................150
stew, hearty (*Dinty Moore* Microwave), 1 cup .........................240
**Beef entree, frozen,** 1 pkg., except as noted:
brisket, sliced (*Stouffer's* Homestyle), 10 oz.............................370
broccoli and (*Stouffer's Skillet Sensations*), ½ of 25-oz. pkg. 320
Burgundy, w/garlic mashed potato (*Michelina's*), 8.5 oz. .........300
Cantonese, w/rice (*Yu Sing*), 8 oz.............................................270
cheddar (*Stouffer's Skillet Sensations*), ½ of 25-oz. pkg. ........600
chipped, creamed (*Banquet* Hot Sandwich Toppers), 4 oz. ......120
chipped, creamed (*Freezer Queen* Cook-in-Pouch), 4 oz..........100
chipped, creamed (*Stouffer's*), ½ cup ......................................160
cured, shaved, cream sauce w/(*Michelina's*), 8 oz. .................420
enchilada, see "Enchilada entree"
fiesta, and rice (*Lean Cuisine Skillet Sensations*), ½ of
    24-oz. pkg. .........................................................................300
ginger, w/rice (*Yu Sing*), 8 oz. .................................................290
Hunan (*Lean Cuisine Everyday Favorites*), 8.5 oz. ...................240
macaroni (*Healthy Choice* Entree), 8.2 oz. ..............................220
mesquite, w/rice (*Lean Cuisine Cafe Classics*), 9 oz. ..............290
nacho bake (*Ortega* Family Fiesta Meals), ¼ pkg., 9 oz...........400
Oriental (*Lean Cuisine Cafe Classics*), 9.25 oz. .......................210
Oriental, and peppers (*Yu Sing*), 8 oz......................................290

**Beef entree, frozen (*cont.*)**

oven roasted (*Lean Cuisine Cafe Classics*), 9.25 oz. ...............260
patty:
    char-broiled (*Freezer Queen*), 9.5 oz. ...............................270
    char-broiled (*Freezer Queen* Family), 1 patty w/gravy .........180
    char-broiled, gravy and (*Morton*), 9 oz. .............................310
    char-broiled, mushroom gravy and (*Banquet* Family),
      1 patty w/gravy.................................................................250
    onion gravy and (*Freezer Queen* Family), 1 patty
      w/gravy .............................................................................260
    w/vegetables, country style (*Banquet*), 9.5 oz. .................350
    Western style (*Banquet*), 9.5 oz. ......................................360
pepper steak, green (*Stouffer's* Homestyle), 10.5 oz. ..............270
pepper steak, Oriental (*Healthy Choice* Entree), 9.5 oz. ............260
pepper steak, w/rice (*Michelina's*), 8 oz. ................................270
pepper steak, w/rice (*Michelina's*), 8.5 oz. .............................280
peppercorn (*Lean Cuisine Cafe Classics*), 8.75 oz. ....................260
and peppers (*Freezer Queen*), 8.5 oz. ....................................210
pie (*Banquet*), 7 oz. ............................................................400
pie (*Marie Callender's*), 9.5-oz. pie .......................................680
pie (*Stouffer's*), 10-oz. pie ...................................................440
pie, potato topped (*Swanson*), 12 oz. ....................................450
portobello (*Lean Cuisine Cafe Classics*), 9 oz. .........................220
pot roast (*Freezer Queen*), 9.25 oz. .......................................140
pot roast (*Lean Cuisine Cafe Classics*), 9 oz............................210
pot roast (*Marie Callender's* Skillet Meals), ½ of 22-oz. pkg. ....290
pot roast (*Michelina's*), 10 oz. ..............................................280
pot roast (*Stouffer's Hearty Portions*), 16 oz. ..........................360
pot roast (*Stouffer's* Homestyle), 8⅞ oz. ................................260
pot roast, gravy (*Marie Callender's* Old Fashion), 15 oz. ..........500
pot roast, Yankee (*Banquet*), 9.4 oz.......................................230
roast (*Marie Callender's*), 14.5 oz. ........................................390
Salisbury steak:
    (*Banquet*), 9.5 oz.............................................................380
    (*Freezer Queen*), 8.5 oz. .................................................300
    (*Freezer Queen* Family), 1 patty w/gravy ...........................160
    (*Lean Cuisine Cafe Classics*), 9.5 oz. ................................280
    (*Lean Cuisine Hearty Portions*), 15.5 oz..............................300
    (*Michelina's*), 8 oz............................................................330

(*Stouffer's Hearty Portions*), 16 oz. ......................................570

(*Stouffer's* Homestyle), 9⅝ oz..............................................360

brown gravy and (*Banquet* Family), 1 patty w/gravy...........240

and gravy, shells and cheese (*Michelina's*), 10.5 oz............440

gravy and (*Banquet* Hot Sandwich Toppers), 4-oz. bag......210

gravy and (*Freezer Queen* Cook-in-Pouch), 5 oz. ................150

gravy and (*Morton*), 9 oz....................................................310

sirloin, and gravy (*Marie Callender's*), 14 oz. .....................550

savory (*Lean Cuisine Skillet Sensations*), ½ of 24-oz. pkg. .....290

sirloin, peppercorn (*Michelina's*), 8.5 oz. ...........................290

sirloin, roasted (*Michelina's* Supreme), 8 oz. ......................240

sirloin, sliced, in gravy w/noodles (*Boston Market*), 14 oz. .....420

sliced (*Banquet*), 9 oz. .......................................................270

sliced, brown gravy and (*Banquet* Family), 2 slices w/gravy....140

sliced, gravy and (*Banquet* Hot Sandwich Toppers), 4 oz...........70

sliced, gravy and (*Freezer Queen*), 9 oz.................................140

sliced, gravy and (*Freezer Queen* Cook-in-Pouch), 4 oz. ...........60

steak, chicken fried (*Banquet*), 10 oz. ..................................420

steak, chicken fried, w/gravy (*Marie Callender's*), 15 oz. ..........650

steak, country fried (*Stouffer's Hearty Portions*), 16 oz. ..........560

steak, country fried, and gravy, mashed potato (*Marie
   Callender's* Family), 1 patty w/gravy and ½ cup potato ......550

stew, hearty (*Banquet* Family Size), 1 cup ...............................170

Stroganoff:

(*Lean Cuisine Hearty Portions* Homestyle), 14.25 oz..........350

(*Marie Callender's* Skillet Meals), ½ of 22-oz. pkg..............310

(*Marie Callender's* Skillet Meals), ¼ of 35-oz. pkg. .............250

(*Stouffer's* Homestyle), 9¾ oz..............................................360

(*Stouffer's Skillet Sensations*), ¼ of 40-oz. pkg...................340

and noodles (*Marie Callender's*), 13 oz. ..............................600

teriyaki (*Lean Cuisine Skillet Sensations*), ½ of 24-oz. pkg. ....280

teriyaki (*Yu Sing*), 8 oz.......................................................240

tips, Français (*Healthy Choice* Entree), 9.5 oz..........................300

tips, in mushroom sauce (*Marie Callender's*), 13 oz. ..............430

tips, Southern (*Lean Cuisine Cafe Classics*), 8.75 oz. ..............270

and tomatoes, chunky (*Stouffer's* Homestyle), 10 oz. ..............290

tortilla bake (*Ortega* Family Fiesta Meals), 10 oz., ¼ pkg.........400

**Beef gravy,** in jars, ¼ cup:

(*Boston Market* Classic) ............................................................30

**Beef gravy (*cont.*)**
(*Franco-American*) ...............................................30
(*Franco-American* Slow Roasted).........................25
(*Franco-American* Fat Free/Slow Roasted Fat Free)......20
(*Heinz* Savory) ..................................................20
**Beef hash, canned,** 1 cup, except as noted:
corned (*Libby's*)...............................................420
corned (*Mary Kitchen*), 7.5-oz. can ....................370
corned (*Mary Kitchen* 50% Less Fat)...................280
corned (*Stagg*) ...............................................450
corned or roast (*Mary Kitchen*)...........................390
**Beef hash, refrigerated,** corned (*Jones Dairy Farm*), 2 oz. ....100
**Beef lunch meat,** 2 oz., except as noted:
(*Carl Buddig*), 2.5-oz. pkg................................100
(*Carl Buddig*), 9 slices, 2 oz. ............................75
(*Healthy Deli* 97% Fat Free Well Done) ................70
corned (*Carl Buddig*), 2.5-oz. pkg......................100
corned (*Carl Buddig*), 9 slices, 2 oz....................75
corned (*Healthy Choice*)....................................60
corned (*Healthy Deli* 95% Fat Free).....................80
corned (*Sara Lee* Deli), 3 slices, 1.6 oz................45
corned, brisket, cooked (*Russer*)........................80
Italian style, medium rare (*Healthy Choice*)............60
London broil, flame seared (*Healthy Deli* 96% Fat Free) ..........70
peppered (*Sara Lee* Deli Choice), 3 slices, 2.2 oz.......70
roast (*Russer*) ..................................................80
roast (*Sara Lee* Deli Choice), 2 slices, 1.6 oz. .......50
roast, Cajun style (*Healthy Choice*) ....................60
roast, flame roasted, medium or rare (*Sara Lee*) ......70
roast, medium (*Healthy Choice*)..........................60
roast, peppered (*Sara Lee*).................................70
roast, top round, Italian style or seasoned (*Healthy Deli*) ..........70
roast, top round, medium or rare (*Sara Lee*).............80
**Beef pie,** see "Beef entree, frozen"
**Beef sandwich/pocket,** frozen, 1 pc.:
barbecue (*Hormel Quick Meal*), 4.5 oz. .................370
and cheddar (*Hot Pockets*), 4.5 oz..........................350
cheese steak (*Deli Stuffs*), 4.5 oz...........................350
cheeseburger (*Hormel Quick Meal*), 4.8 oz. ..............400

cheeseburger, bacon (*Hormel Quick Meal*), 5 oz.....................420
cheeseburger or fajita (*Hot Pockets*), 4.5 oz..........................330
hamburger (*Hormel Quick Meal*), 4.3 oz. ..............................350
jalapeno steak and cheese (*Hot Pockets*), 4.5 oz. ................310
Philly steak (*Healthy Choice Meals To Go*), 6.1 oz. ...............310
Philly steak and cheese (*Croissant Pockets*), 4.5 oz. ............350
Philly steak and cheese (*Lean Pockets*), 4.5 oz.....................290
Philly steak and cheese (*Toaster Breaks* Melts), 2.2 oz. ..........190
potato top (*Mrs. Paterson's Aussie Pie*), 5.5 oz. ....................340
**Beef seasoning mix:**
pot roast/sauerbraten (*Knorr Recipe Classics*), 1 tbsp...............35
stew (*Adolph's Meal Makers*), 1 tbsp. ...................................10
stew/goulash (*Knorr Recipe Classics*), 1⅓ tbsp.........................40
**Beef stew,** see "Beef entree"
**Beer,** 12 fl. oz.:
regular................................................................................146
light....................................................................................100
**Beet,** fresh:
raw (*Frieda's*), ½ cup, 3 oz..................................................35
raw, 2"-diam. beet, 2.9 oz.....................................................35
boiled, drained, 2 beets, 2" diam., 3.5 oz. .............................44
boiled, drained, sliced, ½ cup ...............................................38
**Beet, canned:**
all styles (*S&W*), ½ cup .......................................................30
sliced (*Del Monte*), ½ cup ...................................................35
Harvard (*Seneca*), ½ cup .....................................................90
pickled, sliced (*Del Monte*), ½ cup .......................................80
**Beet greens,** fresh, boiled, drained, 1" pcs., ½ cup .................20
**Berry drink:**
red (*Capri Sun All Natural*), 6.76 fl. oz. ...............................100
punch (*Tropicana*), 8 fl. oz.................................................130
**Berry juice blend** (*Mott's*), 8 fl. oz.....................................140
**Biscuit,** buttermilk (*Awrey's* Country/Round), 2-oz. pc...........200
**Biscuit, refrigerated,** 1 pc., except as noted:
(*Grands!* Homestyle) ..........................................................180
buttermilk or corn (*Grands!*) ...............................................190
buttermilk (*Grands!* Reduced Fat).........................................170
buttermilk or country (*Pillsbury*), 3 pieces............................150
flaky (*Grands!*) ..................................................................200

**Biscuit, refrigerated (*cont.*)**
flaky layers (*Hungry Jack*) ........................................100
flaky layers (*Hungry Jack Butter Tastin'*) .................100
flaky layers, buttermilk (*Hungry Jack*) ....................100
flaky layers, honey butter (*Hungry Jack*) ..................110
Southern style (*Grands!*) ..........................................190
**Biscuit mix** (see also "Baking mix"):
(*Arrowhead Mills*), ¼ cup ........................................120
(*Hodgson Mill Kentucky Kernel*), ¼ cup...................171
buttermilk (*"Jiffy"*), ⅙ pkg.* ..................................160
**Black bean:**
dry (*Frieda's*), ⅓ cup, 3 oz. ....................................120
dry, turtle (*Arrowhead Mills*), ¼ cup........................150
boiled, ½ cup............................................................113
**Black bean, canned** (see also "Refried beans"), ½ cup:
(*Allens*) ...................................................................100
(*Green Giant/Joan of Arc*).......................................100
(*Progresso*) .............................................................110
(*Walnut Acres Organic Farms*)................................110
seasoned (*Trappey's*) ..............................................120
**Black bean dip,** see "Bean dip"
**Black bean sauce,** garlic or shiitake (*Annie Chun's*),
    1 tbsp. ..................................................................25
**Blackberry,** fresh, 1 cup............................................75
**Blackberry, canned,** in heavy syrup (*Oregon*), ½ cup.............120
**Blackberry syrup** (*Knott's Berry Farm*), ¼ cup .........210
**Black-eyed peas:**
immature, see "Cowpeas"
mature (*Frieda's*), ⅓ cup, 3 oz. ...............................130
**Black-eyed peas, canned,** ½ cup:
(*Shari Ann's* Organic) .............................................100
fresh shell (*Allens/East Texas Fair/Dorman*).............120
fresh shell, w/jalapenos (*Trappey's*) ........................120
mature (*Allens*)........................................................110
mature, w/bacon (*Allens/Sunshine/Trappey's*) ..........120
mature, w/bacon and jalapeno (*Trappey's*)................110
**Black-eyed peas,** frozen, ½ cup:
(*Birds Eye*)...............................................................110
(*Seabrook Farms*) ....................................................110

**Blintz,** frozen:

apple (*Empire Kosher*), 2 pcs., 4.4 oz. ...................................220

blueberry or potato (*Empire Kosher*), 2 pcs., 4.4 oz. ..............190

cheese or cherry (*Empire Kosher*), 2 pcs., 4.4 oz. .................200

potato (*Ratner's*), 2.2-oz. pc. ...............................................110

**Blood sausage,** .9-oz. slice..................................................95

**Bloody Mary mix,** bottled:

(*D. L. Jardine's* Red Snapper), 3 fl. oz. ................................25

(*Mr & Mrs T*), 8 fl. oz. ...........................................................40

**Blueberry,** fresh, 1 cup .........................................................81

**Blueberry,** canned:

in light syrup (*Oregon*), ½ cup ............................................110

in heavy syrup (*S&W*), ⅓ cup ..............................................70

**Blueberry, dried** (*Frieda's*), ¼ cup ....................................140

**Blueberry syrup** (*Smucker's*), ¼ cup.................................210

**Bluefish,** meat only:

raw, 4 oz. .............................................................................141

baked, broiled, or microwaved, 4 oz. ...................................180

**Bockwurst,** raw, 2.3-oz. link................................................200

**Bocconcini dish, mix** (*Land O Lakes International Pasta
   Collection*), 1 cup*...........................................................340

**Bologna** (see also "Turkey bologna"), 2 oz., except as noted:

(*Boar's Head* Lower Sodium) .............................................150

(*Healthy Deli* 95% Fat Free/95% Fat Free German).............70

(*Oscar Mayer* Thick Cut).....................................................190

(*Russer*) ..............................................................................180

(*Russer Light*) .....................................................................120

(*Russer* Wunderbar German) ..............................................190

beef (*Hebrew National* Lean), 4 slices, 2 oz. .......................90

beef (*Johnsonville*)..............................................................140

beef (*Russer*) ......................................................................180

beef (*Russer Light*) .............................................................120

beef, pork and beef, or garlic (*Boar's Head*) ......................150

garlic (*Oscar Mayer*), 1.4-oz. slice.....................................130

garlic (*Russer*) ....................................................................180

jalapeno pepper (*Russer*) ...................................................170

Lebanon (*Russer*) ...............................................................100

ring (*Johnsonville*) ..............................................................140

turkey, pork, and beef (*Healthy Choice*), 1-oz. slice ...........30

**Bok choy,** see "Cabbage, bok choy"

**Boniato** (*Frieda's*), 3 oz. .................................................................100

**Borage,** fresh, raw, 1" pcs., 1 cup ...............................................19

**Bouillon,** 1 pkt., except as noted:

beef/beef flavor:

    (*MBT/Wyler's* Broth) ................................................................15

    (*MBT/Wyler's* Very Low Sodium Instant Broth) ....................15

beef or beef and French onion (*Wyler's Shakers*), 1 tsp. ...............5

beef/beef flavor or chicken/chicken flavor:

    (*Herb-Ox*), 1 cube ....................................................................5

    (*Herb-Ox* Instant Broth & Seasoning) .....................................5

    (*Herb-Ox* Instant Broth & Seasoning Low Sodium) ..............10

    (*Wyler's*), 1 cube .....................................................................5

    (*Wyler's Shakers* Reduced Sodium), 1 tsp. ...........................10

chicken/chicken flavor:

    (*MBT/Wyler's* Instant/Very Low Sodium Broth) ....................15

    garlic herb, parsley, or Southwest (*Wyler's Shakers*), 1 tsp....5

    plain or tomato (*Doña Maria*), 1 tsp. ....................................10

vegetable (*Herb-Ox*), 1 cube ...........................................................5

**Bow-tie pasta dish, mix:**

and beans, w/savory herb sauce (*Knorr*), ⅔ cup .....................260

cheese, Italian (*Lipton* Pasta & Sauce), 1 cup* ........................300

w/chicken flavored vegetable sauce (*Knorr*), ⅓ cup ................110

and red lentils (*Marrakesh Express*), 1 cup* ............................220

**Bow-tie pasta entree,** frozen, 9.5-oz. pkg.:

and chicken (*Lean Cuisine Cafe Classics*) ................................220

creamy tomato sauce (*Lean Cuisine Everyday Favorites*) ........260

**Boysenberry,** fresh, see "Blackberry"

**Boysenberry, canned,** in light syrup (*Oregon*), ½ cup ............120

**Boysenberry syrup** (*Smucker's*), ¼ cup ..................................210

**Bran,** see "Cereal, ready-to-eat" and specific grains

**Bratwurst:**

(*Boar's Head*), 4-oz. link ............................................................300

fresh, raw (*Johnsonville* Lower Fat), 3.35-oz. link ....................250

fresh, grilled, 3-oz. link:

    all flavors, except cheddar and honey garlic (*Johnsonville*) ..290

    cheddar (*Johnsonville*) ...........................................................300

    honey garlic (*Johnsonville*) ....................................................280

fresh, pan-fried (*Johnsonville*), 2.47-oz. patty .........................240

fresh, pork, cooked, 3-oz. link.................................................226
cooked (*Johnsonville* Brat Bites), 6 links, 2 oz. .......................200
cooked (*Johnsonville/Johnsonville* Stadium), 2.72-oz. link......250
smoked (*Johnsonville*), 2.7-oz. link.....................................240
**Braunschweiger** (see also "Liverwurst"), 2 oz.:
chub (*Jones Dairy Farm* Light) .............................................100
chub (*Jones Dairy Farm* Original 8 oz.) ................................160
chub, 20% bacon (*Jones Dairy Farm*) ...................................150
chub, w/onion (*Jones Dairy Farm*)........................................160
chunk (*Jones Dairy Farm* Light)............................................90
chunk (*Jones Dairy Farm* Original)........................................180
chunk (*Russer*) ....................................................................170
**Brazil nuts,** shelled, 1 oz., 6–8 kernels................................186
**Bread:**
(*Arnold Health Nut*), 1.3-oz. slice .......................................110
black (*Wild's*), 1.4-oz. slice.................................................100
bran (*Arnold Bran'nola* Original), 1.3-oz. slice.......................100
buttermilk (*Arnold* Country), 1.3-oz. slice..............................110
buttermilk (*Pepperidge Farm Farmhouse*), 1.5-oz. slice...........110
cinnamon (*Arnold*), 1-oz. slice.............................................100
cinnamon (*Pepperidge Farm* Swirl), 1-oz. slice .......................90
Italian (*Arnold Bakery Light*), 2 slices, 1.5 oz...........................80
Italian (*Pepperidge Farm*), 1.1-oz. slice..................................90
Italian (*Pepperidge Farm* Light Style), .7-oz. slice .....................45
multigrain, 7 (*Arnold*), 1.3-oz. slice......................................100
multigrain, 7 (*Pepperidge Farm*), 1.4-oz. slice........................100
multigrain, 7 (*Pepperidge Farm* Light Style), .7-oz. slice............45
multigrain, 9 (*Pepperidge Farm*), 1.2-oz. slice.........................90
multigrain, 12 (*Arnold/Arnold Bran'nola*), 1.3-oz. slice............110
multigrain, crunchy (*Pepperidge Farm*), 1.2-oz. slice................90
multigrain, nutty (*Arnold Bran'nola*), 1.3-oz. slice ..................110
multigrain, whole (*Wild's*), 1-oz. slice ....................................70
oat (*Arnold Bran'nola* Country), 1.3-oz. slice...........................110
oat, crunchy (*Pepperidge Farm*), 1.4-oz. slice ........................100
oat, honey (*Pepperidge Farm*), 1.2-oz. slice ............................90
oat bran (*Arnold*), 2 slices, 2.3 oz........................................180
oatnut (*Arnold*), 1.3-oz. slice...............................................110
oatmeal (*Arnold Bakery Light*), 2 slices, 1.5 oz.........................80
oatmeal (*Pepperidge Farm* Light Style), .7-oz. slice ..................45

**Bread (*cont.*)**

oatmeal (*Pepperidge Farm* Old Fashioned), 1.2-oz. slice............80
oatmeal (*Wild's* European Style), 1-oz. slice ..............................70
oatmeal, soft (*Pepperidge Farm Farmhouse*), 1.5-oz. slice ......110
pita, onion (*Sahara*), 2-oz. pc. ..................................................160
pita, white (*Sahara*), 2-oz. pc. ..................................................150
pita, white or whole wheat (*Cedarlane* Low Fat), 2-oz. pc. .......150
pita, white or whole wheat (*Sahara* Mini), 1-oz. pc...................70
pita, whole wheat (*Sahara*), 2-oz. pc.........................................140
potato (*Arnold* Country), 1.3-oz. slice .......................................100
potato, golden (*Pepperidge Farm*), 1.4-oz. slice ......................110
potato, golden (*Pepperidge Farm Farmhouse*), 1.5-oz. slice....110
pumpernickel (*Arnold*), 1.1-oz. slice............................................80
pumpernickel (*Pepperidge Farm* Dark), 1.1-oz. slice .................80
pumpernickel (*Wild's* Hearty), 1.4-oz. slice...............................100
pumpernickel (*Wild's* Westphalian), 1-oz. slice............................70
raisin cinnamon (*Pepperidge Farm* Swirl), 1-oz. slice ...............80
raisin cinnamon (*Sun•Maid* Swirl), 1-oz. slice ...........................80
rye (*Arnold* Real Jewish Melba Thin), 2 slices, 1.4 oz. .............110
rye (*Wild's* Bauernbrot), 1.3-oz. slice..........................................80
rye (*Wild's* Party), 3 slices, 1.1 oz..............................................80
rye, seeded (*Arnold* Real Jewish), 1.1-oz. slice .........................80
rye, seeded or seedless (*Levy's* Real Jewish), 1.1-oz. slice........90
rye, seedless (*Pepperidge Farm* Deli), 1-oz. slice ......................80
sunflower (*Wild's*), 1.4-oz. slice .................................................100
wheat (*Arnold Bakery Light*), 2 slices, 1.5 oz. ............................80
wheat (*Pepperidge Farm* Light Style), .7-oz. slice......................45
wheat (*Pepperidge Farm* Old Fashioned), 1.2-oz. slice..............90
wheat (*Pepperidge Farm* Very Thin), 3 slices, 1.6 oz...............120
wheat, sesame (*Pepperidge Farm*), 1.4-oz. slice ......................100
wheat, whole (*Arnold Brick Oven* 100%), 2 slices, 1.7 oz. .......130
wheat, whole (*Pepperidge Farm* 100% Stone Ground), 1.2-oz.
   slice ........................................................................................90
wheat, whole (*Pepperidge Farm* 100% Thin), .9-oz. slice ..........60
wheat, winter (*Arnold Best*), 1.1-oz. slice....................................90
white (*Arnold Brick Oven* Big Slice), 1.2-oz. slice......................90
white (*Arnold Brick Oven* Original), 2 slices, 1.7 oz.................130
white (*Arnold Bakery Light*), 2 slices, 1.5 oz. ............................80
white (*Pepperidge Farm* Original), .9-oz. slice ...........................70

white (*Pepperidge Farm* Sandwich), 2 slices, 1.6 oz. ...............130
white (*Pepperidge Farm* Toasting), 1.1-oz. slice .........................90
white (*Pepperidge Farm* Very Thin), 3 slices, 1.6 oz. ...............120
white (*Pepperidge Farm* Farmhouse), 1.5-oz. slice...................110
**Bread, frozen or refrigerated:**
(*Pillsbury* Homestyle), 1/9 loaf......................................................150
French loaf (*Pillsbury*), 1/5 loaf ..................................................150
garlic (*Marie Callender's* Original), 2-oz. pc. ...........................190
garlic, Parmesan/Romano (*Marie Callender's*), 2-oz. pc...........200
**Bread crumbs or cubes,** dry:
(*Arnold* All-Purpose/Italian), 1/4 cup............................................110
plain, dry, 1 cup...........................................................................127
Italian (*Contadina*), 1/4 cup .......................................................100
**Bread mix** (see also "Bread mix, sweet" and "Muffin mix"):
cheese-herb or 9 grain (*Hodgson Mill* European), 1/4 cup.........130
corn (*Arrowhead Mills*), 1/4 cup .................................................120
corn (*Hodgson Mill Kentucky Kernel* Sweet), 1/4 cup .................120
corn, jalapeno (*Hodgson Mill*), 1/4 cup ......................................100
multigrain or rye (*Arrowhead Mills*), 1/3 cup...............................160
potato or caraway rye (*Hodgson Mill* Wholesome), 1/4 cup ......120
spelt or white (*Arrowhead Mills*), 1/3 cup...................................150
white or honey whole wheat (*Hodgson Mill*), 1/4 cup.................120
**Bread mix, sweet** (see also "Muffin mix"), 1/12 loaf\*, except as
  noted:
banana or lemon poppy seed (*Betty Crocker* Quick) ................170
chocolate chip swirl (*Pillsbury* Quick Bread & Coffee Cake Mix),
  1/16 loaf\* ..................................................................................170
cinnamon streusel (*Betty Crocker* Quick), 1/14 loaf\* ..................180
cinnamon swirl (*Pillsbury* Quick Bread & Coffee Cake Mix).....220
cranberry (*Pillsbury* Quick Bread Mix) .....................................160
cranberry orange (*Betty Crocker* Quick)....................................180
gingerbread, whole wheat (*Hodgson Mill*), 1/4 cup dry .............110
**Breadfruit,** fresh, raw, 1/4 small, approx. 3.5 oz. ......................99
**Breadfruit seeds,** roasted, 1 oz. ...............................................59
**Breadnut tree seeds,** dried, 1 tbsp............................................37
**Breadstick:**
all varieties (*Burns & Ricker Crispini*), 5 pcs., 1.1 oz...............120
all varieties (*Real Torino*), 5 pcs., .5 oz......................................60
all varieties (*Stella D'oro* Snack Stix), 4 pcs...............................70

**Breadstick (*cont.*)**

original or onion (*Stella D'oro*), 1 pc..........................................40

sesame (*Stella D'oro*), 1 pc.........................................................50

**Breadstick, frozen or refrigerated,** 2 pcs.:

(*Pillsbury*) .................................................................................140

garlic, w/topping (*Pillsbury*) .....................................................180

**Breakfast sandwich/pocket,** frozen (see also "Sausage
   sandwich"), 1 pc.:

cheese, egg, and ham or sausage (*Pillsbury Toaster
   Scrambles*), 1.7 oz...............................................................180

egg, sausage, cheese pocket (*Croissant Pockets*), 4.5 oz........340

Western (*Pillsbury Toaster Scrambles*), 1.7 oz.........................170

**Broad bean:**

(*Frieda's* Fava), ¾ cup, 3 oz......................................................290

dried, skinless (*Frieda's* Habas), ½ cup, 3 oz. .........................100

mature, dry, 1 cup .....................................................................517

mature, boiled, 1 cup.................................................................187

**Broad bean, canned** (*Progresso* Fava), ½ cup .........................110

**Broccoli,** fresh:

raw (*Andy Boy*), 1 medium stalk .................................................45

raw (*Dole*), 1 medium stalk, 5.3 oz..............................................45

raw, baby (*Mann's Broccolini*), 8 stalks, 3 oz. ............................35

raw, florets (*Mann's Broccoli Wokly*), 4 oz..................................30

raw, florets (*Mann's Broccoli Wokly* Stir-Fry), 4 oz.....................35

raw, chopped, 1 cup ...................................................................25

boiled, drained, 1 medium stalk, 7½–8" long..............................50

**Broccoli, Chinese,** cooked, 1 cup .............................................19

**Broccoli, frozen:**

(*Birds Eye/Freshlike* Stir Fry), 1 cup...........................................30

spears (*Birds Eye*), 3 pcs. ..........................................................25

spears (*Freshlike*), 2 pcs. ...........................................................25

spears (*Green Giant*), 3.5 oz., about 3 pcs. ...............................25

spears, in butter sauce (*Green Giant*), 4 oz., about 3 pcs. .........50

florets (*Birds Eye* Deluxe), 5 pcs. ...............................................25

florets (*Seabrook Farms* Petite), 4 pcs........................................25

florets, baby (*Birds Eye*), 1 cup..................................................25

chopped (*Birds Eye*), ⅓ cup.......................................................25

cuts (*Birds Eye*), ½ cup..............................................................25

cuts (*Freshlike*), 1 cup................................................................25

in cheese sauce (*Birds Eye*), ½ cup................................................70
in cheese sauce (*Freezer Queen*), ⅔ cup...............................80
**Broccoli-cheese pocket,** frozen, 1 pc.:
(*Amy's*), 4.5 oz. ...............................................................270
(*Pepperidge Farm*), 3.7 oz.................................................230
**Broccoli combination,** fresh, 4 oz.:
carrots (*Mann's*) ...............................................................35
cauliflower, baby carrots (*Mann's* Vegetable Medley) .................35
**Broccoli combination,** frozen, ½ cup, except as noted:
(*Birds Eye/Freshlike* Baby Blend), 1 cup ..............................70
beans, onions, red peppers (*Birds Eye*)................................25
carrots, water chestnuts (*Birds Eye*)....................................30
cauliflower (*Birds Eye*) ......................................................20
cauliflower, carrots (*Birds Eye*) ...........................................25
cauliflower, carrots, in cheese sauce (*Birds Eye*)....................70
cauliflower, red peppers (*Birds Eye*) ....................................20
corn, red peppers (*Birds Eye*) .............................................50
potatoes, carrots (*Birds Eye* French Country Style), ⅔ cup .....110
red peppers, onions, mushrooms (*Birds Eye*)..........................25
**Broccoli dish,** frozen:
au gratin (*Stouffer's*), ½ cup ..............................................100
pancake (*Dr. Praeger's*), 1.3-oz. pc. ....................................70
pasta, cauliflower, carrots, in cheese sauce (*Freezer Queen*),
⅔ cup.........................................................................120
pie (*Amy's*), 7.5-oz. pie.....................................................430
**Broccoli rabe,** fresh (*Frieda's*), 3 oz................................25
**Broccoli rabe,** frozen (*Seabrook Farms* Raab), 1 cup.............25
**Broccoli sprout,** fresh (*BroccoSprouts*), 1 oz., ½ cup.............10
**Broth,** see "Bouillon" and "Soup"
**Brown gravy,** w/onions (*Franco-American*), ¼ cup...................25
**Brown gravy mix,** w/ or w/out onion (*Knorr*), ¼ cup\* .............20
**Brownie,** 1 pc., except as noted:
(*Hostess Brownie Bites*), 3 pcs., 1.3 oz.................................170
(*Little Debbie* Cosmic), 2.2 oz.............................................270
(*Little Debbie* Lights), 1.9 oz. ............................................190
chocolate (*Awrey's* Decadent), 1.9 oz. .................................220
chocolate peanut (*Awrey's* Sensation), 1.9 oz.........................230
fudge (*Little Debbie* Singles), 2.5 oz. ...................................310
fudge nut (*Awrey's*), 1.8 oz. ...............................................210

**Brownie, frozen or refrigerated:**
chocolate, bar (*Nestlé Tollhouse*), 1/12 of 18-oz. pkg. ...............180
fudge (*Pillsbury One-Step*), 1/12 pkg. .........................................120
walnut (*Nestlé Tollhouse*), 1/12 of 18-oz. pkg. ...........................170
**Brownie mix\*:**
(*Arrowhead Mills*), 1.1-oz pc. .....................................................110
(*Arrowhead Mills* Fat/Wheat Free), 1.1-oz pc. ............................120
caramel (*Pillsbury* Swirl), 1/14 pkg. ............................................120
cheesecake (*Pillsbury* Swirl), 1/18 pkg. ......................................110
chocolate, dark (*Betty Crocker* Pouch), 1/9 pkg. .........................190
chocolate, dark, fudge (*Betty Crocker* Supreme), 1/20 pkg. ........170
chocolate, double (*Pillsbury*), 1/16 pkg. ......................................150
chocolate, German (*Betty Crocker* Supreme), 1/20 pkg. ..............200
chocolate chunk (*Betty Crocker* Supreme), 1/20 pkg. ..................180
frosted (*Betty Crocker* Supreme), 1/20 pkg. .................................210
fudge (*Betty Crocker* Pouch), 1/9 pkg. .........................................190
fudge (*Betty Crocker* Supreme 19.8 oz.), 1/20 pkg. ....................170
fudge (*Betty Crocker* Supreme 15 oz.), 1/12 pkg. ........................190
fudge (*Betty Crocker* Supreme Original), 1/20 pkg. ......................160
fudge ("*Jiffy*"), 1/6 pkg. ...............................................................160
fudge (*Pillsbury*), 1/18 pkg. .........................................................190
fudge, hot (*Betty Crocker* Supreme), 1/20 pkg. ...........................170
fudge, hot (*Pillsbury* Swirl), 1/14 pkg. .........................................170
turtle (*Betty Crocker*), 1/20 pkg. .................................................170
walnut (*Betty Crocker* Supreme), 1/20 pkg. .................................180
**Bruschetta,** pesto, mozzarella, and tomato
(*Cedarlane*), 1.3-oz. pc. ...............................................................100
**Brussels sprouts,** fresh:
raw (*Dole*), 1 cup ...........................................................................40
raw, 1 sprout, .7 oz. ...........................................................................8
boiled, drained, 1/2 cup ...................................................................30
**Brussels sprouts,** frozen:
(*Birds Eye/Freshlike*), 6 pcs. .........................................................35
(*Birds Eye* Deluxe), 11 pcs. ...........................................................35
(*Freshlike* Select), 5 pcs. ...............................................................35
(*Seabrook Farms*), 7 pcs. ...............................................................20
baby, in butter sauce (*Green Giant*), 2/3 cup ................................60
**Buckwheat flour** (*Hodgson Mill*), 1/3 cup ..................................160

**Buckwheat groats:**
(*Arrowhead Mills*), ¼ cup ........................................................140
roasted, dry, 1 cup ...................................................................567
roasted, cooked, 1 cup ............................................................155
**Bulgur** (see also "Tabouli"):
dry (*Arrowhead Mills*), ¼ cup .................................................150
dry, w/soy grits (*Hodgson Mill*), ¼ cup .................................120
cooked, 1 cup ..........................................................................151
**Bun,** see "Roll"
**Bun, sweet,** 1 pc.:
cinnamon roll (*Awrey's* Homestyle), 3 oz..............................270
cinnamon roll (*Little Debbie*), 4 oz........................................470
honey (*Hostess*), 4 oz.............................................................460
honey (*Little Debbie*), 4 oz.....................................................520
honey (*Little Debbie*), 3 oz.....................................................390
honey (*Morton*) .......................................................................270
honey, mini (*Morton*) ..............................................................160
**Bun, sweet, frozen,** cinnamon (*Sara Lee* Deluxe), 1 pc...........370
**Burbot,** meat only:
raw, 4 oz. .................................................................................102
baked, broiled, or microwaved, 4 oz. ......................................130
**Burdock root:**
(*Frieda's* Gobo Root), ¾ cup, 3 oz. .........................................60
boiled, drained, 1" pcs., 1 cup ................................................110
**Burger,** see "Beef sandwich/pocket"
**Burger, vegetarian,** frozen, 1 pc.:
(*Amy's* All American), 2.5 oz...................................................170
(*Tofutti Quit Beef'n*), 2.5 oz. ..................................................140
(*Yves* Burger Burger), 3 oz.....................................................119
Bombay or California (*Dr. Praeger's*), 2.8 oz...........................100
California or Texas (*Amy's* Veggie), 2.5 oz.............................130
w/cheese (*Dr. Praeger's* Royale), 3 oz...................................120
w/"cheese," nondairy (*Tofutti Quit Beef'n*), 2.5 oz................180
Chicago (*Amy's* Veggie), 2.5 oz.............................................160
***Burger King,*** 1 serving:
breakfast dishes:
    biscuit.................................................................................300
    biscuit w/egg ....................................................................380
    biscuit w/sausage.............................................................490

**Burger King** breakfast dishes (*cont.*)

biscuit w/sausage, egg, and cheese ................................620
cini-minis, w/out vanilla icing, 4 rolls ...............................440
*Croissan'wich,* w/sausage and cheese.............................450
*Croissan'wich,* w/sausage, egg, and cheese.....................530
French toast sticks, 5 pcs. ..............................................440
hash browns, large .........................................................410
hash browns, small..........................................................240

breakfast components:

bacon.................................................................................40
ham .................................................................................35
*A.M. Express* dip .............................................................80
*A.M. Express* jam, grape or strawberry ...........................30
vanilla icing, 1 oz..............................................................110
*Land O Lakes* whipped classic blend...............................65

sandwiches:

bacon cheeseburger........................................................400
bacon double cheeseburger.............................................620
*Big King*.........................................................................640
*BK Big Fish*....................................................................720
*BK Broiler* chicken .........................................................530
cheeseburger...................................................................360
chicken ............................................................................710
chicken w/out mayo..........................................................500
Chick'N Crisp....................................................................460
Chick'N Crisp w/out mayo.................................................360
double cheeseburger........................................................580
*Double Whopper* ............................................................920
*Double Whopper* w/out mayo .........................................760
*Double Whopper* w/cheese ...........................................1010
*Double Whopper* w/cheese, w/out mayo ..........................850
hamburger........................................................................320
*Whopper*.........................................................................660
*Whopper* w/out mayo .....................................................510
*Whopper* w/cheese.........................................................760
*Whopper* w/cheese, w/out mayo ....................................600
*Whopper Jr.*....................................................................400
*Whopper Jr.* w/out mayo .................................................320

*Whopper Jr.* w/cheese..............................................450
*Whopper Jr.* w/cheese, w/out mayo ..................470
sandwich condiments:
   *Bull's Eye* barbecue sauce, .5 oz..................20
   ketchup, .5 oz.............................................15
   King sauce, .5 oz........................................70
   tartar sauce, 1.5 oz. ................................260
*Chicken Tenders:*
   4 pcs. ........................................................180
   5 pcs. ........................................................230
   8 pcs. ........................................................350
dipping sauces, 1 oz.:
   barbecue.....................................................35
   honey flavored/honey mustard .....................90
   ranch ........................................................170
   sweet and sour...........................................45
side orders:
   fries, king size .........................................590
   fries, medium ...........................................400
   fries, small................................................250
   onion rings, king size ...............................600
   onion rings, medium..................................380
dessert and shakes:
   Dutch apple pie .........................................300
   shake, chocolate, medium .........................440
   shake, chocolate, small..............................330
   shake, vanilla, medium...............................430
   shake, vanilla, small ..................................330
   shake, syrup added, chocolate, medium ....570
   shake, syrup added, chocolate, small.........390
   shake, syrup added, strawberry, medium....550
   shake, syrup added, strawberry, small ......390
**Burrito,** frozen or refrigerated, 1 pc.:
bean and cheese (*Las Campanas*), 4 oz......270
bean and cheese (*Patio*), 5 oz. ....................300
beans, rice and cheese (*Cedarlane*), 5.9 oz..........260
beef, red hot (*Las Campanas*), 4 oz. ............300
beef and bean (*Las Campanas*), 4 oz. ..........310
beef and bean, green chili (*Las Campanas*), 4 oz. ...................300

**Burrito (*cont.*)**
beef and bean, hot or red hot w/chilies (*Patio*), 5 oz..............320
beef and bean, medium (*Patio*), 5 oz........................................310
beef and bean, mild (*Patio*), 5 oz. ...........................................330
chicken (*Las Campanas*), 4 oz. ...............................................200
chicken (*Patio*), 5 oz................................................................290
vegetable, roasted, and cheese (*Cedarlane*), 6 oz. ...................330
**Burrito dinner mix:**
(*Chi-Chi's* Dinner Kit), 2 shells and seasoning.......................300
(*Ortega*), 1 tortilla and ⅛ pkt. seasoning...............................150
bean (*Taco Bell Home Originals*), 1 burrito*............................200
**Burrito entree** (see also "Burrito"), chicken, con queso
 (*Healthy Choice* Entree), 10.55 oz. .....................................350
**Burrito seasoning mix:**
(*Chi-Chi's* Fiesta), ¼ pkg. .........................................................40
(*Lawry's* Spices & Seasonings), 1 tbsp. ....................................30
**Butter** (see also "Margarine"), 1 tbsp.:
(*Land O Lakes*)............................................................................100
(*Land O Lakes* Light) ...................................................................50
(*Land O Lakes Ultra Creamy*)......................................................110
whipped (*Land O Lakes*) ...............................................................70
whipped (*Land O Lakes* Light) .....................................................35
**Butter beans,** see "Lima beans"
**Buttercup squash** (*Frieda's*), ¾ cup, 3 oz. ...............................30
**Butterfish,** meat only:
raw, 4 oz. ....................................................................................166
baked, broiled, or microwaved, 4 oz. ........................................212
**Butternut squash,** fresh, baked, cubed, 1 cup............................82
**Butternut squash, frozen,** boiled, drained, mashed, 1 cup........94
**Butterscotch baking chips** (*Hershey's*), 1 tbsp.........................80
**Butterscotch topping,** 2 tbsp.:
(*Kraft*) .........................................................................................130
(*Smucker's* Spoonable Toppings)...............................................130
(*Smucker's* Sundae Syrup).........................................................110
caramel (*Smucker's* Special Recipe Topping) ...........................130

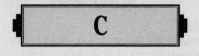

# C

**FOOD AND MEASURE**                                    **CALORIES**

**Cabbage,** fresh:
raw, 2-lb. head ....................................................................218
raw, shredded, ½ cup..............................................................9
boiled, drained, shredded, ½ cup.........................................17
**Cabbage, bok choy,** fresh:
raw (*Frieda's*), 1 cup, 3 oz...................................................10
raw, baby (*Frieda's*), ⅔ cup, 3 oz.......................................10
boiled, drained, shredded, ½ cup.........................................10
**Cabbage, mustard** (*Frieda's* Gai Choy), 1 cup, 3 oz.........20
**Cabbage, napa,** fresh, cooked, 1 cup.................................13
**Cabbage, pe-tsai,** raw, shredded, ½ cup..............................6
**Cabbage, red,** ½ cup:
raw, shredded .......................................................................10
boiled, drained, shredded ......................................................16
**Cabbage, savoy,** boiled, drained, shredded, ½ cup...........18
**Cabbage, Tuscan** (*Frieda's*), ⅔ cup, 3 oz.........................20
**Cabbage entree,** stuffed, frozen (*Lean Cuisine Everyday
    Favorites*), 9.5-oz. pkg. ..................................................210
**Cake** (see also "Cheesecake"), ¹⁄₁₆ cake, except as noted:
banana, frosted (*Entenmann's*), ⅛ cake.............................290
banana, sheet (*Awrey's*), ¹⁄₂₄ cake....................................350
Black Forest torte (*Awrey's* 8"), ¹⁄₁₂ cake..........................370
carrot, cream cheese iced, 2 layer (*Awrey's* 9") ..............390
carrot, sheet (*Awrey's* Supreme), ¹⁄₂₄ cake.......................400
cherries cordial (*Awrey's* Marquise 9").............................250
chocolate (*Awrey's* Marquise Killer 9")..............................280
chocolate, creme filled, frosted (*Entenmann's*), ⅛ cake ..........300
chocolate, double, torte (*Awrey's* 8"), ¹⁄₁₂ cake................340
chocolate, German, 3 layer (*Awrey's* 9") ..........................370
chocolate, tropical (*Awrey's* Marquise 9") .........................230
chocolate chip crumb loaf (*Entenmann's*), ⅛ cake ..................250
chocolate fudge, chocolate frosted (*Entenmann's*), ⅛ cake .....260
chocolate peanut (*Awrey's* Marquise Fantasy 9")................330

**Cake** (*cont.*)

coconut butter cream, yellow, 3 layer (*Awrey's* 9")...................390
coffee cake (*Entenmann's* Light Fat Free), ⅑ cake ...................210
crumb (*Entenmann's* Ultimate), ⅒ cake..............................250
devil's food, marshmallow frosted (*Entenmann's*), ⅛ cake......280
espresso, French (*Awrey's* Marquise 9")...............................330
golden loaf (*Entenmann's* Light Fat Free), ⅛ cake..................130
golden, fudge frosted (*Entenmann's*), ⅛ cake.......................280
lemon (*Awrey's* Marquise Whisper 9")..................................270
lemon or orange, butter cream, 3 layer (*Awrey's* 9") ...............340
loaf (*Entenmann's* All Butter), ⅙ cake..................................210
marble (*Entenmann's* All Butter), ⅛ cake..............................190
peach, Georgia (*Awrey's* Marquise 9").................................260
pound (*Awrey's* Golden), ⅙ cake ........................................250
raisin or sour cream loaf (*Entenmann's*), ⅛ cake...................220
raspberry (*Awrey's* Marquise Extraordinaire 9").....................370
raspberry nut (*Awrey's* Marquise 9")....................................290
red velvet (*Awrey's* Marquise 9")..........................................310
sponge, not iced, sheet (*Awrey's*), 1/24 cake.........................180
yellow, yellow iced, 2 layer (*Awrey's* 8")..............................300

**Cake, frozen** (see also "Cheesecake, frozen or refrigerated"),
   ⅛ cake, except as noted:

carrot (*Mrs. Smith's*), ⅙ cake .............................................300
chocolate, double, layer (*Sara Lee*).....................................260
chocolate, German, layer (*Sara Lee*)....................................280
chocolate fudge, 3 layer (*Pepperidge Farm*) ........................150
chocolate mousse (*Sara Lee*), ⅕ cake.................................400
coffee cake, butter streusel, crumb, or raspberry
   (*Sara Lee*), ⅙ cake .....................................................220
coffee cake, cheese (*Sara Lee* Reduced Fat), ⅙ cake..............180
coffee cake, pecan (*Sara Lee*), ⅙ cake ................................230
coconut, fudge/golden or vanilla layer (*Sara Lee*) ..................260
devil's food or fudge stripe, 3 layer (*Pepperidge Farm*)...........250
golden, 3 layer (*Pepperidge Farm*).......................................250
pound (*Sara Lee* All Butter), ¼ cake ...................................320
pound (*Sara Lee* All Butter Family Size), ⅙ cake...................310
pound (*Sara Lee* Reduced Fat), ¼ cake ...............................280
pound, chocolate swirl (*Sara Lee*), ¼ cake............................330
pound, strawberry swirl (*Sara Lee*), ¼ cake...........................290

strawberry shortcake (*Sara Lee*) ........................................180
**Cake, mix\*** (see also "Cheesecake, mix"):
angel food (*Pillsbury*), $\frac{1}{12}$ cake ....................................140
angel food (*SuperMoist* Easy), $\frac{1}{4}$ cake ......................170
angel food, chocolate swirl or confetti
   (*SuperMoist*), $\frac{1}{12}$ cake.....................................150
angel food, white (*SuperMoist* One-Step), $\frac{1}{12}$ cake ...........140
banana (*Pillsbury Moist Supreme*), $\frac{1}{12}$ cake....................250
butter pecan (*SuperMoist*), $\frac{1}{12}$ cake ..............................240
butter recipe (*Pillsbury Moist Supreme*), $\frac{1}{12}$ cake................260
carrot (*SuperMoist*), $\frac{1}{10}$ cake ......................................320
cherry chip (*SuperMoist*), $\frac{1}{10}$ cake...............................300
chocolate (*Pillsbury Moist Supreme*), $\frac{1}{12}$ cake................260
chocolate, butter recipe or chip (*SuperMoist*), $\frac{1}{12}$ cake...........250
chocolate, w/fudge swirls (*SuperMoist*), $\frac{1}{9}$ cake.............210
chocolate, German, or fudge (*SuperMoist*), $\frac{1}{12}$ cake .............270
chocolate, milk (*SuperMoist*), $\frac{1}{12}$ cake..........................240
devil's food (*SuperMoist*), $\frac{1}{12}$ cake ..............................270
devil's food (*Sweet Rewards*), $\frac{1}{12}$ cake ........................200
fudge marble (*SuperMoist*), $\frac{1}{10}$ cake.............................290
gingerbread (*Betty Crocker* Classic), $\frac{1}{8}$ cake ..................230
lemon (*Pillsbury Moist Supreme*), $\frac{1}{12}$ cake ....................250
lemon (*SuperMoist*), $\frac{1}{12}$ cake......................................240
pineapple or party swirl (*SuperMoist*), $\frac{1}{12}$ cake ..............250
pineapple upside-down (*Betty Crocker* Classic), $\frac{1}{6}$ cake..........400
pound (*Betty Crocker* Classic), $\frac{1}{8}$ cake ..........................260
rainbow chip (*SuperMoist*), $\frac{1}{10}$ cake .............................300
red velvet (*Duncan Hines Moist Deluxe*), $\frac{1}{12}$ cake ..................240
spice (*SuperMoist*), $\frac{1}{12}$ cake.......................................240
strawberry (*SuperMoist*), $\frac{1}{12}$ cake................................250
strawberry swirl (*SuperMoist*), $\frac{1}{10}$ cake .......................300
vanilla, French (*Pillsbury Moist Supreme*), $\frac{1}{12}$ cake ..............250
vanilla, French or golden (*SuperMoist*), $\frac{1}{12}$ cake ..............240
white (*SuperMoist*), $\frac{1}{12}$ cake ......................................230
white (*Sweet Rewards*), $\frac{1}{12}$ cake.................................190
white, sour cream (*SuperMoist*), $\frac{1}{10}$ cake......................280
yellow (*Pillsbury Moist Supreme*), $\frac{1}{12}$ cake....................250
yellow, butter recipe (*SuperMoist*), $\frac{1}{12}$ cake..................260
yellow, golden (*"Jiffy"*), $\frac{1}{5}$ cake....................................220

**Cake mix (*cont.*)**
yellow, w/fudge swirl (*SuperMoist*), 1/10 cake ...........................210
**Cake, snack:**
apple (*Little Debbie* Flips), 1.2 oz. ...................................150
banana (*Little Debbie* Twins), 2.2 oz. ...............................250
blueberry (*Little Debbie* Loaves), 2 oz...............................220
Boston creme (*Drake's*), 1.5 oz. ......................................180
chocolate:
   (*Little Debbie* Snack Cakes), 2.5 oz. ...........................310
   creme filled (*Drake's Devil Dogs*), 1.6 oz................180
   creme filled (*Drake's Yodels*), 2 pcs., 2.2 oz...........290
   creme filled (*Drake's Ring-Dings*), 2 pcs., 2.7 oz. ..............330
   creme filled (*Hostess Ho-Hos*), 3 pcs., 3 oz........................380
   creme filled (*Hostess Suzy-Q's*), 2-oz. ...........................230
   creme filled (*Little Debbie* Swiss Cake Rolls), 2.2 oz. .........270
   peanut butter filled (*Drake's Funny Bones*), 2 pcs.,
     2.5 oz. ..........................................................................300
chocolate chip cake (*Little Debbie*), 2.4 oz. ...............................310
coconut (*Little Debbie* Rounds), 1.2 oz................................150
coffee cake (*Drake's*) 1.2 oz. ........................................140
coffee cake (*Drake's* Mini), 4 pcs., 1.76 oz. ............................210
coffee cake (*Little Debbie* Big Snack), 3.4 oz. ........................370
coffee cake, apple (*Little Debbie*), 2.1 oz. ...............................230
coffee cake, crumb (*Hostess*), 1.1 oz......................................140
cupcake:
   chocolate, creme filled (*Hostess*), 1.8 oz..............................180
   chocolate, creme filled (*Little Debbie*), 1.6 oz. ...................180
   chocolate or golden, creme filled (*Drake's Yankee/ Sunny
     Doodles*), 2 pcs., 2 oz. ..............................................220
   golden, creme filled, chocolate iced (*Hostess*), 1.9 oz. ........200
   lemon or orange, creme filled (*Little Debbie*), 1.7 oz..........210
   orange, creme filled, orange iced (*Hostess*), 1.5 oz. ...........160
devil's food (*Little Debbie* Devil Cremes), 1.7 oz....................190
devil's food (*Little Debbie* Devil Squares), 2.2 oz.....................270
fudge cake, frosted (*Little Debbie*), 1.5 oz. ...............................200
fudge rounds (*Little Debbie*), 1.2 oz. ......................................140
fudge rounds (*Little Debbie* Big Snacks), 2 oz.........................240
golden, creme filled (*Hostess Twinkies*), 1.5 oz......................150
golden, creme filled (*Hostess Twinkies* Low Fat), 1.5 oz.........130

golden, creme filled (*Little Debbie* Golden Cremes), 1.5 oz......150
lemon or raspberry (*Little Debbie* Angel Cakes), 1.6 oz. .........130
marshmallow (*Little Debbie* Supremes), 1.1 oz. .......................130
nutty bars (*Little Debbie*), 2.1 oz. .............................................330
oatmeal (*Little Debbie* Lights), 1.3 oz. ....................................130
oatmeal and creme (*Little Debbie*), 1.3 oz. ..............................170
peanut butter bars (*Little Debbie*), 1.9 oz. ...............................170
peanut clusters (*Little Debbie*), 1.4 oz. ...................................190
pecan spin wheels (*Drake's*), 1 oz............................................100
strawberry shortcake rolls (*Little Debbie*), 2.2 oz.....................230
**Calabaza** (*Frieda's*), ½ cup, 3 oz. ..........................................10
**Calves' liver,** see "Liver"
**Camouflage melon** (*Frieda's*), 1 cup .........................................50
**Candy:**
almond, chocolate covered (*Hershey's*), 11 pcs., 1.3 oz. .........210
(*Baby Ruth*), 2.1-oz. bar ...........................................................270
(*Bittyfinger*), 2 bars, 1.34 oz.....................................................170
(*Buncha Crunch*), 1.4-oz. pkg....................................................200
(*Butterfinger*), 2.1-oz. bar ........................................................270
(*Butterfinger BB's*), 1.7-oz. pkg. ...............................................220
butterscotch (*Land O Lakes*), 3 pcs., .6 oz. ...............................70
caramel (*Hershey's* Classic), 6 pcs., 1.3 oz. .............................160
caramel, chocolate coated (*Milk Duds*), 1.8-oz. box.................240
caramel, chocolate coated (*Rolo*), 1.9-oz. pkg..........................260
caramel, chocolate filled (*Hershey's* Classic), 6 pcs., 1.3 oz. ...160
caramel fudge (*Hershey's Sweet Escapes*), .7-oz. bar ................70
caramel and milk chocolate (*Nestlé Treasures*), 3 pcs...............170
coconut, chocolate coated (*Mounds*), 1.9-oz. pkg. ..................250
coconut, chocolate coated, almonds (*Almond Joy*),
    1.7-oz. pkg. .........................................................................240
chocolate, assorted (*Hershey's* Miniatures), 2.25-oz. pkg. ........350
chocolate, assorted (*Hershey's* Pot of Gold), 1.5 oz. .................210
chocolate, candy coated (*M&M's*), 1.7-oz. bag.........................240
chocolate, candy coated, almond (*M&M's*), 1.3-oz. bag ..........200
chocolate, candy coated, crispy (*M&M's*), 1.5-oz. bag.............200
chocolate, candy coated, peanut (*M&M's*), 1.75-oz. bag .........250
chocolate, dark (*Dove*), 1.3-oz. bar...........................................200
chocolate, dark (*Special Dark*), 1.4-oz. bar ..............................220
chocolate, dark (*Special Dark* Miniatures), 5 pcs., 1.5 oz.........230

**Candy** (*cont.*)

chocolate, dark, almond (*Hershey's Nuggets*), 4 pcs., 1.4 oz...220
chocolate, milk:

    (*Cadbury's* Dairy Milk), 9 blocks, 1.4 oz..............................220
    (*Dove*), 1.3-oz. bar..............................................................200
    (*Hershey's*), 1.5-oz. bar ....................................................230
    (*Hershey's Hugs/Hugs and Kisses*), 9 pcs., 1.4 oz. ............220
    (*Hershey's Kisses*), 1.5-oz. pkg. .......................................230
    (*Hershey's Nuggets*), 4 pcs., 1.4 oz...................................210
    (*Nestlé*), 1.45-oz. bar.........................................................220
    (*Symphony*), 1.5-oz. bar ...................................................230
    almond (*Cadbury's*), 9 blocks, 1.4 oz.................................220
    almond (*Hershey's*), 1.4-oz. bar ........................................230
    almond (*Hershey's Kisses*), 9 pcs., 1.4 oz. ........................230
    almond (*Hershey's Nuggets*), 4 pcs., 1.3 oz. ......................210
    almond and toffee (*Symphony*), 1.5-oz. bar ......................230
    caramel (*Caramello*), 1.2-oz. bar ......................................170
    cookie (*Hershey's Cookies 'n' Mint*), 1.5-oz. bar ................230
    crisps (*Cadbury's Krisp*), 9 blocks, 1.4 oz. .........................200
    nut and raisin (*Cadbury's* Fruit & Nut), 9 blocks, 1.4 oz. ....210
    nut and raisin (*Chunky*), 1.4-oz. bar ..................................210
    peanut (*Mr. Goodbar*), 1.7-oz. bar......................................270
    raisin and almond (*Hershey's Nuggets*), 4 pcs., 1.4 oz. .....190
    toffee and almond (*Hershey's Nuggets*), 4 pcs., 1.4 oz. .....210
chocolate, white, cookie (*Hershey's Cookies 'n' Creme*
    *Nuggets*), 4 pcs., 1.3 oz. ..................................................190
chocolate, white, crisps (*Nestlé White Crunch*), 1.4-oz. bar ....220
chocolate truffle (*Hershey's* Pot of Gold), 3 pcs., 1.5 oz. .........210
cinnamon (*Mexican Hats/Red Hot Dollars*), 1.4 oz...................140
cookie bar, caramel (*Twix*), 1-oz. bar......................................140
cookie bar, peanut (*Twix*), 2 bars, 1.8 oz. ..............................280
fruit flavor, all flavors:

    chews (*ChewMongous*), .6-oz. pc. ......................................60
    chews (*Jolly Rancher*), 2-oz. pkg.......................................210
    chews (*LifeSavers*), 11 pcs. ..............................................150
    gummed (*Amazin' Fruit*), 1.5-oz. bag .................................140
    gummed (*GummiSavers* Five Flavor/Wild Berries), 1.5 oz..140
    gummed (*GummiSavers Crystal Craze*), 1.5-oz. pkg. .........130
    gummed (*Jolly Rancher Gummis*), 1.7-oz. pkg.................150

gummed (*Jujubes*), 1.5-oz. box..............................130
gummed (*Jujyfruits*), 2.1-oz. box .......................200
jellies (*Chuckles*), 4 pcs., 1.6 oz. ....................150
jellies (*Jolly Rancher* Jolly Jellies), 1.3-oz. pkg. ..................110
gum, chewing, 1 pc.:
   all varieties (*Fruit Stripe*)................................10
   all varieties (*LifeSavers Ice Breakers*).....................5
   (*CareFree/CareFree* Sugarless)..........................5
   (*Stick Free* Sugarless Peppermint) .....................10
gumdrops, 10 pcs., 1.3 oz. .................................140
hard, all flavors (*Jolly Rancher*), 3 pcs., .6 oz ..........70
hard, all flavors (*LifeSavers* Bag), 4 pcs. ..............60
hard, all flavors (*TasteTations*), 3 pcs., .6 oz. ..........60
hard, all fruit flavors (*LifeSavers* Roll), 2 pcs...........20
honey (*Bit-O-Honey*), 1.7-oz. bar.........................190
jellybeans (*Jolly Rancher* Jolly Beans), 25 pcs., 1.4 oz. ..........130
licorice (*Diamond*), 10 pcs., 1.4 oz.......................120
licorice (*Switzer* Bites), 18 pcs., 1.4 oz. ...............130
licorice (*Twizzlers* Bites), 16 pcs., 1.4 oz. ............130
licorice (*Twizzlers* Twists), 2.5-oz. pkg.................240
licorice, candy coated (*Good & Fruity*), 1.75-oz. pkg...........180
licorice, candy coated (*Good & Plenty*), 1.75-oz. pkg. ........170
licorice, cherry (*Nibs*), 27 pcs., 1.4 oz...................140
licorice, chocolate (*Twizzlers* Twists), 3 pcs., 1.5 oz..........150
licorice, strawberry (*Twizzlers* Twists), 1.7-oz. pkg...........170
lollipop (*LifeSavers* Popsicles Swirled), 1 pop.............45
lollipop, all flavors (*Jolly Rancher*), .6-oz. pop ...........60
malted milk balls (*Whoppers*), .75-oz. pkg. .............100
(*Mars* Almond), 1.75-oz. bar...............................240
marshmallow (*Kraft Jet-Puffed*), 5 pcs....................110
(*Milky Way*), 2-oz. bar ....................................270
(*Milky Way* Lite), 1.6-oz. bar .............................170
(*Milky Way* Midnight), 1.75-oz. bar........................220
mint, chocolate (*Frango*), 4 pcs., 1.4 oz. ................210
mint, spearmint, or wintergreen (*LifeSavers* Roll), 3 pcs. ..........20
(*Mocha Crunch*), 1.3-oz. bar...............................200
(*Nestlé Turtles*), 2 pcs., 1.16 oz. .......................160
nonpareils (*Sno-Caps*), 2.3-oz. pkg. ......................300
(*Oh Henry!*), .9-oz. bar....................................120

**Candy** (*cont.*)

(*100 Grand*), 1.5-oz. pkg. ....................................................190
peanut butter (*Hershey's Sweet Escapes*), .7-oz bar..................90
peanut butter, candy coated (*Reese's Pieces*), 1.6-oz. pkg.......230
peanut butter and chocolate (*5th Avenue*), 2-oz. bar...............280
peanut butter, milk chocolate (*Nestlé Treasures*), 4 pcs. ..........240
peanut butter cookie cup (*Reese's*), .6-oz. pkg.......................90
peanut butter cup (*Reese's*), 1.2-oz. pkg. ..............................180
peanut and caramel (*PayDay*), 1.8-oz. bar..............................260
peanuts, chocolate coated (*Goobers*), 1.38-oz. pkg. ...............210
peppermint, chocolate coated (*York*), 1.4-oz. patty.................160
peppermint, chocolate coated (*York* Bites), 15 pcs., 1.4 oz. ....150
pretzel, milk chocolate (*Flipz*), 8 pcs., 1 oz..............................130
(*Snickers*), 2.1-oz. bar........................................................280
(*Snickers* Munch), 1.4-oz. bar..............................................230
raisins, chocolate covered (*Raisinets*), *1.58-oz. pkg.*..............*190*
*raisins, chocolate covered, semisweet* (Nestlé), 1⅓ tbsp...........70
(*Reese's NutRageous*), 1.9-oz. bar........................................290
taffy, all flavors (*Mighty Bite*), 5 pcs. ...................................170
(*3 Musketeers*), 2.1-oz. bar.................................................260
toffee (*Skor*), 1.4-oz. bar....................................................210
(*Top Secret*), 2.2-oz. bar....................................................320
wafer, chocolate (*Hershey's Sweet Escapes*), .7-oz bar .............80
wafer, chocolate coated (*Kit Kat*), 1.5-oz. bar........................220
(*Whatchamacallit*), 1.7-oz. bar.............................................240
(*Zagnut*), 1.7-oz. bar.........................................................230
(*Zero*), 1.8-oz. bar.............................................................230
**Cannellini bean,** see "Kidney bean"
**Cannelloni dinner,** frozen (*Amy's*), 9 oz.............................330
**Cannelloni entree,** frozen, cheese (*Lean Cuisine
  Everyday Favorites*), 9⅛-oz. pkg. ......................................230
**Cantaloupe,** fresh:
(*Dole*), ¼ medium ...............................................................50
cubed, 1 cup ........................................................................56
**Capers,** in jars (*Crosse & Blackwell*), 1 tbsp. .......................5
**Capon,** roasted, meat w/skin, 4 oz......................................260
**Caponata,** see "Eggplant appetizer"
**Cappuccino,** see "Coffee, flavored, mix"
**Carambola,** fresh, sliced, 1 cup............................................36

**Carambola, dried** (*Frieda's* Starfruit), ⅓ cup ...........................140
**Caramel topping,** 2 tbsp.:
(*Hershey's Chocolate Shoppe* Fat Free)................................100
(*Kraft*) .................................................................................120
(*Smucker's* Microwave Topping Fat Free/Sundae Syrup) .........110
(*Smucker's Magic Shell*) .......................................................220
hot (*Smucker's* Spoonable Toppings) ....................................120
**Caraway seed,** 1 tsp. ...............................................................7
**Cardamom,** ground, 1 tsp. .......................................................6
**Cardoon,** fresh, raw (*Frieda's*), 1 cup, 3 oz. ...........................15
**Carissa,** fresh, raw, trimmed, 1 fruit, .7 oz. ...........................12
**Carnival squash** (*Frieda's*), ¾ cup, 3 oz. ...............................30
**Carob drink mix,** powder, 1 tbsp. ...........................................45
**Carp,** meat only:
raw, 4 oz. ...............................................................................144
baked, broiled, or microwaved, 4 oz. ....................................184
**Carrot,** fresh:
raw (*Frieda's* Gold), ⅔ cup, 3 oz. .........................................35
raw, whole (*Dole*), 1 carrot, 7" X 1¼" diam, 2.8 oz. ...................35
raw, whole, baby, peeled (*Mann's*), 3 oz. ...............................38
raw, whole, baby, peeled, cut (*Green Giant*), 3 oz. ...................35
raw, crinkle cut, baby (*Mann's*), 3 oz. ....................................35
boiled, drained, sliced, ½ cup ...............................................35
**Carrot, canned or in jars,** ½ cup, except as noted:
baby (*Greenleaf*) ...................................................................21
baby (*Twin Tree Gardens* Belgian), 20 pcs., 4.5 oz. ...............21
baby (*Reese's*) .......................................................................15
sliced (*Allens/Crest Top*) .......................................................35
sliced (*Del Monte*) .................................................................35
sliced or French style (*S&W*) ................................................30
**Carrot, frozen:**
whole, baby (*Birds Eye*), ½ cup ............................................40
whole or sliced (*Freshlike*), ⅔ cup ........................................35
sliced (*Birds Eye*), ½ cup .....................................................35
honey glazed, sliced (*Green Giant*), 1 cup ............................90
**Carrot–fruit juice blend** (*Welch's* Tropical Carrot
     Sensation), 8 fl. oz. ..........................................................120
**Casaba,** fresh, raw, cubed, 1 cup ............................................44
**Cassava** (see also "Yuca root"), fresh, 14.4-oz. root .............653

**Cashew:**
(*Beer Nuts* Select), 1 oz...............................................170
(*Planters* Fancy/Halves/Halves Lightly Salted), 1 oz. ...............170
(*Planters* Salted), 1-oz. pkg..........................................160
dry or oil roasted, 1 oz., 18 medium....................................163
honey roasted (*Planters*), 1-oz. pkg. .................................150
**Cashew butter** (*Arrowhead Mills*), 2 tbsp............................160
**Catfish,** channel, meat only:
farmed, raw, 4 oz.......................................................153
farmed, baked, broiled, or microwaved, 4 oz.............................172
wild, raw, 4 oz.........................................................108
wild, baked, broiled, or microwaved, 4 oz...............................119
**Cauliflower,** fresh:
raw (*Andy Boy*), ⅙ medium head..........................................25
raw (*Dole*), ⅙ medium head, 3.5 oz. ....................................25
raw, florets (*Mann's Cauliettes*), 4 oz. ...............................30
boiled, drained, 3 florets, 1.9 oz......................................12
green, raw, 1 cup........................................................20
green, cooked, 1" pcs., ½ cup............................................20
**Cauliflower, frozen:**
(*Birds Eye*), ½ cup ....................................................20
florets (*Freshlike*), 4 pcs............................................20
boiled, drained, 1" pcs., 1 cup.........................................34
in cheese sauce (*Birds Eye*), ½ cup....................................80
in cheese sauce (*Green Giant*), ½ cup..................................60
**Cavatappi dish, mix,** sun-dried tomato basil pesto (*Land O
    Lakes International Pasta Collection*), 1 cup* .....................330
**Caviar** (see also "Roe"), black or red, 1 oz.........................71
**Caviar spread,** Greek (*Krinos* Taramosalata), 1 tbsp. ..............90
**Cayenne,** see "Pepper, seasoning"
**Celeriac,** fresh:
raw (*Frieda's*), ¾ cup, 3 oz...........................................35
boiled, drained, pcs., 1 cup ...........................................42
**Celery,** fresh:
raw, strips, 1 cup......................................................20
raw, diced, 1 cup.......................................................19
boiled, drained, 2 stalks, 2.7 oz.......................................14
boiled, drained, diced, 1 cup ..........................................27
**Celery seed,** dried, 1 tsp...........................................8

**Cellophane noodle,** see "Noodle, Chinese"
**Celtuce,** fresh, raw, 1 leaf, .3 oz. .................................................1
**Cereal, ready-to-eat** (see also specific grains):
amaranth flakes (*Arrowhead Mills*), 1 cup .....................128
bran (*Kellogg's All-Bran* Original), ½ cup ......................80
bran (*Kellogg's All-Bran Bran Buds*), ⅓ cup ...................80
bran (*Kellogg's All-Bran Extra Fiber*), ½ cup ..................50
bran (*Nabisco 100% Bran*), ⅓ cup .................................80
bran, raisin (*Kellogg's/Kellogg's Raisin Bran Crunch*), 1 cup....190
bran, raisin (*Total*), 1 cup ...........................................170
bran, raisin (*Wheaties* Raisin Bran), 1 cup ....................180
bran flakes (*Arrowhead Mills*), 1 cup ..............................90
bran flakes (*Kellogg's Complete* Wheat Bran), ¾ cup..........90
bran flakes (*Post*), ¾ cup ...........................................100
buckwheat flakes, maple (*Arrowhead Mills*), 1 cup ..........160
corn (*Corn Chex*), 1 cup .............................................110
corn (*Kellogg's Corn Pops*), 1 cup ...............................120
corn flakes (*Arrowhead Mills*), 1 cup .............................130
corn flakes (*Country*), 1 cup .......................................110
corn flakes (*Kellogg's Corn Flakes*), 1 cup ....................100
corn flakes (*Kellogg's Honey Crunch Corn Flakes*), ¾ cup........120
corn flakes (*Post Toasties*), 1 cup ................................100
corn flakes (*Total*), 1⅓ cup .........................................110
corn flakes, frosted (*Kellogg's Frosted Flakes*), ¾ cup .............120
corn or millet, puffed (*Arrowhead Mills*), 1 cup...........................60
corn and rice (*Kellogg's Crispix*), 1 cup .......................110
granola (*Kellogg's* Low Fat w/Raisins), ⅔ cup .....................220
granola (*Kellogg's* Low Fat w/out Raisins), ½ cup ...............190
granola, fruit (*Nature Valley*), ⅔ cup .............................210
kamut, puffed (*Arrowhead Mills*), 1 cup...........................50
kamut flakes (*Arrowhead Mills*), 1 cup ...........................110
multigrain (see also "granola," above):
   (*Banana Nut Crunch*), 1 cup ...................................250
   (*Basic 4*), 1 cup..................................................200
   (*Cinnamon Toast Crunch*), ¾ cup .............................130
   (*Cranberry Almond Crunch*), 1 cup ...........................220
   (*Fiber One*), ½ cup..................................................60
   (*Golden Grahams*), ¾ cup .....................................120
   (*Grape-Nuts*), ½ cup.............................................200

**Cereal, ready-to-eat (*cont.*)**

| | |
|---|---|
| (*Honey Nut Clusters*), 1 cup | 210 |
| (*Honeycomb*), 1⅓ cups | 110 |
| (*Kellogg's Apple Jacks/Froot Loops*), 1 cup | 120 |
| (*Kellogg's Müeslix*), ⅔ cup | 200 |
| (*Kellogg's Product 19*), 1 cup | 100 |
| (*Kix*), 1⅓ cups | 120 |
| (*Multi-Grain Cheerios*), 1 cup | 110 |
| (*Team Cheerios*), 1 cup | 120 |
| (*Total* Whole Grain), ¾ cup | 110 |
| (*Trix*), 1 cup | 120 |
| (*Waffle Crisp*), 1 cup | 130 |
| all varieties (*Fruit & Fibre*), 1 cup | 210 |
| flakes (*Arrowhead Mills*), 1 cup | 110 |
| flakes (*Grape-Nuts*), ¾ cup | 100 |
| flakes (*Healthy Choice*), ¾ cup | 110 |
| flakes (*Kellogg's Smart Start*), 1 cup | 180 |
| flakes (*Kellogg's Special K Plus*), 1 cup | 210 |

oat:

| | |
|---|---|
| (*Alpha-Bits*), 1 cup | 130 |
| (*Apple Cinnamon Cheerios*), ¾ cup | 120 |
| (*Cheerios*), 1 cup | 110 |
| (*Frosted Cheerios/Honey Nut Cheerios*), 1 cup | 120 |
| (*Honey Nut Bunches of Oats*), ¾ cup | 120 |
| (*Lucky Charms*), 1 cup | 120 |
| almonds (*Honey Nut Bunches of Oats*), ¾ cup | 130 |
| almonds (*Oatmeal Crisp*), 1 cup | 220 |
| apple cinnamon (*Barbara's* Toasted O's), ¾ cup | 110 |
| apple cinnamon raisin (*Oatmeal Crisp*), 1 cup | 210 |
| honey nut (*Barbara's* Toasted O's), ¾ cup | 120 |
| shredded (*Barbara's* Shredded Spoonfuls), ¾ cup | 120 |
| shredded, bite size (*Barbara's*), 1¼ cups | 220 |
| oat bran (*Kellogg's Cracklin' Oat Bran*), ¾ cup | 190 |
| oat bran flakes (*Arrowhead Mills*), 1 cup | 140 |
| oat bran flakes (*Kellogg's Complete*), ¾ cup | 110 |
| rice (*Kellogg's Cocoa Krispies*), ¾ cup | 120 |
| rice (*Kellogg's Razzle Dazzle Rice Krispies*), ¾ cup | 110 |
| rice (*Kellogg's Rice Krispies*), 1¼ cups | 120 |
| rice (*Kellogg's Rice Krispies Treats*), ¾ cup | 120 |

rice (*Rice Chex*), 1¼ cups.................................................120
rice flakes (*Arrowhead Mills*), 1 cup .......................80
spelt flakes (*Arrowhead Mills*), 1 cup....................100
wheat (*Wheat Chex*), 1 cup.....................................180
wheat, puffed (*Arrowhead Mills*), 1 cup...................60
wheat, puffed (*Golden Crisp*), ¾ cup ....................110
wheat, shredded (*Nabisco Honey Nut* Bite Size), 1 cup...........200
wheat, shredded (*Nabisco Original*), 2 pcs............160
wheat, shredded (*Nabisco Original Spoon Size*), 1 cup ...........170
wheat, shredded, frosted (*Nabisco* Bite Size), 1 cup ...............190
wheat, shredded, sweetened (*Arrowhead Mills*), 1 cup ...........200
wheat, whole, biscuits:
   (*Kellogg's Frosted Mini-Wheats* Bite Size), 24 pcs..............200
   (*Kellogg's Frosted Mini-Wheats* Original), 5 pcs. ...............180
   strawberry (*Kellogg's Mini-Wheats*), ¾ cup .......................170
wheat flakes (*Frosted Wheaties*), ¾ cup ...................................110
wheat flakes (*Wheaties*), 1 cup .................................................110
**Cereal, cooking/hot,** dry:
(*Arrowhead Mills Bear Mush*), ¼ cup .......................................160
barley (*Arrowhead Mills Bits O Barley*), ⅓ cup..........................140
couscous, 1 cont.:
   apple cinnamon (*Marrakesh Express Cocorico!*)................260
   banana or peach (*Marrakesh Express Cocorico!*)...............280
   blueberry (*Marrakesh Express Cocorico!*) ........................270
   strawberry (*Marrakesh Express Cocorico!*) ......................250
multigrain:
   banana nut bread (*Harvest Mornings*), 1 pkt. ....................150
   blueberry muffin or raspberry (*Harvest Mornings*), 1 pkt...140
   4 grain, plus flax (*Arrowhead Mills*), ¼ cup .......................150
   7 grain (*Arrowhead Mills*), ⅓ cup .....................................140
   7 grain, wheat free (*Arrowhead Mills*), ¼ cup....................120
oats/oatmeal:
   plain (*Arrowhead Mills*), 1-oz. pkt. .....................................110
   cranberry (*Arrowhead Mills* Instant), 1.23-oz. pkt. .............130
   maple (*Maypo*), ½ cup ......................................................210
   maple apple (*Arrowhead Mills* Instant), 1.23-oz. pkt. .........130
rice (*Arrowhead Mills Rice and Shine*), ¼ cup ..........................150
rice (*Cream of Rice/Creme de Arroz*), ¼ cup ............................170
rice (*Lundberg* Purely Organic), ⅓ cup .....................................190

**Cereal, cooking/hot (*cont.*)**
rice, almond, sweet (*Lundberg*), ⅓ cup ....................................200
rice, cinnamon raisin (*Lundberg*), ⅓ cup ...............................190
wheat (*Cream of Wheat* 10/2½/1 Minute), 3 tbsp. ..................120
wheat (*Cream of Wheat* Instant Original), 1 pkt.......................100
wheat (*Wheat Hearts*), ¼ cup....................................................130
wheat (*Wheatena*), ⅓ cup .........................................................160
wheat, all varieties, except original (*Cream of Wheat*
    Instant), 1 pkt........................................................................130
**Cereal bar,** see "Granola and cereal bar"
**Chayote,** boiled, drained, 1" pcs., 1 cup .....................................38
**Cheese** (see also "Cheese food" and "Cheese product"), 1 oz.,
    except as noted:
American, processed, white or yellow:
    (*Kraft* Deluxe) ....................................................................100
    (*Kraft* Deluxe Singles), ¾-oz. slice.........................................80
    (*Kraft* Singles), ¾-oz. slice.....................................................70
    (*Land O Lakes* 50% Reduced Fat Light).................................70
    (*Land O Lakes/Land O Lakes* Reduced Salt) ......................110
    sharp (*Kraft Old English*) ...................................................100
American and Swiss, processed (*Land O Lakes* Loaf)..............100
blue ..............................................................................................100
brick (*Land O Lakes*) ................................................................100
Brie................................................................................................95
Camembert ...................................................................................85
caraway.......................................................................................107
cheddar:
    (*Cracker Barrel New York Aged Reserve*) ...........................120
    (*Land O Lakes*) .................................................................110
    all varieties (*Cracker Barrel* Reduced Fat)............................90
    medium or mild (*Kraft/Kraft Off the Block*) .......................110
    medium or mild, shredded (*Kraft*), ¼ cup ...........................100
    mild (*Kraft Marbled*) ..........................................................110
    sharp (*Cracker Barrel* Reduced Fat Vermont)......................90
    sharp or extra sharp (*Cracker Barrel*) ...............................120
    sharp or extra sharp (*Kraft/Kraft Off the Block*) ...............120
    sharp, marbled (*Cracker Barrel*).......................................110
cheddar, shredded (*Kraft*), ¼ cup.............................................110
cheddar, shredded (*Kraft* Reduced Fat), ¼ cup ........................80

cheddar, shredded (*Kraft Free*), ¼ cup .....................40
cheddar–Monterey jack (*Kraft Marbled*) ................100
cheddar–Monterey jack, shredded (*Kraft*), ¼ cup ...................100
cheddar-mozzarella (*Kraft Marbled*)........................100
*Chedarella* (*Land O Lakes*) .....................................100
Cheshire.....................................................................110
Colby (*Cracker Barrel* Reduced Fat) .........................80
Colby (*Kraft*)............................................................110
Colby (*Land O Lakes*) ..............................................110
Colby or Colby jack (*Land O Lakes*) .........................110
Colby, longhorn (*Sara Lee*)......................................110
Colby, longhorn, jack (*Sara Lee*) .............................100
Colby Monterey jack (*Kraft/Kraft Marbled/Off the Block*) .........110
Colby and Monterey jack, shredded (*Kraft*), ¼ cup ..................100
cottage, ½ cup:
    4%, large curd (*Knudsen*).................................130
    4%, large or small curd (*Breakstone's*) .............120
    4%, small curd (*Knudsen*).................................120
    2%, large or small curd (*Breakstone's*) ...............90
    2%, small curd (*Knudsen*).................................100
    1.5%, w/pineapple (*Knudsen*).............................120
    1%, plain or garden salad (*Light n' Lively*) ...........80
    1%, peach and pineapple (*Light n' Lively*) ...........110
    nonfat (*Breakstone's Free/Light n' Lively Free*) ....80
cottage cheese, dry curd (*Breakstone's*), ¼ cup.........................45
cream cheese (*Organic Valley*)..................................90
cream cheese (*Philadelphia*) ...................................100
cream cheese (*Philadelphia Free*) .............................30
cream cheese, chives (*Philadelphia*)..........................90
cream cheese, soft, 2 tbsp.:
    (*Philadelphia*)...................................................100
    (*Philadelphia Light*)............................................70
    plain or garden vegetables (*Philadelphia Free*).....................30
    apple cinnamon, pineapple, or salmon (*Philly Flavors*).......100
    cheesecake, chive and onion, garden vegetable, honey
      nut, or strawberry (*Philly Flavors*) .....................110
    jalapeno (*Philly Flavors* Light)...............................60
    roasted garlic or raspberry (*Philly Flavors* Light) ..................70
    strawberries (*Philadelphia Free*) ...........................45

**Cheese (*cont.*)**

cream cheese, whipped (*Philadelphia*), 2 tbsp. ..........................70
Edam..............................................................................................101
feta...................................................................................................75
feta, crumbled, 1 cup....................................................................395
fontina...........................................................................................110
Gjestost (*Ski Queen*) ..................................................................130
goat, four pepper or garlic and herbs (*Montchevré*) ................70
goat, mild, or w/basil and roasted garlic (*Chavrie*), 1.1 oz........50
goat, semisoft type ......................................................................103
goat, soft type................................................................................76
Gouda ...........................................................................................101
grated (*Kraft Free*), 2 tsp. .........................................................152
grated, garlic herb or red pepper (*Kraft Parm Plus!*), 2 tsp. ......15
Gruyère .........................................................................................117
Havarti (*Sara Lee*)......................................................................120
Havarti, plain, dill or jalapeno (*Boar's Head*) ..........................110
Italian style, finely shredded, all varieties (*Kraft*), ⅓ cup .........100
jalapeno jack, processed (*Land O Lakes* Loaf)..........................100
Limburger (*Knirps*).......................................................................80
mascarpone (*Bel Gioioso*) ..........................................................124
Mexican style, finely shredded, all varieties (*Kraft*), ⅓ cup......120
Monterey, processed (*Kraft* Singles), ¾-oz. slice ......................70
Monterey jack (*Cracker Barrel* Reduced Fat)...............................80
Monterey jack (*Kraft/Kraft Off the Block*)...................................110
Monterey jack (*Sara Lee*) ..........................................................100
Monterey jack, plain or jalapeno (*Boar's Head*).........................100
Monterey jack, w/ or w/out hot peppers (*Land O Lakes*) .........110
Monterey jack w/jalapeno (*Kraft*) ..............................................110
Monterey jack, shredded (*Kraft*), ¼ cup ....................................100
mozzarella (see also "string," p. 47):
    (*Boar's Head*)........................................................................90
    (*Sara Lee* Deli), ¾-oz. slice.................................................60
    whole milk................................................................................80
    whole milk, low moisture........................................................90
    part skim, low moisture (*Kraft/Kraft Off the Block*) .............80
    part skim, low moisture (*Kraft* Slices), 1.5-oz. slice............120
    part skim, low moisture (*Land O Lakes*) .............................80
    part skim, low moisture (*Sara Lee*) .....................................80

shredded (*Healthy Choice* Fancy), ¼ cup ...............................50
shredded (*Kraft Free*), ¼ cup.....................................................45
shredded (*Kraft* Reduced Fat), ⅓ cup.......................................80
shredded, whole milk, low moisture (*Kraft*), ⅓ cup ...........100
shredded, part skim, low moisture (*Kraft*), ⅓ cup................90
Muenster (*Land O Lakes*).........................................................100
Muenster (*Sara Lee*)................................................................100
Muenster, shredded, ¼ cup.......................................................121
Neufchâtel (*Organic Valley*) ......................................................70
Neufchâtel (*Philadelphia*) ...........................................................70
Parmesan...................................................................................111
Parmesan, grated (*Di Giorno*), 2 tsp.......................................20
Parmesan, grated (*Di Giorno* 100%), 2 tsp...........................25
Parmesan, grated (*Land O Lakes*), 1 tbsp..............................35
Parmesan, grated or shredded (*Kraft* 100%), 2 tsp.................20
Parmesan, shredded (*Di Giorno* 100%), 2 tsp.........................20
pimento, processed (*Kraft* Deluxe Singles)..............................100
pimento, processed (*Kraft* Singles), ¾-oz. slice .........................70
pizza blend, shredded:
   4 cheese (*Kraft*), ¼ cup.......................................................90
   cheddar and mozzarella (*Kraft* Reduced Fat), ⅓ cup............90
   low moisture mozzarella and cheddar (*Kraft*), ⅓ cup.........120
Port de Salut...............................................................................100
provolone (*Land O Lakes*)..........................................................100
provolone, picante/sharp (*Boar's Head*) ..................................100
provolone, smoke flavor (*Kraft* Slices), 1.5-oz. slice ..............150
provolone, smoked (*Sara Lee* Deli), ¾-oz. slice .......................80
ricotta (*Breakstone's*), ¼ cup ...................................................110
ricotta, whole milk, ½ cup.........................................................216
ricotta, part skim, ½ cup ..........................................................170
Romano ......................................................................................110
Romano, grated (*Di Giorno* 100%), 2 tsp...............................25
Romano, grated (*Kraft* 100%), 2 tsp......................................20
Romano, shredded (*Di Giorno* 100%), 2 tsp. ........................20
Roquefort...................................................................................105
sharp, processed (*Kraft* Singles), ¾-oz. slice ...........................70
string, part skim, low moisture (*Kraft Handi-Snacks*)................80
Swiss (*Kraft*) .............................................................................110
Swiss (*Kraft Deli-Thin* Slices/*Kraft* Slices), .8-oz. slice ..............90

**Cheese** *(cont.)*

Swiss (*Kraft* Slices/*Kraft* Slices Aged), 1.5-oz. slice ................170
Swiss (*Land O Lakes*) ...................................................................110
Swiss (*Land O Lakes* 50% Reduced Fat Light)............................80
Swiss, baby (*Cracker Barrel*) .......................................................110
Swiss, baby (*Land O Lakes* Loaf/Wheel)....................................110
Swiss, processed (*Kraft* Deluxe Singles).....................................90
Swiss, shredded (*Kraft*), ⅓ cup..................................................100
Swiss, shredded, fine (*Kraft*), ⅓ cup..........................................110
Tilsit ...............................................................................................96

**"Cheese," nondairy,** 1 oz.:

American, roasted garlic, or mozzarella (*Tofutti*)........................70
cheddar, shredded (*Tofutti Better Than Cheddar*)......................70
cream cheese (*Tofutti Better Than Cream Cheese*)....................80
cream cheese (*Tofutti Better Than Cream Cheese* Low Fat) .......40

**Cheese dip,** 2 tbsp.:

jalapeno and cheddar (*Frito-Lay*) ...............................................50
cheddar, mild (*Frito-Lay*).............................................................60
salsa (*Chi-Chi's*)..........................................................................90
salsa (*D. L. Jardine's* Queso Loco/Caliente) ..............................40
salsa (*Pace* Picante con Queso) ................................................90
salsa, medium or mild (*Taco Bell Home Originals*)....................45
and salsa, medium or mild (*Cheez Whiz*) ................................100

**Cheese entree,** frozen, cheddar and chicken bake (*Stouffer's*),
   11.5-oz. pkg. ...........................................................................450

**Cheese fondue,** see "Fondue"

**Cheese food** (see also "Cheese" and "Cheese product"):

American (*Land O Lakes* Slices), ¾-oz. slice..............................70
American (*Land O Lakes* Slices), ⅔-oz. slice .............................60
American, white or yellow (*Kraft* Reduced Fat), ¾ oz.................50
cheddar, medium or mild (*Kraft* Cheddary Melts), 1 oz............110
cheddar, shredded (*Kraft* Cheddary Melts), ¼ cup ...................120
w/garlic or jalapeno peppers (*Kraft*), 1 oz. ................................90
Italian herb, jalapeno, onion, pepperoni, or salami
   (*Land O Lakes*), 1 oz................................................................90
shredded (*Velveeta*), ¼ cup.......................................................130
shredded (*Velveeta* Mild Mexican), ¼ cup .................................120

**Cheese pocket,** grilled (*Toaster Pockets* Melts), 2.2-oz. pc. ....190

**Cheese product** (see also "Cheese food"):
(*Cheez Whiz Light*), 2 tbsp.............................................80
(*Velveeta Light*), 1 oz. ...............................................60
American, white or yellow (*Kraft Free*), ¾ oz. ...........30
American flavor (*Light n' Lively*), ¾ oz......................45
cheddar, sharp (*Kraft Free*), ⅔ oz. .............................35
Swiss flavor (*Kraft Free*), ¾ oz. ................................30
**Cheese sauce,** 2 tbsp.:
plain or jalapeno (*Cheez Whiz*)....................................90
mild salsa or squeezable (*Cheez Whiz*).....................100
**Cheese sauce, cooking,** see also "Pasta sauce," ¼ cup:
Alfredo (*Ragú Cheese Creations!* Classic)..................120
Alfredo, light Parmesan (*Ragú Cheese Creations!*) ..................80
cheddar, double (*Ragú Cheese Creations!*) ..................110
4 cheese or garlic-Parmesan (*Ragú Cheese Creations!*)..........120
Romano, cream tomato (*Ragú Cheese Creations!*)....................60
**Cheese spread** (see also "Cheese"), 2 tbsp., except as noted:
(*Land O Lakes Golden Velvet*).......................................80
(*Velveeta/Velveeta* Mexican), 1 oz. ............................90
American, cheddar, or cheddar and bacon (*Easy Cheese*)........100
bacon (*Kraft*) ...............................................................90
blue (*Kraft Roka*) .........................................................80
cheddar baseball or nacho (*Easy Cheese*).....................90
cheddar-cream cheese, all varieties (*Cracker Barrel*) ...............80
feta, w/garlic and chives (*Cypress*), 1 oz. ...................110
Limburger (*Mohawk Valley*) ..........................................80
olive and pimento (*Kraft*) ............................................70
pimento (*Kraft*).............................................................80
pineapple (*Kraft*) .........................................................70
sharp (*Kraft Old English*)..............................................90
**Cheeseburger,** see "Beef sandwich/pocket"
**Cheesecake** (*Entenmann's* Deluxe French), ⅕ cake.................460
**Cheesecake, frozen or refrigerated:**
(*Baby Watson*), ⅙ cake .................................................270
(*Carousel* New York Cheese Cake), 3-oz. cake.........................230
(*Jell-O* Original), 3.3-oz. cont. ....................................160
(*Sara Lee* 25% Reduced-Fat), ¼ cake....................................310
(*Sara Lee* Original), ¼ cake ..........................................350
cherry (*Sara Lee*), ¼ cake ............................................350

**Cheesecake, frozen or refrigerated (*cont.*)**

chocolate chip (*Sara Lee*), ¼ cake ...............................410
chocolate dipped praline pecan or toasted almond crunch
   (*Sara Lee Cheesecake Bites*), .8-oz. pc. ...............90
French (*Sara Lee*), ⅙ cake .......................................350
fudge brownie (*Sara Lee Cheesecake Singles*), 3.9-oz. pc. ......390
strawberry (*Jell-O*), 3.5-oz. cont. ..............................150
strawberry (*Sara Lee*), ¼ cake ...................................330
strawberry, French (*Sara Lee*), ⅙ cake ..........................320
strawberry (*Sara Lee Cheesecake Singles*), 3.9-oz. pc. ...........370
**Cheesecake mix,** ⅛ cake\*, except as noted:
(*Betty Crocker* Original) .........................................400
(*Jell-O* No Bake Homestyle/Real), ⅙ cake\* .......................360
cherry or strawberry (*Jell-O* No Bake) ...........................340
chocolate chip (*Betty Crocker*) ..................................410
strawberry swirl (*Betty Crocker*) ................................380
strawberry swirl (*Jell-O* No Bake Reduced Fat) ...................250
**Cherimoya,** fresh, raw, trimmed, 1 fruit, 1.2 lbs. ............514
**Cherries jubilee,** canned (*Lucky Leaf*), 2.3 oz., ⅑ can ........80
**Cherry,** fresh, 1 cup:
(*Dole*) ..........................................................90
sour, red, w/pits .................................................52
sweet, w/pits .....................................................84
sweet, pitted ....................................................104
**Cherry, candied,** red (*S&W*), 1 pc. ...........................15
**Cherry, canned,** ½ cup, except as noted:
sour, red, in heavy syrup, 1 cup .................................233
sweet, pitted:
   Bing, in heavy syrup (*Oregon*), ½ cup ....................110
   dark, in heavy syrup (*Del Monte*), ½ cup .................100
   dark, in heavy syrup (*Oregon*), ½ cup ....................100
   dark, in heavy syrup (*S&W*), ½ cup .......................140
   Royal Anne, pitted, in heavy syrup (*Oregon*), ½ cup .......110
tart, red, pitted, in water (*Oregon*), ⅔ cup .....................60
**Cherry, dried:**
bing (*Frieda's*), ¼ cup .........................................120
tart (*Frieda's*), ⅓ cup .........................................150
**Cherry, maraschino,** green or red, w/liquid, 1 oz. .............33

**Cherry drink:**
(*Kool-Aid Bursts*), 6.76 fl. oz.............................................100
(*Kool-Aid Splash*), 8 fl. oz. ..........................................100
wild (*Capri Sun All Natural*), 6.76 fl. oz. ...................110
**Cherry drink mix,** regular or black (*Kool-Aid*), 8 fl. oz. ..........100
**Cherry juice blend** (*Mott's*), 8 fl. oz. ........................120
**Cherry syrup,** cherries jubilee (*Hershey's Chocolate*
    *Shoppe*), 2 tbsp. ..................................................110
**Chervil, dried,** 1 tsp.........................................................1
**Chestnut,** in jars, roasted (*Minerve*), 4 whole, 1 oz...................50
**Chestnut, Chinese,** 1 oz.:
dried, shelled ..............................................................103
boiled or steamed .........................................................44
roasted.........................................................................68
**Chestnut, European:**
raw, peeled, 1 oz...........................................................56
roasted, 1 cup.............................................................350
**Chestnut, Japanese:**
dried, ¼ cup.................................................................140
roasted, 1 oz.................................................................57
**Chicken** (see also "Capon"), fresh, 4 oz., except as noted:
broiler or fryer, roasted:
    meat w/skin..............................................................271
    meat only ................................................................215
    meat only, chopped or diced, 1 cup .....................266
    skin only, 1 oz. ........................................................129
    dark meat, w/skin...................................................287
    dark meat only ........................................................232
    light meat, w/skin...................................................252
    light meat only ........................................................196
    light meat only, chopped or diced, 1 cup .............242
    breast, meat w/skin.................................................223
    breast, meat only .....................................................187
    breast, meat only, chopped or diced, 1 cup ..........231
    drumstick, meat w/skin...........................................245
    drumstick, meat only ..............................................197
    leg, meat w/skin......................................................263
    leg, meat only..........................................................217
    thigh, meat w/skin...................................................280

**Chicken (*cont.*)**

thigh, meat only ................................................................237
wing, meat w/skin ............................................................329

roasting, roasted:

meat w/skin .....................................................................253
meat only .........................................................................189
meat only, chopped or diced, 1 cup ..............................234
dark meat only ................................................................202
dark meat only, chopped or diced, 1 cup ......................249
light meat only .................................................................174
light meat only, chopped or diced, 1 cup ......................214

stewing, stewed:

meat w/skin .....................................................................323
meat only .........................................................................269
meat only, chopped or diced, 1 cup ..............................332
dark meat only ................................................................296
dark meat only, chopped or diced, 1 cup ......................361
light meat only .................................................................242
light meat only, chopped or diced, 1 cup ......................298

**Chicken, canned,** 2 oz.:

(*Hormel* Chunk) ...................................................................70
breast (*Hormel* Chunk No Salt) .........................................60
breast, chunk, in water (*Swanson* Premium).....................60

**Chicken, frozen or refrigerated,** 3 oz., except as noted:

whole, cooked:

dark (*Perdue/Perdue Oven Stuffer/Perdue* Cut Up/Split).....210
dark, all styles except honey roasted (*Perdue* Rotisserie)...180
dark, honey roasted (*Perdue* Rotisserie) .....................200
dark, roasted, toasted garlic (*Perdue*) .........................190
white (*Perdue/Perdue Oven Stuffer*) .............................170
white, all styles (*Perdue* Rotisserie) .............................140
white, roasted, toasted garlic (*Perdue*)........................160
quarters, breast (*Perdue*)...............................................170
quarters, leg (*Perdue*).....................................................220

whole, barbecued (*Empire* Kosher), 5 oz. ......................280
bites (*Country Skillet*), 5 pcs. ..........................................270

breast, cooked:

whole (*Perdue*) ...............................................................160
whole (*Perdue Oven Stuffer*).........................................150

boneless, skinless (*Perdue Fit 'N Easy*)..............................110
boneless, skinless (*Perdue Oven Stuffer*) ...........................120
quarter, oven roasted (*Boston Market*), 6-oz. pkg. .............180
split, roasted (*Perdue*), 6.8-oz. pc. ...................................370
split, skinless, roasted (*Perdue*), 5.8-oz. pc. ......................250
breast, carved, cooked (*Perdue Short Cuts*), ½ cup.................100
breast, crispy baked, 1 pc.:
　(*Butterball* Original)................................................180
　Italian (*Butterball*) .................................................190
　lemon pepper or Parmesan (*Butterball*)............................200
　Southwestern (*Butterball*) .........................................170
breast, seasoned, raw, boneless, 4-oz. breast:
　roasted (*Chicken By George*).......................................110
　Cajun, teriyaki, Italian bleu cheese, lemon oregano, or
　　mesquite barbecue (*Chicken By George*)........................130
　Caribbean grill (*Chicken By George*)................................150
　lemon herb (*Chicken By George*) ..................................120
　mustard dill or tomato herb (*Chicken By George*) ..............140
breast, seasoned, cooked, boneless:
　Italian style, lemon pepper, teriyaki, or roasted garlic
　　herb (*Perdue*) ..................................................90
　cutlet, thin sliced, roasted garlic thyme, or tomato herb
　　w/basil (*Perdue* Thin Sliced) ....................................90
breast cutlet, breaded, cooked:
　(*Perdue* Fully Cooked), 3.5-oz. pc..................................240
　(*Perdue* Fully Cooked Homestyle)....................................120
　Italian style (*Perdue* Fully Cooked) ................................130
breast quarter, cooked (*Perdue*)......................................170
breast strips, breaded, cooked:
　hot and spicy (*Perdue Kick'n Chicken*) ..............................110
　original or barbecue (*Perdue Kick'n Chicken*) ......................120
breast tenderloin, cooked:
　boneless, skinless (*Perdue Fit 'N Easy*)..............................100
　boneless, skinless (*Perdue* Individually Frozen)..................100
　breaded (*Perdue* Fully Cooked)......................................170
　breaded (*Perdue* Fully Cooked Individually Frozen).............200
breast tenders (*Banquet* Original), 3 pcs...........................250
breast tenders (*Country Skillet*), 3 pcs. ...........................240
breast tenders, baked (*Banquet* Fat Free), 3 pcs....................120

**Chicken, frozen or refrigerated (*cont.*)**

breast tenders, baked (*Butterball*), 3 pcs.....................................170
breast tenders, Southern (*Banquet*), 3 pcs. ............................260
chunks (*Country Skillet*), 5 pcs. .............................................270
cutlets, raw (*Empire* Kosher), 4 oz.........................................110
drumstick, cooked (*Perdue*), 2.2-oz. pc..................................110
fillet, breaded and battered (*Empire* Kosher), 4 oz...................240
fried (*Country Skillet*).............................................................270
fried, bone-in (*Banquet* Original/*Banquet* Southern)................280
fried, breast, breaded and battered (*Empire* Kosher)................170
fried, chunks, Southern fried (*Country Skillet*), 5 pcs. ..............270
fried, country, bone-in (*Banquet*).............................................270
fried, cut up, assorted (*Empire* Kosher) ...................................200
fried, drum and thigh (*Empire* Kosher) .....................................240
fried, honey barbecue, skinless, bone-in (*Banquet*) .................230
fried, hot 'n spicy, bone-in (*Banquet*) .....................................260
fried, patty, Southern (*Country Skillet*), 1 patty .......................190
fried, skinless, bone-in (*Banquet*) ...........................................220
leg, roasted (*Perdue*), 5.6-oz. pc............................................370
leg and thigh, oven roasted (*Boston Market*), 6-oz. pkg. .........290
nuggets (*Banquet* Original), 6 pcs............................................270
nuggets (*Country Skillet*), 10 pcs. ...........................................280
nuggets, battered and breaded (*Empire* Kosher) ......................180
nuggets, breast (*Banquet*), 7 pcs. ...........................................280
nuggets, breast, breaded, cooked (*Perdue* Fully Cooked/Fully
    Cooked Golden Brown), 5 pcs. ..........................................240
nuggets, breast, and cheese (*Perdue* Fully Cooked), 5 pcs. .....270
nuggets, breast, mozzarella cheese (*Banquet*), 6 pcs. .............280
nuggets, Southern (*Banquet*), 5 pcs.........................................160
patty (*Banquet* Original/Southern), 1 patty...............................190
patty (*Country Skillet*), 1 patty ...............................................190
patty, breast, baked (*Banquet* Fat Free), 1 patty.......................100
patty, breast, honey barbecue, grilled (*Banquet*), 1 patty.........110
patty, breast, honey mustard, grilled (*Banquet*), 1 patty ..........120
thigh, cooked:
    roasted (*Perdue*/*Perdue* Skin-Up), 3.2-oz. pc.....................240
    boneless, skinless (*Perdue* Individually Frozen),
        3.7-oz. pc..................................................................180

fajita (*Perdue*), 2.4-oz. pc. .....................................................120
   3 pepper (*Perdue Short Cuts* Cooked Carved), ½ cup........130
wing, roasted (*Perdue*), 2 pcs. ...............................................210
wing, roasted (*Perdue Kick'n Wings*) ................................180
wing, barbecue or teriyaki, cooked (*Perdue Kick'n Wings*) ......200
wing, firehouse big (*Banquet*), 2 pcs. ...............................190
wing, herb roasted, cooked (*Perdue Kick'n Wings*) ..................190
wing, honey barbecue (*Banquet*), 4 pcs. ...........................380
wing, hot 'n spicy (*Banquet*), 4 pcs. ...................................180
wing, hot and spicy, cooked (*Perdue Kick'n Wings*).................190
wing, smokehouse big (*Banquet*), 2 pcs. ...........................200
wingette, roasted (*Perdue*), 3 pcs. .....................................210
wingette, roasted (*Perdue Oven Stuffer*), 3 pcs. ......................220
**Chicken, ground,** cooked:
(*Perdue Fit 'N Easy*), 3 oz. ..................................................170
(*Perdue Fit 'N Easy* Burgers), 3-oz. pc. ...............................160
breast (*Perdue Fit 'N Easy*), 3 oz. .......................................80
**Chicken dinner,** frozen, 1 pkg.:
Alfredo, broccoli (*Healthy Choice* Meal), 11.5 oz. ....................300
Cantonese (*Healthy Choice* Meal), 10.75 oz. .............................280
country breaded (*Healthy Choice* Meal), 10.25 oz. ...................350
country herb (*Healthy Choice* Meal), 12.15 oz. .........................320
Dijon (*Healthy Choice* Meal), 11 oz. .....................................270
fried (*Swanson Hungry Man* Classic), 16.5 oz. ..........................790
fried (*Banquet Extra Helping*), 14.7 oz. ..................................910
fried, boneless, white (*Banquet Extra Helping*), 13 oz. .............690
fried, boneless, white (*Swanson*), 11 oz. ...............................430
fried, boneless, white (*Swanson Hungry-Man*), 13.75 oz.........660
honey glazed (*Healthy Choice* Meal), 10 oz. ...........................270
mesquite, barbecue (*Healthy Choice* Meal), 10.5 oz. ................310
nuggets (*Swanson*), 11 oz. .................................................590
parmigiana (*Healthy Choice* Meal), 11.5 oz. ............................330
roast (*Healthy Choice* Meal), 11 oz. .....................................230
roast, boneless (*Swanson Hungry-Man*), 15.25 oz. .................500
sesame (*Healthy Choice* Meal), 10.8 oz. ...............................360
stir-fry, w/vegetables (*Healthy Choice* Meal), 11 oz. .................360
sweet and sour (*Healthy Choice* Meal), 11 oz. ..........................360
teriyaki (*Healthy Choice* Meal), 11 oz. ..................................270
white meat, boneless (*Swanson*), 11 oz. ...............................430

**Chicken dinner, frozen (*cont.*)**
white meat, boneless (*Swanson Hungry-Man*), 13.75 oz. ........660
**Chicken entree, canned or packaged:**
and dumplings (*Dinty Moore*), 7.5-oz. can ...............................200
and dumplings (*Dinty Moore* Microwave), 1 cup....................200
and noodles (*Dinty Moore American Classics*), 1 bowl ...........270
w/potato (*Dinty Moore American Classics*), 1 bowl.................240
stew (*Dinty Moore*), 1 cup.......................................................220
stew, and dumplings (*Dinty Moore*), 1 cup..............................260
**Chicken entree, frozen** (see also "Chicken, frozen or
    refrigerated"), 1 pkg., except as noted:
and almonds, w/rice (*Yu Sing*), 9 oz. .....................................300
à la king (*Freezer Queen* Cook-in-Pouch), 4 oz. .....................60
à la king (*Michelina's*), 8 oz....................................................280
à la king (*Stouffer's*), 11.5 oz. ...............................................370
à l'orange (*Lean Cuisine Café Classics*), 9 oz............................230
Alfredo:
    (*Lean Cuisine Skillet Sensations*), ½ of 24-oz. pkg............280
    (*Marie Callender's* Skillet Meals), ½ of 23-oz. pkg.............490
    (*Stouffer's Skillet Sensations*), ½ of 25-oz. pkg..................450
    and broccoli (*Banquet*), 1 cup..........................................270
baked (*Lean Cuisine Cafe Classics*), 8⅝ oz. ............................240
basil cream sauce (*Lean Cuisine Cafe Classics*), 8.5 oz. ..........260
and biscuits (*Freezer Queen* Family), 1 cup .............................200
barbecue sauce (*Lean Cuisine Hearty Portions*), 13⅞ oz. ........380
breast:
    (*Stouffer's Hearty Portions*), 15⅛ oz...................................500
    (*Stouffer's* Homestyle), 10 oz. ..........................................360
    baked (*Stouffer's* Homestyle), 8⅞ oz...................................260
    in barbecue sauce (*Stouffer's* Homestyle), 10 oz. ...............500
    country glazed (*Healthy Choice* Entree), 10.55 oz...............350
    fried (*Stouffer's* Homestyle), 8⅞ oz.....................................360
    grilled, and rice pilaf (*Marie Callender's*), 11.75 oz. ...........360
    strips, breaded (*Healthy Choice* Entree), 8 oz. ....................270
    in wine sauce (*Lean Cuisine Cafe Classics*), 8.5 oz. ............210
broccoli, creamy, cheese and rice (*Banquet* Family), 1 cup......280
and broccoli pasta bake (*Stouffer's*), ⅕ of 40-oz. pkg.............340
cacciatore (*Michelina's*), 8 oz. ................................................270
carbonara (*Lean Cuisine Cafe Classics*), 9 oz. .........................280

cheese, 3 (*Lean Cuisine Skillet Sensations*),
½ of 24-oz. pkg............................................................370
chow mein (*Lean Cuisine Everyday Favorites*), 9 oz.........240
chow mein, w/rice (*Yu Sing*), 8.75 oz............................270
cordon bleu (*Marie Callender's*), 13 oz. .......................610
country bake (*Healthy Choice* Bowl), 9.5 oz. ................230
creamed (*Stouffer's*), 6.5 oz. ......................................250
croquettes (*Freezer Queen* Family), 1 patty and gravy.............160
and dumplings (*Marie Callender's*), 14 oz......................390
and dumplings (*Stouffer's* Homestyle), 10 oz...................340
enchilada, see "Enchilada"
escalloped, and noodles (*Stouffer's*), 10 oz. .................460
fajita bake (*Ortega* Family Fiesta Meals), 10 oz., ¼ pkg............320
fettuccine (see also "Fettuccine entree"):
 Alfredo (*Healthy Choice* Entree), 8.5 oz......................280
  (*Lean Cuisine Everyday Favorites*), 9.25 oz. ..............270
  (*Stouffer's Hearty Portions*), 16.75 oz. .....................640
  (*Stouffer's* Homestyle), 10.5 oz. ..............................350
 w/broccoli (*Lean Cuisine Hearty Portions*), 13⅝ oz. .........390
fiesta (*Healthy Choice* Bowl), 9.5 oz.............................220
fiesta (*Lean Cuisine Cafe Classics*), 9.25 oz..................270
fingers (*Banquet*), 7.1 oz. ...........................................740
Florentine (*Lean Cuisine Everyday Favorites*), 8 oz..........220
Florentine (*Lean Cuisine Hearty Portions*), 13.25 oz.........380
fried (*Banquet* Original), 9 oz. ....................................470
fried, country, and gravy (*Marie Callender's*), 16 oz. ..........620
fried, white meat (*Banquet*), 8.75 oz. .........................480
fried, white meat, boneless (*Banquet*), 8.25 oz. ...........840
garlic (*Lean Cuisine Skillet Sensations*), ½ of 24-oz. pkg. ......340
garlic lemon, w/rice (*Healthy Choice* Bowl), 9.5 oz............300
garlic, Milano (*Healthy Choice* Entree), 9.5 oz. ............260
garlic, w/rice (*Yu Sing*), 8 oz......................................240
garlic, roasted, w/potato, vegetables, and sauce (*Oven
 Sensations*), ½ of 24-oz. pkg. ...................................320
ginger, w/rice (*Yu Sing*), 8 oz......................................250
glazed (*Lean Cuisine Cafe Classics*), 8.5 oz...................240
glazed (*Lean Cuisine Hearty Portions*), 13 oz.................330
glazed (*Marie Callender's*), 13 oz. ...............................490
glazed, Oriental (*Lean Cuisine Hearty Portions*), 14 oz............370

**Chicken entree, frozen (*cont.*)**

glazed, w/rice (*Michelina's*), 8 oz. ..............................250
glazed, w/rice (*Michelina's*), 9.5 oz. ...........................300
grilled:
   (*Banquet*), 9.9 oz. .................................................330
   (*Lean Cuisine Cafe Classics*), 9⅜ oz. ....................250
   Alfredo, w/broccoli (*Michelina's*), 10 oz. ...............400
   w/barbecue glaze and potato (*Boston Market*), 15.1 oz. ....430
   and mashed potato (*Marie Callender's*), 10 oz. ...................340
   w/mashed potato (*Healthy Choice* Entree), 8 oz..................180
   in mushroom sauce (*Marie Callender's*), 14 oz. .................480
   and penne (*Lean Cuisine Hearty Portions*), 14 oz. .............360
   salsa (*Lean Cuisine Cafe Classics*), 8⅞ oz. ........................270
   Sonoma (*Healthy Choice* Entree), 9 oz. ...............................230
   Southwestern (*Marie Callender's*), 14 oz...........................410
   and vegetables (*Stouffer's Skillet Sensations*),
      ½ of 25-oz. pkg.................................................400
herb (*Marie Callender's* Skillet Meals), ½ of 24-oz. pkg. ..........290
herb, and roasted potato (*Lean Cuisine Skillet Sensations*),
   ½ of 24-oz. pkg.................................................270
herb roasted (*Lean Cuisine Cafe Classics*), 8 oz. ......................190
herb roasted (*Michelina's*), 10 oz. .............................................260
herb roasted, and potato (*Marie Callender's*), 14 oz. .................580
homestyle (*Stouffer's Skillet Sensations*), ½ of 25-oz. pkg......390
honey barbecue, w/rice (*Michelina's*), 8.5 oz. ...........................290
honey mustard (*Healthy Choice* Entree), 9.5 oz. .......................290
honey mustard (*Lean Cuisine Cafe Classics*), 8 oz. ...................270
honey roasted (*Lean Cuisine Cafe Classics*), 8.5 oz. .................270
honey roasted (*Marie Callender's*), 14 oz..................................440
imperial (*Freezer Queen*), 8.5 oz. .............................................220
Italiano (*Michelina's*), 7.5 oz......................................................240
lo mein (*Yu Sing*), 8.5 oz. .........................................................220
Mandarin (*Healthy Choice* Entree), 10 oz...................................280
Mandarin (*Lean Cuisine Everyday Favorites*), 9 oz. ...................260
Mandarin, w/rice (*Yu Sing*), 8 oz. .............................................300
Marsala, w/garlic mashed potato (*Michelina's*), 8.5 oz. ............280
medallions, cheese sauce (*Lean Cuisine Cafe Classics*),
   9⅜ oz..................................................................300
Mediterranean (*Lean Cuisine Cafe Classics*), 10.5 oz. ..............260

Mexicali bake (*Ortega* Family Fiesta Meals), 10 oz., ¼ pkg. .....330
(*Michelina's* Littles), 5.5 oz......................................................310
and noodles (*Marie Callender's*), 13 oz. ...................................520
nuggets (*Banquet*), 6.75 oz. ....................................................430
nuggets (*Freezer Queen* Family), 6 pcs. ..................................250
nuggets (*Morton*), 7 oz. ...........................................................340
Oriental (*Lean Cuisine Skillet Sensations*), ¼ of 40-oz. pkg. ....280
patty, breaded (*Morton*), 16.75 oz...........................................290
Parmesan (*Lean Cuisine Cafe Classics*), 10⅞ oz. ....................300
parmigiana (*Banquet*), 9.5 oz...................................................320
parmigiana (*Stouffer's* Homestyle), 12 oz. ...............................460
parmigiana, breaded (*Marie Callender's*), 16 oz.......................660
parmigiana, breaded (*Michelina's*), 10 oz. ...............................410
and pasta, homestyle (*Healthy Choice* Entree), 9 oz................270
and pasta, Southwestern (*Healthy Choice* Bowl), 9.5 oz. .........320
pasta, w/vegetables, marinara sauce (*Empire* Kosher), 1 cup ..140
pasta primavera (*Banquet*), 9.5 oz...........................................320
in peanut sauce (*Lean Cuisine Cafe Classics*), 9 oz. ................260
pesto, w/penne (*Michelina's*), 8 oz...........................................250
piccata (*Lean Cuisine Cafe Classics*), 9 oz. .............................270
piccata, w/rice (*Michelina's*), 9 oz. ..........................................330
pie/pot pie:
    (*Banquet*), 7-oz. pie.............................................................380
    (*Empire* Kosher), 1 pie........................................................440
    (*Lean Cuisine Everyday Favorites*), 9.5-oz. pie ...................300
    (*Marie Callender's*), 9.5-oz. pie ..........................................680
    (*Stouffer's*), 10-oz. pie ........................................................520
    (*Stouffer's Hearty Portions*), 16-oz. pie ..............................590
    (*Swanson*), 7-oz. pie............................................................410
    au gratin (*Marie Callender's*), 9.5-oz. pie............................690
    and broccoli (*Banquet*), 7-oz. pie........................................350
    and broccoli (*Marie Callender's*), 9.5-oz. pie ......................670
    colonial (*Healthy Choice* Bowl), 9.5 oz. ..............................310
    potato topped (*Swanson*), 12-oz. pie ..................................440
primavera (*Lean Cuisine Skillet Sensations*), ½ of
    24-oz. pkg. ..........................................................................320
primavera, w/spirals (*Michelina's*), 8 oz...................................250
and rice, w/broccoli and cheese (*Marie Callender's* Skillet
    Meals), ½ of 25-oz. pkg......................................................440

**Chicken entree, frozen (*cont.*)**

and rice, savory (*Stouffer's Skillet Sensations* Homestyle),
    ¼ of 40-oz. pkg.............................................................................300
and rice, spicy sauce and (*Michelina's*), 8 oz............................240
roast, and vegetables (*Marie Callender's* Skillet Meals),
    ½ of 25-oz. pkg............................................................................260
roast (*Lean Cuisine Everyday Favorites*), 8⅛ oz.......................260
roast, w/mushrooms (*Lean Cuisine Hearty Portions*),
    12.5 oz. .......................................................................................330
sesame (*Healthy Choice* Entree), 9.75 oz.................................250
sliced, gravy and (*Freezer Queen* Cook-in-Pouch), 4 oz. ...........60
Sorrentino, w/linguine (*Michelina's*), 8.5 oz.............................310
sweet and sour (*Freezer Queen*), 8.5 oz...................................280
sweet and sour (*Marie Callender's*), 14 oz. ..............................570
sweet and sour, w/rice (*Yu Sing*), 8.5 oz. ................................340
teriyaki:
    (*Marie Callender's*), 13 oz. ....................................................510
    (*Marie Callender's* Skillet Meals), ½ of 24-oz. pkg................340
    (*Stouffer's Skillet Sensations*), ½ of 25-oz. pkg. ..................320
    w/rice (*Healthy Choice* Bowl), 9.5 oz.....................................270
    w/rice (*Michelina's*), 8.5 oz. ..................................................290
tetrazzini (*Michelina's*), 8 oz. ....................................................320
vegetable and, stir-fry (*Michelina's*), 8 oz. ...............................200
and vegetables (*Freezer Queen*), 8 oz. ....................................170
and vegetables (*Freezer Queen* Deluxe Family), 1 cup..............220
and vegetables (*Lean Cuisine Cafe Classics*), 10.5 oz. .............240
and vegetables, w/linguine (*Freezer Queen* Deluxe Family),
    1 cup ...........................................................................................250
and vegetables, Marsala (*Healthy Choice* Entree), 11.5 oz. ......240
in wine sauce (*Lean Cuisine Cafe Classics*), 8⅛ oz..................220
**"Chicken" entree, vegetarian,** frozen, ½ pkg., 5 oz.:
Szechuan (*Cedarlane* Veggie Chick'n) .......................................220
teriyaki (*Cedarlane* Veggie Chick'n) ...........................................220
**Chicken entree mix, packaged,** 1 cup\*, except as noted:
cheddar and broccoli (*Chicken Helper*) ......................................300
cheddar and mozzarella (*Chicken Helper Oven Favorites*),
    8.4 oz.\*.......................................................................................320
cheese, 4 (*Chicken Helper*) .......................................................310
fettucine Alfredo or Parmesan pasta (*Chicken Helper*).............290

fried rice (*Chicken Helper*) ........................................260
garlic, creamy roasted (*Chicken Helper*)..............................290
and penne, Alfredo, three cheese (*Lipton Sizzle and Stir*)........410
potatoes au gratin (*Chicken Helper Oven Favorites*),
    8.1 oz.* ..........................................................270
and rice, creamy (*Chicken Helper Oven Favorites*), 8 oz.* .......290
and rice, herb (*Chicken Helper*) ....................................260
and rice, lemon garlic (*Lipton Sizzle and Stir*)...........................350
and rice, teriyaki stir fry (*Lipton Sizzle and Stir*) ......................360
Southwestern (*Chicken Helper*) ...............................................240
and stuffing (*Chicken Helper*) ..................................................290
stuffing and gravy (*Chicken Helper Oven Favorites*
    Homestyle), 8 oz.* .................................................................300
**Chicken gravy,** ¼ cup:
(*Boston Market* Roasted) ................................................30
(*Franco-American*)......................................................40
(*Franco-American* Fat Free) ................................................15
(*Franco-American* Slow Roast) ..............................................25
(*Heinz* Classic Fat Free) .....................................................20
(*Heinz* Home Style Fat Free) .................................................25
giblet (*Franco-American*) ......................................................30
**Chicken gravy mix,** roasted (*Knorr*), 1 tbsp. or ¼ cup* ..........30
**Chicken liver pâté,** see "Pâté"
**Chicken lunch meat,** breast, 2 oz., except as noted:
(*Carl Buddig*), 2.5-oz. pkg. .....................................110
(*Carl Buddig*), 9 slices, 2 oz. ...............................................85
(*Carl Buddig* Premium Lean Slices), 2.5-oz. pkg. ......................60
barbecue (*Boar's Head Bar B Q Sauce Basted*) ..........................60
browned (*Healthy Choice*), 2 oz. ...........................................60
grilled (*Louis Rich Carving Board*), 2 slices, 1.6 oz. ..................45
mesquite (*Healthy Choice*), 2 oz. ...........................................60
oven roasted (*Healthy Choice*) ...............................................45
oven roasted (*Louis Rich*), 1-oz. slice......................................35
oven roasted (*Sara Lee* Deli), 3 slices......................................50
oven roasted, rotisserie flavor (*Sara Lee*).................................50
oven roasted or smoked (*Healthy Choice Deli Thin Deli
    Traditions*), 6 slices, 1.9 oz. ..............................................60
skinless (*Healthy Choice*), 2 oz. ...........................................45
smoked (*Healthy Choice*), 1-oz. slice.......................................30

**Chicken lunch meat (*cont.*)**
smoked, hickory (*Boar's Head*)....................................................60
smoked, honey (*Carl Buddig* Premium Lean), 2.5-oz. pkg.........70
smoked, honey roast (*Healthy Choice Deli Thin Savory*
   *Selections*), 6 slices, 1.9 oz. ..................................................70
**Chicken pie,** see "Chicken entree, frozen"
**Chicken salad,** packaged:
w/crackers (*Bumble Bee*), 3.5-oz. pkg. .....................................230
w/out crackers (*Bumble Bee*), 2.9 oz. .......................................140
**Chicken sandwich/pocket,** frozen, 1 piece:
(*Mrs. Paterson's Aussie Pie*), 5.5 oz. .......................................380
breaded (*Hormel Quick Meal*), 4.3 oz........................................340
and broccoli (*Healthy Choice Meals To Go*), 6.1 oz. .................310
broccoli (*Lean Pockets* Supreme), 4.5 oz. ................................280
broccoli and cheddar (*Croissant Pockets*), 4.5 oz. ...................320
and cheddar, w/broccoli (*Hot Pockets*), 4.5 oz. .......................310
fajita (*Lean Pockets*), 4.5 oz......................................................260
grilled (*Hormel Quick Meal*), 4.7 oz...........................................310
Parmesan (*Lean Pockets*), 4.5 oz..............................................300
**Chicken sauce,** 2 tbsp.:
Dijon or teriyaki (*Lawry's* Weekday Gourmet)............................40
fajita (*Lawry's* Weekday Gourmet)...............................................20
orange glaze liquid (*Lawry's* Weekday Gourmet) ........................30
**Chicken sauce, cooking,** ½ cup:
cacciatore (*Ragú Chicken Tonight*) .............................................70
French, country (*Ragú Chicken Tonight*) ...................................120
honey mustard (*Ragú Chicken Tonight*) ......................................60
mushroom, creamy (*Ragú Chicken Tonight*)................................80
sweet and sour (*Ragú Chicken Tonight*).....................................150
**Chicken seasoning mix:**
Dijonne (*Knorr Recipe Classics*), 1 tbsp. ...................................30
California citrus (*Lawry's* Spices & Seasonings), 1 tsp. .............25
**Chicken seasoning and coating mix:**
(*Hodgson Mill Don's Chuck Wagon* Baking), ¼ cup....................95
(*Shake 'n Bake* Original Recipe), ⅛ pkt......................................40
barbecue, honey mustard or tangy honey (*Shake 'n Bake*),
   ⅛ pkt.......................................................................................45
buffalo wing (*Shake 'n Bake*), ⅒ pkt. ..........................................40
extra crispy (*Oven Fry*), ⅛ pkt. ...................................................60

home style flour (*Oven Fry*), ⅛ pkt................................................40

hot and spicy or Italian (*Shake 'n Bake*), ⅛ pkt. .........................40

**Chicken spread,** canned, 1 tbsp. ...............................................25

*Chick-fil-A,* 1 serving:

chicken soup, hearty breast of .................................................110

chicken dishes:

    *Chick-fil-A* char-grilled chicken garden salad.......................190

    *Chick-fil-A* chicken Caesar salad.............................................230

    *Chick-fil-A* chicken nuggets, 8 pcs. ......................................290

    *Chick-fil-A Chick-n-Strips,* 4 pcs............................................230

    *Chick-fil-A Chick-n-Strips* salad ............................................370

    *Chick-fil-A* char-grilled chicken sandwich ..............................280

    *Chick-fil-A* char-grilled chicken club sandwich.......................390

    *Chick-fil-A* chicken salad sandwich ........................................320

    *Chick-fil-A* chicken sandwich.................................................290

side items:

    carrot and raisin salad, cup....................................................150

    *Chick-fil-A* waffle potato fries................................................290

    cole slaw, cup.........................................................................130

    tossed salad ...........................................................................80

dipping sauces:

    barbecue sauce .......................................................................45

    honey mustard sauce...............................................................45

    Dijon honey mustard sauce ......................................................60

    Polynesian sauce....................................................................110

salad dressings:

    basil vinaigrette .....................................................................250

    blue cheese ...........................................................................230

    buttermilk ranch.....................................................................220

    Dijon honey mustard, fat free ..................................................70

    house.....................................................................................190

    Italian, light.............................................................................20

    spicy or Thousand Island.......................................................210

desserts:

    *Chick-fil-A* cheesecake, plain ................................................300

    *Chick-fil-A* lemon pie............................................................280

    fudge nut brownie..................................................................350

    *Icedream,* 1 cone .................................................................140

**Chickpeas,** see "Garbanzo beans"
**Chicory, witloof,** fresh, raw:
(*Frieda's* Belgian Endive), 2 cups, 3 oz.........................................15
1 head, 1.9 oz. .............................................................................9
**Chicory greens,** fresh, raw, chopped, 1 cup .............................41
**Chicory root,** fresh, raw, 1" pcs., ½ cup.....................................33
**Chili,** canned or packaged, 1 cup, except as noted:
w/beans (*Hormel*), 7.5-oz. can ................................................230
w/beans (*Stagg Chili Laredo/Country Brand*) ...........................320
w/beans (*Stagg Chunkero*) .......................................................300
w/beans (*Stagg Classic/Dynamite Hot*) .....................................330
w/beans (*Stagg Silverado*) .......................................................230
w/beans, hot (*Hormel*), 7.4-oz. can ..........................................230
w/beans, regular, chunky or hot (*Hormel*)..................................270
w/beans, regular or hot (*Hormel* Microcup Meals)..................220
w/out beans (*Hormel* Microcup Meals)......................................190
w/out beans (*Stagg Double Barrel Beef*) ...................................340
w/out beans (*Stagg Steak House*)..............................................330
w/out beans, regular or hot (*Hormel*).........................................210
chicken, w/beans (*Greene's Farm*) ...........................................230
chicken, w/beans (*Stagg Ranch House*) ....................................290
chicken, w/out beans (*Stagg Chicken Grande*) .........................250
macaroni (*Hormel* Microcup Meals Chili Mac) .........................200
turkey, w/beans (*Hormel*) .........................................................210
turkey, w/beans (*Stagg Ranchero*) ............................................240
turkey, w/out beans (*Hormel*)....................................................190
vegetarian (*Hormel*) .................................................................200
vegetarian (*Stagg Vegetable Garden*) .......................................200
vegetarian, all varieties (*Amy's*)................................................190
vegetarian, regular or spicy (*Shari Ann's* Organic) ...................230
vegetarian, 3 bean (*Greene's Farm*)...........................................150
**Chili bean,** canned, ½ cup:
(*Campbell's*)..............................................................................130
Mexican (*Allen/Brown Beauty*)..................................................120
spicy (*Green Giant/*Joan of Arc) ..............................................110
**Chili dip:**
(*Fritos*), 6 oz. ...........................................................................200
cheese (*Fritos*), 1.2 oz. ..............................................................45
**Chili dinner,** frozen, w/cornbread (*Amy's*), 10.5-oz. pkg. ........320

**Chili entree,** frozen, 1 pkg.:

bean, 3, w/rice (*Lean Cuisine Everyday Favorites*), 10 oz........250

w/beans (*Stouffer's*), 8¾ oz........................................290

black bean, w/green tomatoes, rice (*Michelina's*), 8 oz. ..........310

black bean, w/rice (*Michelina's*), 10 oz. ......................400

and cornbread (*Healthy Choice* Bowl), 9.5 oz.................350

and cornbread (*Marie Callender's*), 16 oz. ..................560

w/macaroni (*Michelina's* Chili-Mac), 8 oz. ..................290

**Chili pepper,** see "Pepper, chili"

**Chili powder,** 1 tsp..........................................................8

**Chili sauce,** tomato:

(*Heinz*), 1 tbsp..................................................................15

(*Del Monte*), 1 tbsp. .......................................................20

**Chili seasoning mix,** dry:

(*Adolph's Meal Makers*), 1 tbsp. ....................................30

(*D. L. Jardine's* Texas Chili Fixins/Chili Works), 3 tbsp. ..............60

(*Shotgun Willie's* Kit), 3 tbsp.........................................50

**Chimichanga entree,** frozen (*Banquet*), 9.5 oz.......................500

**Chitterlings,** pork, simmered, 4 oz. ...................................344

**Chives,** fresh, raw, chopped, 1 tbsp. ...............................<1

**Chives, freeze-dried,** ¼ cup.............................................3

**Chocolate,** see "Candy"

**Chocolate, baking:**

(*Nestlé Choco Bake*), .5 oz. ............................................80

bar, bittersweet, semisweet or unsweetened (*Baker's*), .5 oz. ....70

bar, semisweet (*Nestlé*), .5 oz. .......................................70

bar, sweet (*Baker's German*), .5 oz. ................................60

bar, unsweetened (*Nestlé*), .5 oz. ...................................80

bar, white (*Nestlé*), .5 oz. ..............................................80

chips or morsels, 1 tbsp., except as noted:

   (*Hershey's* Bake Shoppe Reduced Fat)...............................60

   milk (*Nestlé* Morsels) ...................................................70

   milk or semisweet (*Hershey's* Real)..................................80

   mint or raspberry (*Hershey's*).........................................80

   semisweet or mint (*Nestlé* Morsels)................................70

   white (*Nestlé* Premier) ..................................................80

chunks, semisweet (*Nestlé*), 1 tbsp. ...............................70

**Chocolate drink** (*Hershey's*), 8-fl.-oz. box.........................130

**Chocolate drink mix,** powder, 2 tbsp.:
(*Nesquik*)....................................................................................90
(*Nesquik* No Sugar)..................................................................40
**Chocolate milk,** 1 cup:
(*Hershey's*)..............................................................................230
(*Hershey's* Fat Free)..............................................................150
(*Hershey's* Reduced Fat)........................................................190
(*Nesquik*)................................................................................230
(*Nesquik* Fat Free)..................................................................160
**Chocolate shake** (*Hershey's*), 1 cont.................................230
**Chocolate syrup,** 2 tbsp., except as noted:
(*Hershey's*), 2-oz. pouch .......................................................150
(*Hershey's* Lite)........................................................................50
(*Hershey's Special Dark*)........................................................110
(*Nesquik*)................................................................................100
malt (*Hershey's*), 2-oz. pouch ...............................................140
mint (*Hershey's Chocolate Shoppe* Sundae Fat Free)..............110
**Chocolate topping,** 2 tbsp.:
(*Hershey's* Shell)....................................................................230
(*Smucker's* Sundae Syrup)....................................................110
chocolate or chocolate fudge (*Smucker's Magic Shell*)...........220
fudge (*Hershey's Chocolate Shoppe* Fat Free) .........................100
fudge or crisps (*Hershey's* Shell) ..........................................190
fudge (*Smucker's* Spoonable) ................................................130
fudge (*Smucker's* Spoonable Light) .........................................90
fudge or hot fudge (*Hershey's*) ..............................................130
fudge or hot fudge (*Smucker's* Microwave)..............................130
fudge, double chocolate (*Hershey's*) ......................................120
fudge, hot (*Smucker's* Special Recipe/Spoonable) ...................140
**Chorizo:**
(*Fiorucci* Cantimpalo), 1 oz. ...................................................130
beef, raw (*Aidell's* Mexican), 3.5-oz. link................................400
**Chow chow relish** (*Crosse & Blackwell*), 1 tbsp.........................10
**Chutney,** 1 tbsp.:
apple curry (*Crosse & Blackwell*) ..............................................25
cranberry (*Crosse & Blackwell*) .................................................40
mango, all varieties except Major Grey's (*Patak's*).....................60
mango, Major Grey's (*Crosse & Blackwell*) .................................60

mango, Major Grey's (*Patak's*) ....................................................50
mango and lime (*Patak's*) ...........................................................50
**Cilantro,** fresh, raw, 1 cup ........................................................11
**Cinnamon,** ground, 1 tsp. ............................................................6
**Cisco,** meat only, raw, 4 oz. ....................................................112
**Citrus drink blends,** 8 fl. oz.:
punch (*Florida's Natural Growers' Pride*) ...............................130
punch (*Minute Maid*) ...............................................................120
punch (*Tropicana*) ....................................................................140
**Clam,** mixed species, meat only:
raw, 1 large, .7 oz. ....................................................................15
raw, 4 oz. ....................................................................................84
1 cup w/liquid ...........................................................................168
breaded, fried, 20 small, 6.6 oz. ..............................................380
boiled, poached, or steamed, 20 small, 6.7 oz. ......................281
boiled, poached, or steamed, 4 oz. .........................................168
**Clam, canned,** ¼ cup, except as noted:
whole, baby, drained (*Bumble Bee*), ⅓ of 10-oz. can ...............50
chopped or minced (*Neptune* Fancy Atlantic Surf) ...................20
chopped, ocean (*Chincoteague*) .................................................30
chopped or minced, ocean (*Neptune* Atlantic Ocean) ...............30
chopped, sea (*Chincoteague*) .....................................................25
**Clam chowder,** see "Soup"
**Clam dip,** 2 tbsp.:
(*Breakstone's* Chesapeake/*Kraft* Premium) ..............................50
(*Kraft*) .........................................................................................60
**Clam entree,** frozen:
breaded, fried (*Howard Johnson*), 5-oz. pkg. ..........................350
breaded, fried (*Chincoteague* Premium), 3 oz. ........................265
breaded, fried (*Mrs. Paul's/Van de Kamp's*), 18 pcs., 3 oz. ......250
on the half shell (*Chincoteague* Premium), 2 pcs. ....................20
stuffed (*Chincoteague* Premium), 1 pc. ...................................130
**Clam juice:**
ocean (*Chincoteague*), 8 fl. oz. ..................................................10
sea (*Chincoteague*), 4 fl. oz. .......................................................15
**Clam sauce,** canned, ½ cup:
red (*Olde Cape Cod*) .................................................................100
red (*Progresso*) ...........................................................................80
white (*Chincoteague* Premium) .................................................120

**Clam sauce** (*cont.*)
white (*Colavita*) .................................................................90
white (*Progresso* 12-oz. jar) ..........................................150
white, w/garlic and herbs (*Progresso* 15-oz. can) ...................140
**Cloves, ground,** 1 tsp. ............................................................7
**Cobbler,** frozen:
apple (*Marie Callender's*), ¼ of 17-oz. pkg. ............................370
apple (*Mrs. Smith's* 32 oz.), ⅛ cobbler ...............................270
berry (*Marie Callender's*), ¼ of 17-oz. pkg. ............................370
blackberry or peach (*Mrs. Smith's* 32 oz.), ⅛ cobbler ............260
cherry (*Marie Callender's*), ¼ of 17-oz. pkg. ..........................380
cherry (*Mrs. Smith's* 32 oz.), ⅛ cobbler ...............................280
peach (*Marie Callender's*), ¼ of 17-oz. pkg. ..........................360
**Cocktail sauce,** see "Seafood sauce"
**Cocoa,** baking, 1 tbsp.:
(*Hershey's*) .....................................................................20
(*Nestlé*) .........................................................................15
**Cocoa mix,** dry, 1.2-oz. pkt., except as noted:
(*Hershey's*), 1 tbsp. .............................................................30
(*Hershey's* Classic), 1-oz. pkt. ........................................120
(*Hershey's* Goodnight Hug/Kiss) .......................................150
all flavors (*Land O Lakes Cocoa Classics*), 1 pkt. .....................160
almond or mint (*Hershey's* Collection) ..............................150
chocolate, Dutch (*Hershey's* Collection) ............................160
chocolate, Dutch (*Hershey's* Collection Fat Free) ...................50
w/marshmallows (*Hershey's* Classic), 1-oz. pkt. ..................120
raspberry or Irish creme (*Hershey's* Collection) .....................150
vanilla, French (*Carnation*), 1-oz. pkt. ..............................120
vanilla, French (*Hershey's* Collection) ................................140
vanilla, French (*Hershey's* Collection Fat Free) .......................50
**Coconut,** fresh, shelled, raw:
(*Dole*), 1 cup, not packed .................................................283
(*Frieda's* White/Young), ¼ cup .........................................140
shredded, 1 cup ...............................................................283
**Coconut, canned or packaged:**
(*Baker's Angel Flake*), 2 tbsp. ............................................70
flaked, sweetened, 1 cup .................................................341
w/almond bits (*Almond Joy*), 1 tbsp. ..................................60
**Coconut cream,** canned, 1 tbsp. .......................................37

**Coconut milk,** canned:
(*A Taste of Thai*), ¼ cup................................................110
(*A Taste of Thai* Lite), ⅓ cup .................................................45
**Cod, Atlantic,** meat only:
raw, 4 oz. ................................................................93
baked, broiled, or microwaved, 4 oz. .......................................119
**Cod, Atlantic, canned,** 4 oz..............................................119
**Cod, Pacific,** meat only:
raw, 4 oz. ................................................................93
baked, broiled, or microwaved, 4 oz. .......................................119
**Cod entree,** frozen:
au gratin (*Oven Poppers*), 5-oz. pc. ......................................220
fillet (*Mrs. Paul's* Premium), 4.2-oz. pc. ................................260
fillet, breaded (*Van de Kamp's* Premium), 4-oz. pc....................220
stuffed, w/broccoli and cheese (*Oven Poppers*),
   5-oz. pc. ....................................................150
**Coffee,** brewed, regular or decaffeinated, 6 fl. oz. ......................5
**Coffee, flavored, mix,** 8 fl. oz.*, except as noted:
all flavors (*General Foods International* Sugar/Fat Free) .............25
all flavors, except latte cappuccino frothé (*Nescafé*), 3 tbsp. ......80
cafe Français (*General Foods International*) ...............................60
cafe Vienna (*General Foods International*)...................................70
cafe Vienna (*General Foods International* Sugar Free).................30
cappuccino:
   all flavors (*Land O Lakes Cappuccino Classics*), 1 pkt........130
   all flavors, except iced and mocha (*Maxwell House*) .............90
   iced (*Land O Lakes DownTown Café*), 1 pkt. .......................60
   iced (*Maxwell House*) ...............................................180
   Italian (*General Foods International*) ..............................60
   mocha (*Maxwell House*) ...............................................100
   mocha or vanilla (*Maxwell House* Sugar Free) .....................60
   orange (*General Foods International*)................................70
chocolate, Viennese (*General Foods International*) ....................50
French vanilla or Irish cream (*General Foods International*) ......60
hazelnut Belgian (*General Foods International*) .........................70
*Kahlua Cafe* (*General Foods International*) ..............................60
latte cappuccino frothé (*Nescafé*), 3 tbsp. ...............................90
mocha, Suisse (*General Foods International*)..............................60

**Coffee, iced,** 8 fl. oz.:

café latte (*Blue Luna*)..............................................................130

café mocha (*Blue Luna* Lite).......................................................70

**Coffee creamer,** see "Creamer, nondairy"

**Coffee substitute,** cereal grain (*Postum*), 8 fl. oz.* ..................10

**Cole slaw,** refrigerated, 4 oz.:

(*Blue Ridge Farms*)....................................................................130

(*Chef's Express*)........................................................................190

**Cole slaw dressing,** see "Salad dressing"

**Collard greens,** fresh:

raw, chopped, 1 cup ....................................................................11

boiled, drained, chopped, 1 cup .................................................49

**Collard greens, canned** (*Allens/Sunshine*), ½ cup ..................30

**Collard greens, frozen,** chopped:

(*Birds Eye*), 1 cup .....................................................................30

(*Seabrook Farms*), ½ cup ..........................................................30

**Cookie:**

all varieties (*Pepperidge Farm Spritzers*), 5 pcs., 1.1 oz..........140

all varieties (*Stella D'oro* Breakfast Treats), .8-oz. pc...............100

almond (*Frieda's*), 2 pcs., 1 oz.................................................170

almond (*Stella D'oro Almond Toast*), 2 pcs., 1 oz.....................110

almond (*Stella D'oro* Chinese Dessert), 1.2-oz. pc. ..................170

animal:

    (*Barnum's Animals*), 10 pcs. ..............................................140

    chocolate chip (*Keebler*), 7 pcs., 1 oz. ...............................130

    frosted (*Keebler*), 6 pcs., 1 oz. ...........................................130

    iced or sprinkled (*Keebler*), 6 pcs., 1.1 oz. ........................150

apple (*Newtons* Fat Free), 2 pcs.................................................90

apple cinnamon (*Newtons* Cobblers Fat Free), 1 pc. ..................70

arrowroot (*National* Biscuit), 1 pc. .............................................20

biscotti:

    (*Almondina* Choconut), 4 pcs., 1.1 oz. ...............................140

    (*Real Torino* Amaretti), 6 pcs., 1.1 oz. ...............................120

    almond, mini (*Real Torino*), 4 pcs., 1.1 oz. ........................140

    cashews (*Stella D'oro*), 7-oz. pc. ........................................110

    chocolate (*Nonni's* Decadence), 1.2-oz. pc.........................130

    chocolate or chocolate almond (*Real Torino*), 1.1-oz. pc....140

    chocolate or hazelnut (*Stella D'oro*), .8-oz. pc. ..................100

chocolate almond, mini (*Real Torino*), 4 pcs., 1.1 oz..........140
chocolate almond, chocolate chunk, or French vanilla
   (*Stella D'oro*), .8-oz. pc..................................................90
fudge dipped, all varieties (*Stella D'oro*), 1 pc....................120
butter:
   (*Keebler*), 5 pcs., 1.1 oz.................................................150
   (*Keebler Cookie Stix*), 5 pcs., 1.2 oz..............................160
   dark chocolate topped (*Carr's Imperials*), 2 pcs., 1 oz........150
   milk chocolate topped (*Carr's Imperials*), 2 pcs., 1 oz........140
butter sandwich, fudge filled (*E. L. Fudge*), 2 pcs., .9 oz..........120
cappuccino crisps (*Murray* Sugar Free), 4 pcs., 1.1 oz. ..........150
cappuccino sandwich (*Café Cremes*), 2 pcs. .....................160
caramel (*SnackWell's* Delights), 1 pc. .................................70
caramel bar (*Little Debbie*), 1.2 oz. ...................................160
chocolate (*Stella D'oro* Castelets), 2 pcs., 1 oz.................130
chocolate crisps (*SnackWell's*), 18 pcs..............................130
chocolate wafer (*Nabisco Famous Wafers*), 5 pcs....................140
chocolate wafer (*Nilla* Reduced Fat), 8 pcs. .........................110
chocolate wafer (*Real Torino*), 2 pcs., .9 oz........................130
chocolate chip/chunk:
   (*Grandma's* Big Homestyle), 1.4-oz. pc. ...........................190
   (*Grandma's* Tiny Bites), 12 pcs........................................280
   (*Chips Ahoy!*), 3 pcs. ....................................................160
   (*Chips Ahoy!* Mini), 5 pcs................................................150
   (*Chips Ahoy!* Reduced Fat), 3 pcs. ...................................140
   (*Keebler Chips Deluxe*), .5-oz. pc......................................80
   (*Keebler Chips Deluxe* Chocolate Lovers), .6-oz. pc..............90
   (*Keebler Chips Deluxe* Rainbow/Soft 'n Chewy), .6-oz. pc....80
   (*Keebler Cookie Stix*), 4 pcs, 1 oz. ...................................130
   (*Keebler Soft Batch*), .6-oz. pc..........................................80
   (*Little Debbie*), 1.3 oz. ...................................................180
   (*Murray* Sugar Free), 3 pcs., 1.1 oz..................................150
   (*SnackWell's* Bite Size), 13 pcs.........................................130
   chunk (*Keebler Soft Batch* Homestyle), .9-oz. pc.................130
   chunky (*Chips Ahoy!*), 1 pc................................................80
   crisps (*SnackWell's*), 18 pcs.............................................150
   double (*SnackWell's* Bite Size), 13 pcs..............................130
   double chocolate (*Chips Ahoy!*), 3 pcs. .............................160
   fudge (*Grandma's* Big Homestyle), 1.4-oz. pc...................170

**Cookie, chocolate chip/chunk (*cont.*)**

pecan (*Chips Ahoy!* Mini), 5 pcs. ........................................150
walnut, crunchy (*Keebler Chips Deluxe*), .6-oz. pc. ...............90
chocolate sandwich:
    (*Keebler Droxies*), 3 pcs., 1.1 oz. ..................................140
    (*Murray* Sugar Free), 3 pcs., 1 oz. ..................................120
    (*Oreo*), 3 pcs., 1.2 oz. ......................................................160
    (*Oreo* Minis), 1.5-oz. pkg. ................................................200
    (*Oreo* Minis), 9 pcs. ..........................................................140
    (*Oreo* Reduced Fat), 3 pcs. ..............................................130
    (*SnackWell's*), 2 pcs. ........................................................110
    fudge covered (*Oreo*), 1 pc. ..............................................110
coconut (*Keebler Chips Deluxe*), .6-oz. pc. ...........................80
coconut creme (*SnackWell's*), 2 pcs. ....................................110
coffee creme sandwich (*Peek Freans*), 2 pcs., 1.1 oz. .............110
cranberry biscuit (*Keebler Golden Fruit*), .7-oz. pc. .................80
Danish wedding (*Keebler*), 4 pcs., 1 oz. ................................120
devil's food or golden devil's food (*SnackWell's*), 1 pc. .............50
egg (*Stella D'oro* Jumbo), 2 pcs., .8 oz. ................................90
egg (*Stella D'oro Roman Egg Biscuits*), 1.2-oz. pc. .................140
fig bar (*Little Debbie*), 1.5 oz. ...............................................150
fig bar (*Fig Newtons*), 2 pcs. .................................................110
fig bar (*Fig Newtons* Fat Free), 2.1-oz. pkg. ...........................100
fortune cookie (*Frieda's*), 4 pcs., 1 oz. ..................................120
fudge:
    (*Grandma's* Minis), 9 pcs. ................................................150
    (*Stella D'oro* Swiss), 2 pcs., .9 oz. ..................................130
    double (*Murray* Sugar Free), 3 pcs., 1.2 oz. ....................140
    double, caramel (*Keebler Fudge Shoppe*), 2 pcs., 1.1 oz. ....140
    peanut butter stick (*Keebler Fudge Shoppe*), 3 pcs.,
       1 oz. ............................................................................150
    stick (*Keebler Fudge Shoppe*), 3 pcs., 1 oz. ....................150
    stripe (*Keebler Fudge Shoppe*), 3 pcs., 1 oz. ..................160
    stripe (*Keebler Fudge Shoppe* Reduced Fat), 3 pcs.,
       1 oz. ............................................................................140
fudge sandwich (*Grandma's* Value), 3 pcs. ............................180
fudge sandwich, fudge (*E. L. Fudge*), 2 pcs., .9 oz. ...............120
fudge sandwich, vanilla (*Grandma's* Value), 3 pcs. ...............120
ginger (*Little Debbie*), .7 oz. .................................................90

ginger lemon creme (*Carr's*), 2 pcs., 1 oz.................................140
gingersnap (*Keebler*), 5 pcs., 1.2 oz..................................150
gingersnap (*Murray* Sugar Free), 6 pcs., 1 oz. ...................110
gingersnap (*Nabisco*), 4 pcs. ..........................................120
*Golden Bars* (*Stella D'oro*), 1-oz. pc..............................100
graham:
    (*Keebler Grahams* w/Calcium), 8 pcs., 1 oz. ................130
    (*Nabisco* Grahams), 4 pcs. .....................................120
    chocolate (*Honey Maid*), 8 pcs. ................................120
    chocolate (*Keebler Grahams* w/Calcium), 8 pcs., 1.1 oz.....140
    chocolate, cinnamon, or honey (*Teddy Grahams*),
      24 pcs.......................................................130
    chocolate chip (*Teddy Grahams*), 24 pcs. .................140
    chocolate covered (*Keebler Fudge Shoppe* Deluxe),
      3 pcs., .9 oz...............................................140
    cinnamon (*Keebler Snackin' Grahams*), 21 pcs., 1 oz.........130
    cinnamon sugar or honey (*Elf Grahams*), 16 pcs.,
      1.1 oz........................................................140
    frosted (*Teddy Grahams Dizzy Grizzlies*), 8 pcs. ...........150
    fudge covered (*Fudge Favorites*), 3 pcs....................140
    honey (*Honey Maid*), 8 pcs. ...................................120
    honey (*Keebler Grahams* w/Calcium), 8 pcs., 1.1 oz. .........140
    oatmeal (*Honey Maid* Crunch), 8 pcs. .......................130
ladyfinger (*Real Torino*), 3 pcs., 1 oz. ...............................110
lemon (*Keebler Coolers*), 5 pcs., 1.1 oz. ............................140
lemon crisps (*Murray* Sugar Free), 4 pcs., 1.1 oz. ...............140
lemon sandwich (*Murray* Sugar Free), 3 pcs., 1 oz. ..............120
lime (*Peek Freans* Calypso), 2 pcs. ..................................130
marshmallow, chocolate coated (*Mallomars*), 2 pcs. ............120
marshmallow, chocolate coated (*Pinwheels*), 1 pc..............130
mint, chocolate/fudge covered:
    (*Keebler Fudge Shoppe* Grasshopper), 4 pcs., 1.1 oz.........150
    (*Mystic Mint*), 1 pc. ................................................90
mint creme (*SnackWell's*), 2 pcs.....................................110
molasses (*Grandma's* Big Homestyle), 1.4-oz. pc. ...............160
oat graham (*Carr's* Hob Nobs), 2 pcs., 1 oz.......................140
oatmeal (*Barbara's* Crisp Old Fashioned), .6-oz. pc. ...............70
oatmeal (*Keebler* Country Style), 2 pcs., .8 oz.....................120
oatmeal (*Murray* Sugar Free), 3 pcs., 1.1 oz........................140

**Cookie** (*cont.*)

oatmeal, plain or iced (*Nabisco* Family Favorites), 1 pc.............80
oatmeal raisin (*Grandma's* Big Homestyle), 1.4-oz. pc.............160
oatmeal raisin (*Grandma's* Tiny Bites), 12 pcs.....................280
oatmeal raisin (*Keebler Soft Batch*), .6-oz. pc......................70
oatmeal raisin (*Keebler Soft Batch* Homestyle), .9-oz. pc.........130
oatmeal raisin (*Little Debbie*), 1.3 oz. .............................160
orange creme wafer (*Real Torino*), 2 pcs., .8 oz. ..................130
pastry puff:
   apricot glazed (*Real Torino*), 3 pcs., 1.1 oz. ...............160
   cappuccino chocolate (*Ferrara*), 5 pcs., 1.1 oz...............150
   frosted or chocolate frosted (*Real Torino*), 2 pcs., .8 oz.....140
peach apricot (*Newtons* Cobblers Fat Free), 1 pc. ...................70
peanut caramel cluster (*Keebler Fudge Shoppe*), .7-oz. pc. .....100
peanut creme patty (*Nutter Butter*), 5 pcs. ........................160
peanut butter (*Grandma's* Big Homestyle), 1.4-oz. pc.............190
peanut butter (*Grandma's* Minis), 9 pcs.............................150
peanut butter (*Murray* Sugar Free), 8 pcs., 1 oz....................120
peanut butter chocolate chip (*Grandma's* Big), 1.4-oz. pc........190
peanut butter cups (*Keebler Chips Deluxe*), .6-oz. pc................80
peanut butter chip (*SnackWell's* Bite Size), 13 pcs..................120
peanut butter sandwich (*Grandma's*), 5 pcs. ........................210
peanut butter sandwich (*Nutter Butter*), 2 pcs. .....................130
peanut butter sandwich (*Nutter Butter* Bites), 10 pcs...............150
(*Peek Freans* Nice), 4 pcs., 1.2 oz..................................160
(*Peek Freans* Tropical Cremes), 2 pcs...............................130
rainbow (*Beigel's*), 1.2-oz. pc......................................120
raisin biscuit (*Keebler Golden Fruit*), .7-oz. pc. ....................80
raspberry or strawberry (*Newtons* Fat Free), 2 pcs. .................90
strawberry kiwi (*Newtons* Tropical Fat Free), 2 pcs. .................90
shortbread (*Barbara's* Crisp Traditional), .6-oz. pc...................80
shortbread (*Lorna Doone*), 4 pcs....................................140
shortbread (*Murray* Sugar Free), 8 pcs., 1 oz.......................120
shortbread (*Walkers*), .7-oz. pc....................................100
shortbread, all varieties (*Keebler Sandies*), .6-oz. pc................80
shortbread, almond (*Crookes & Hanson* English), .9-oz. pc. ...120
shortbread, fudge striped (*Fudge Favorites*), 3 pcs. ................160
shortbread, pecan (*Pecanz*), 1 pc. ...................................90
S'mores (*Keebler Fudge Shoppe*), 3 pcs., 1.2 oz.....................160

(*Stella D'oro Angel Wings*), 2 pcs., .9 oz. ...................................140
(*Stella D'oro Anginetti*), 4 pcs., 1.1 oz. ...................................140
(*Stella D'oro Lady Stella* Assortment), 3 pcs., 1 oz. .................130
sugar (*Grandma's* Tiny Bites), 12 pcs. ...................................280
sugar, rainbow (*Keebler Cookie Stix*), 5 pcs., 1.2 oz. ...............150
sugar wafer (*Biscos*), 8 pcs. ...................................................140
sugar wafer, chocolate (*Keebler*), 3 pcs., 1.1 oz. .....................140
sugar wafer, lemon (*Keebler*), 3 pcs., .9 oz. ............................130
sugar wafer, peanut butter (*Keebler*), 4 pcs., 1.1 oz. ...............160
sugar wafer, strawberry or vanilla (*Grandma's*), 3 pcs. ............160
tea biscuit (*Carr's*), 2 pcs., 1 oz. ............................................140
tea biscuit (*Social Tea*), 6 pcs. ...............................................120
tea biscuit, chocolate topped (*Carr's*), 2 pcs., .9 oz. .................130
vanilla (*Grandma's* Minis), 9 pcs. ............................................150
vanilla, creme filled (*Keebler Classic Collection*), .6-oz. pc. ........80
vanilla creme wafer (*Real Torino*), 2 pcs., .9 oz. .......................140
vanilla sandwich (*Café Cremes*), 2 pcs. ...................................160
vanilla sandwich (*Cameo*), 2 pcs., 1 oz. ...................................130
vanilla sandwich (*Grandma's*), 5 pcs. .......................................210
vanilla sandwich (*Grandma's* Value), 3 pcs. ..............................180
vanilla sandwich (*Keebler Vienna Fingers*), 2 pcs., 1 oz. ..........140
vanilla sandwich, creme (*SnackWell's*), 2 pcs. ..........................110
vanilla sandwich, fudge (*Café Cremes*), 2 pcs. .........................200
vanilla wafer (*Keebler* Golden), 8 pcs., 1.1 oz. ..........................150
vanilla wafer (*Keebler* Golden Reduced Fat), 8 pcs., 1.1 oz. ......130
vanilla wafer (*Keebler* Rainbow), 8 pcs. ...................................130
vanilla wafer (*Nilla*), 8 pcs. ......................................................140
vanilla wafer (*Nilla* Reduced Fat), 8 pcs. ..................................120
waffle sandwich, apricot (*Carr's Petits Bijoux*), 4 pcs.,
    1.1 oz. .................................................................................140

**Cookie, frozen or refrigerated:**
chocolate chip:
    (*Nestlé Toll House/Toll House* Big Batch), 1.1-oz. pc. .........140
    (*Nestlé Toll House* Reduced Fat), 1.2-oz. pc. .....................130
    (*Pillsbury*), 1 oz. ..............................................................140
    (*Pillsbury One Step*), ⅒ pkg. ...........................................150
    (*Pillsbury* Ready-to-Bake), 1 pc. .....................................120
    bar (*Nestlé Toll House*), .9-oz. pc. ....................................110
    walnut (*Nestlé Toll House*), .9-oz. pc. ...............................110

**Cookie, frozen or refrigerated, chocolate chip (*cont.*)**
    w/walnuts (*Pillsbury*), 1 oz. ................................................130
    and white fudge (*Nestlé Toll House*), 1.2-oz. pc. ...............150
chocolate chunk (*Nestlé Toll House*), 1.2-oz. pc. .....................150
*M&M's* (*Pillsbury*), 1 oz. .............................................................130
peanut butter chocolate chip (*Nestlé Toll House*),
    1.2-oz. pc. .........................................................................150
rugelach (*Tofutti*), .75-oz. pc. ....................................................130
sugar (*Pillsbury*), 2¼" slices .....................................................130
sugar, bar (*Nestlé Toll House*), .9-oz. pc. ...............................110
**Cookie crumbs:**
crumbs (*Oreo*), 2 tbsp. ................................................................90
crumbs, graham cracker (*Keebler*), 3 tbsp. ...............................80
crumbs, graham cracker (*Nabisco*), 2½ tbsp. ............................70
pieces (*Oreo Crunchies*) ............................................................50
**Coriander,** fresh, see "Cilantro"
**Coriander, dried:**
leaf, 1 tbsp. ...................................................................................5
seed, 1 tsp. ...................................................................................5
**Corkscrew pasta,** see "Pasta"
**Corkscrew pasta dish, mix,** about 1 cup*:
cheese, 4 (*Pasta Roni*) .............................................................410
garlic sauce, creamy (*Pasta Roni*) ...........................................420
**Corn,** fresh, white or yellow:
raw, 1 large ear, 7¾–9" long ....................................................123
raw, kernels, 1 cup .....................................................................132
boiled, drained, kernels, 1 cup ..................................................177
**Corn, canned,** ½ cup, except as noted:
kernel:
    gold and white (*Del Monte* Supersweet) ...............................80
    golden (*Del Monte*) .................................................................90
    golden (*Del Monte* Supersweet No Salt/Sugar) ....................60
    golden (*Del Monte* Supersweet Vac Pack) ...........................70
    golden (*Green Giant*) ..............................................................80
    golden (*Green Giant Niblets*), ⅓ cup .....................................80
    golden (*Greene's Farm* Organic Garden) ..............................60
    golden (*S&W*) .........................................................................90
    white shoepeg (*Green Giant*), ⅓ cup ....................................80

white, sweet (*Del Monte*)......................................................60
w/peppers (*Del Monte* Fiesta Supersweet)..........................50
cream style:
   golden (*Del Monte* Supersweet/Supersweet No Salt)............60
   golden (*Del Monte/Del Monte* No Salt)..................................90
   golden (*Green Giant* 14.75 oz.)...........................................90
   golden (*Green Giant* 8.5 oz.).............................................100
   white (*Del Monte*).................................................................100

**Corn, frozen:**
on the cob, 1 ear:
   (*Birds Eye*)..........................................................................120
   (*Freshlike* 3/4), 5.5-oz. ear.................................................140
   (*Freshlike* 6/8/12/24), 3-oz. ear...........................................80
   (*Green Giant Nibblers*), 2.15-oz. ear...................................70
   (*Green Giant Niblets*), 5-oz. ear.........................................150
kernels:
   (*Birds Eye*), 1/3 cup..............................................................70
   (*Birds Eye* Deluxe), 1/3 cup .................................................60
   (*Green Giant Niblets*), 2/3 cup.............................................80
   (*Seabrook Farms*), 2/3 cup..................................................80
   in butter sauce (*Birds Eye*), 1/2 cup....................................110
   in butter sauce (*Green Giant Niblets*), 2/3 cup....................130
   in herb sauce (*Boston Market*), 10-oz. pkg........................360
   white, shoepeg (*Green Giant*), 1/2 cup..................................70
creamed (*Green Giant*), 1/2 cup.............................................110
**Corn, pickled,** baby (*Haddon House*), 3 pcs., 1 oz. ...................10
**Corn bran,** crude, 1 cup.........................................................170
**Corn chips, puffs and similar snacks,** 1 oz., except as noted:
(*Baked Bugles*), 1½ cups, 1.1 oz. .........................................130
(*Corn Nuts* Original), 1/3 cup..................................................120
(*Fritos/Fritos* King Size/Scoops)............................................160
(*Munchos*)..............................................................................160
all varieties (*Barbara's Thangs*) ............................................120
all varieties (*Fritos Racerz*) ...................................................160
all varieties, except smokin' barbecue (*Bugles*), 1.1 oz. ..........160
barbecue, regular or honey (*Fritos*).......................................150
barbecue, smokin' (*Bugles*), 1⅓ cups, 1.1 oz.......................150
cheese:
   (*Chee•tos* X's and O's) ........................................................160

**Corn chips, puffs and similar snacks, cheese (*cont.*)**
 (*Chee•tos* Zig Zags) ............................................170
 balls, puffed (*Chee•tos*)......................................150
 balls, puffed (*Planters Cheez Mania* White Cheddar) ..........160
 crunchy or puffed (*Chee•tos*)..............................160
 curls (*Chee•tos*) ..............................................150
 curls (*Herr's*) .................................................110
 curls (*Planters Cheez Mania*) ...............................150
 puffs (*Barbara's* Bakes), 1½ cups, 1 oz.............................160
 puffs (*Barbara's* Original/Jalapeno), ¾ cup, 1 oz. ...............150
 chili (*Fritos*) ...................................................160
 hot (*Chee•tos* Flamin') .....................................150
 hot (*Chee•tos* Puff Rods)....................................160
hot (*Fritos Sabrositas* Flamin') ...................................160
lime and chili (*Fritos Sabrositas*)................................150
onion (*Funyons*) .......................................................140
ranch, onion (*Barbara's Onion Zings*) ........................130
sour cream and onion (*Corn Nuts*), ⅓ cup....................130
tortilla:
 (*Doritos* Toasted) ..............................................140
 (*Tostitos* Baked/Baked Bite Size)............................110
 (*Tostitos* Bite Size/Crispy Rounds/Santa Fe Gold).........140
 (*Tostitos* Restaurant Style)...................................150
 (*Tostitos Wow!*) ..................................................90
 (*Santitas*)...........................................................130
 barbecue (*Doritos* Smokey Red)..............................150
 blue corn (*Barbara's/Barbara's* No Salt), 1.1 oz................140
 cheddar quesadilla (*Tostitos* Bake Bite Size) ..................120
 hot (*Doritos* Flamin') ..........................................140
 jalapeno cheddar (*Doritos* 3D's) ............................130
 lime (*Tostitos* Restaurant Style).............................140
 nacho cheese (*Doritos* Cheesier/3D's Cheesier).............140
 nacho cheese (*Doritos Wow!* Cheesier) ....................90
 nacho, spicy (*Doritos*).........................................140
 ranch (*Doritos* Cooler/3D's Cooler)........................140
 salsa (*Barbara's* Pinta) ........................................130
 salsa and cream cheese (*Tostitos* Bake Bite Size)..............120
 salsa verde (*Doritos*)...........................................150
 cream (*Doritos* Sonic)..........................................140

taco (*Doritos* Supreme) ........................................140
white corn (*Herr's* Restaurant Style)..........................140
**Corn chips and dip,** kit:
corn chips and dip, chili or sloppy joe (*Fritos*), ½ kit ...............380
tortilla chips and salsa (*Tostitos*), 1 pkg. ....................320
tortilla chips and salsa con queso (*Tostitos*), 1 pkg...................460
**Corn dog,** see "Frankfurter sandwich"
**Corn flour:**
masa, white or yellow, 1 cup....................................416
whole grain, white or yellow, 1 cup.............................422
yellow, degerminated, 1 cup....................................473
**Corn fritter,** frozen (*Mrs. Paul's*), 1 pc. ....................130
**Corn grits,** dry:
white (*Albers* Hominy), ¼ cup..................................140
white (*Arrowhead Mills*), ¼ cup................................140
yellow (*Arrowhead Mills*), ¼ cup ..............................130
**Corn syrup,** dark or light (*Karo*), 2 tbsp. ...................120
**Cornish hen,** fresh or frozen, ready to cook:
whole, cooked, dark (*Perdue*), 3 oz............................200
whole, cooked, white (*Perdue*), 3 oz. .........................160
whole, split, roasted, dark meat from 1 half (*Perdue*) .............200
whole, split, roasted, white meat from 1 half (*Perdue*).............190
half, roasted, meat w/skin, 4.6 oz. ............................335
half, roasted, meat only, 3.9 oz. .............................147
**Cornmeal** (see also "Corn flour" and "Polenta"):
blue (*Arrowhead Mills*), ¼ cup................................130
white (*Albers*), 3 tbsp. .....................................110
white (*Hodgson Mill* Plain), scant ¼ cup .....................100
yellow (*Arrowhead Mills*), ¼ cup .............................120
yellow (*Hodgson Mill* Plain/Organic), scant ¼ cup .................100
yellow, self-rising (*Hodgson Mill*), ¼ cup......................90
**Cornstarch** (*Argo*), 1 tbsp. ................................30
**Couscous:**
dry (*Frieda's*), ¼ cup .......................................210
cooked, 1 cup .................................................176
**Couscous dish, mix,** 1 cup*:
cranberry (*Marrakesh Express* Calypso) .......................200
lentil curry or olive garlic (*Marrakesh Express*) .................170
mango salsa (*Marrakesh Express*).............................190

**Couscous dish, mix (*cont.*)**
mushroom, wild (*Marrakesh Express*)..............................190
sesame ginger (*Marrakesh Express*)..............................180
toasted, all varieties (*Marrakesh Express* Grande)....................250
tomato, sun-dried, or vegetable (*Marrakesh Express*)..............190
**Couscous salad** (*Cedarlane*), ½ cup..............................140
**Cowpeas,** fresh:
young pods, w/seeds, boiled, drained, 1 cup..............................32
leafy tips, boiled, drained, chopped, 1 cup..............................12
**Cowpeas, canned,** see "Black-eyed peas"
**Cowpeas, frozen,** boiled, drained, 1 cup..............................224
**Crab,** meat only:
Alaska king, raw, 4 oz...............................95
Alaska king, boiled, poached, or steamed, 4 oz. ....................110
blue, raw, 4 oz. ..............................99
blue, boiled, poached, or steamed, 4 oz..............................116
blue, boiled, poached, or steamed, not packed, 1 cup..............138
blue, boiled, poached, or steamed, flaked, 1 cup..............................120
Dungeness, raw, 4 oz..............................98
Dungeness, boiled, poached, or steamed, 4 oz. ....................125
queen, raw, 4 oz..............................102
queen, boiled, poached, or steamed, 4 oz..............................130
**Crab, canned:**
(*Reese*), ½ cup..............................45
lump, drained (*Bumble Bee* Fancy), ½ of 4.25-oz. can..............40
white, drained (*Orleans* Fancy), ½ of 6-oz. can ....................28
**"Crab," imitation,** from surimi, 4 oz. ..............................116
**Crab entree,** frozen:
bites, w/cheese (*Mrs. Paul's/Van de Kamp's*), 4 pcs., 4 oz.......320
cakes, unbreaded (*Chincoteague* Maryland Style), 1 pc. ..........170
cakes, lightly breaded (*Chincoteague* Maryland Style), 4 oz.....280
cakes (*Van de Kamp's*), 2.75-oz. pc. ..............................190
cakes, deviled (*Mrs. Paul's*), 2.9-oz. pc. ..............................180
cakes, mini (*Mrs. Paul's*), 6 pcs., 3.25 oz..............................220
cakes, mini (*Van de Kamp's*), 4 pcs., 4 oz. ..............................260
nuggets, unbreaded (*Chincoteague* Cocktail), 6 pcs..............180
nuggets, lightly breaded (*Chincoteague* Cocktail), 3 oz. ..........210
**Crabapple,** fresh, w/peel, sliced, 1 cup ..............................84

**Cracker:**

all varieties (*Barbara's* Wafer Crisps), 3 pcs., .5 oz....................60
all varieties (*Carr's Cocktail Croissant*), 22 pcs., 1.1 oz. ..........140
all varieties (*Harvest Bakery*), 2 pcs., .6 oz..............................70
all varieties (*Toasteds*), 5 pcs., .6 oz. ....................................80
all varieties (*Wheatables*), 12 pcs., 1.1 oz...............................140
bacon (*Nabisco*), 15 pcs. ........................................................160
biscuit, assorted (*Carr's*), 3 pcs., .6 oz....................................83
biscuit, English (*Carr's* Wheatolo), 1 pc., .5 oz. .........................70
butter/butter flavor:
    (*Hi Ho*), 4 pcs., .5 oz.......................................................70
    (*Hi Ho* Reduced Fat), 5 pcs.............................................70
    (*Keebler Club*), 4 pcs., .5 oz..........................................70
    (*Keebler Club* Reduced Fat), 5 pcs., .6 oz........................70
    (*Ritz/Ritz* Low Sodium), 5 pcs., .6 oz. .............................80
    (*Ritz* Reduced Fat/Whole Wheat), 5 pcs. ..........................70
    (*Ritz Air Crisps*), 24 pcs., 1.1 oz....................................140
    (*Ritz Bits* Sandwich), 10 pcs............................................170
    (*Town House*), 5 pcs., .6 oz............................................80
    (*Town House* Reduced Fat), 5 pcs., .5 oz.........................70
    (*Waverly*), 5 pcs.............................................................70
    (*Carr's Croissant*), 3 pcs., .5 oz.....................................70
cheese:
    (*Barbara's* Bites), 26 pcs., 1.1 oz. ..................................120
    (*Big Cheez-It*), 13 pcs. ..................................................150
    (*Carr's Cocktail Cheddars*), 22 pcs., 1.1 oz. ...................150
    (*Chee•tos* Golden Toast), 1 pkg. ....................................240
    (*Cheese Nips* Reduced Fat), 31 pcs., 1.1 oz. ...................130
    (*Cheese Nips Air Crisps* Original), 32 pcs. .......................130
    (*Cheez-It* Original), 27 pcs., 1.1 oz. ................................160
    (*Cheez-It* Reduced Fat), 29 pcs., 1.1 oz..........................140
    (*Cheez-It Chip-Its*), 29 pcs., 1.1 oz. ...............................130
    (*Ritz Bits*), 14 pcs., 1.1 oz. ...........................................170
    (*SnackWell's* Zesty), 38 pcs. ..........................................130
    (*Tid-Bits*), 32 pcs., 1.1 oz. ............................................160
cheddar (*Better Cheddars*), 22 pcs., 1.1 oz. ..........................150
cheddar (*Better Cheddars* Reduced Fat), 24 pcs., 1.1 oz. ....140
cheddar (*Carr's*), 3 pcs., .5 oz................................................80
cheddar (*Cheese Nips*), 29 pcs................................................150

**Cracker, wheat (*cont.*)**

    cheddar (*Cheese Nips* Xtra), 27 pcs. .....................................140

    cheddar (*Keebler Snax Stix* Zesty), 20 pcs., 1 oz. ...............120

    cheddar (*Sportz*), 40 pcs. ...................................................150

    cheddar or Parmesan (*Goldfish*), 1.1 oz. ............................140

    hot and spicy or white cheddar (*Cheez-It*), 26 pc., 1.1 oz. ..150

    nacho (*Cheez-It*), 1.5-oz. pkg. ..........................................210

    pizza (*Cheese Nips*), 27 pcs. ............................................140

    and sesame (*Twigs*), 15 pcs., 1.1 oz. ................................150

    Swiss (*Nabisco*), 15 pcs., 1 oz. .........................................140

cheese sandwich:

    (*Chee•tos*), 1 pkg. ..........................................................210

    (*Ritz*), 1.38-oz. pkg. ........................................................200

    (*Ritz Bits*), 1.75-oz. pkg. ..................................................270

    bacon (*Chee•tos*), 1 pkg. .................................................190

    cheddar (*Cheese Nips*), 1.38-oz. pkg. ..............................200

    cheddar (*Keebler Club*), 1.3-oz. pkg. ...............................190

    cheddar, toast (*Nabisco*), 1.38-oz. pkg. ...........................200

    cheddar, wheat (*Keebler Club*), 1.3-oz. pkg. ....................200

    jalapeno (*Doritos*), 1 pkg. ...............................................230

    nacho (*Doritos*), 1 pkg. ...................................................240

    peanut butter (*Keebler*), 1.36-oz. pkg. .............................190

(*Chicken in a Biskit*), 12 pcs., 1.1 oz. ...................................160

flatbread, classical or sesame (*Real Torino*), 2 pcs., .9 oz. ......120

graham cracker, see "Cookie"

grain, 5 (*Harvest Crisps*), 13 pcs., 1.1 oz. .............................130

milk (*Royal Lunch*), 1 pc. .......................................................60

(*Munch'ems* Original Baked), 35 pcs., 1.1 oz. .........................130

onion, French (*SnackWell's*), 38 pcs. ....................................130

onion, French (*Triscuit* Thin Crisps), 14 pcs., 1 oz. .................130

oyster/soup (*Krispy*), 17 pcs., .5 oz. ......................................60

oyster/soup (*Premium*), 23 pcs., .5 oz. ...................................60

oyster/soup (*Zesta*), 45 pcs., .6 oz. ........................................70

peanut butter sandwich:

    (*Ritz*), 1.38-oz. pkg. ........................................................190

    (*Ritz Bits*), 1.75-oz. pkg. ..................................................260

    (*Ritz Bits*), 14 pcs., 1.1 oz. ..............................................170

    cheese (*Cheese Nips/Nabisco*), 1.38-oz. pkg. ..................190

    toast (*Keebler*), 1.36-oz. pkg. ..........................................190

pepper, cracked (*SnackWell's*), 5 pcs.............................60
pizza (*Sportz*), 39 pcs. ...........................................150
poppy and sesame (*Carr's*), 4 pcs., .6 oz.....................80
ranch (*Munch'ems* Baked), 33 pcs., 1 oz.....................130
rice, black sesame (*San-J*), 5 pcs., 1 oz. ....................140
rice, brown (*San-J*), 5 pcs., 1 oz. .............................130
rice, brown, tamari (*San-J*), 5 pcs., 1 oz. ...................120
saltine:
   all varieties (*Premium*), 5 pcs., .5 oz. ...................60
   (*Krispy/Krispy* Unsalted Tops), 5 pcs., .5 oz.............60
   (*Krispy/Zesta* Fat Free), 5 pcs., .5 oz. ..................50
   (*Zesta* Original), 5 pcs., .6 oz. .............................60
   (*Zesta* Reduced Sodium/Unsalted Tops), 5 pcs., .6 oz...........70
   whole wheat (*Krispy*), 5 pcs., .5 oz.......................60
seasoned (*Keebler Snax Stix*), 21 pcs., 1 oz. ...............130
sesame and onion (*Monterey*), 3 pcs., .5 oz. ................70
(*Sociables*), 7 pcs., .5 oz. .......................................80
soda/water (*Carr's Table Water*), 6 pcs., .6 oz. .............70
soda/water (*Zesta Export Sodas*), 3 pcs., .6 oz. ............60
sour cream and onion (*Munch'ems* Baked), 28 pcs.,
   1.1 oz. ...........................................................140
sour cream and onion (*Ritz Air Crisps*), 23 pcs., 1.1 oz...........140
vegetable (*Nabisco Thins*), 14 pcs. ...........................160
vegetable, garden (*Harvest Crisps*), 15 pcs., 1.1 oz. ............130
vegetable, roasted (*Monterey*), 3 pcs., .5 oz. ...............60
(*Waverly*), 5 pcs., .5 oz..........................................70
wheat:
   (*Barbara's* Lite Rite Rounds), 5 pcs., .5 oz. ..............55
   (*Keebler Snax Stix* Hearty), 20 pcs., 1 oz. ...............130
   (*Monterey* Hearty), 3 pcs., .5 oz. .........................60
   (*Monterey* Savory), 3 pcs., .5 oz. .........................70
   (*Toasteds* Reduced Fat), 5 pcs., .5 oz......................60
   (*Wheat Thins* Big), 10 pcs., 1.1 oz. ......................140
   (*Wheat Thins* Multi-Grain), 17 pcs., 1.1 oz. .............130
   (*Wheat Thins* Original), 16 pcs., .8 oz. ..................140
   (*Wheat Thins* Reduced Fat), 16 pcs.........................130
   (*Wheat Thins Air Crisps*), 24 pcs., 1 oz....................130
   (*Wheatables* Reduced Fat), 13 pcs., 1 oz. ................130
   (*Wheatsworth*), 5 pcs., .6 oz..............................180

**Cracker (*cont.*)**

    all flavors (*Barbara's Wheatines*), ½"-square, .5 oz.............50

    ranch (*Wheat Thins Air Crisps*), 23 pcs.............................130

    whole (*Carr's*), 2 pcs., .6 oz. ...........................................80

    whole (*Triscuit* Original/Low Sodium/Deli-Style Rye),

        7 pcs., 1.1 oz. ...........................................................140

    whole (*Triscuit* Reduced Fat), 8 pcs., 1.1 oz......................130

    whole (*Triscuit Thin Crisps*), 15 pcs., 1.1 oz. ...................130

    whole, French onion (*Triscuits Thin Crisps*), 14 pcs. ..........130

    whole, garden herb (*Triscuits*), 6 pcs. .............................130

**Cracker meal** (*Nabisco*), ¼ cup.........................................110

**Cranberry,** fresh, raw:

whole (*Dole*), ½ cup..........................................................23

whole (*Ocean Spray*), ½ cup ..............................................30

chopped, 1 cup..................................................................54

**Cranberry, dried,** ⅓ cup:

(*Frieda's*)......................................................................120

sweetened (*Craisins*) .......................................................130

**Cranberry bean,** mature, boiled, 1 cup...............................241

**Cranberry drink blend,** 8 fl. oz., except as noted:

apple (*Cranapple*) ...........................................................160

apple raspberry (*Minute Maid*) .........................................123

(*Cran•Cherry*) .................................................................160

(*Cran•Currant/Cran•Raspberry/Cran•Strawberry*) ...............140

(*Cran•Grape*)..................................................................170

(*Cran•Mango/Cran•Tangerine*)..........................................130

(*Lightstyle Cran•Grape/Cran•Mango/Cran•Raspberry*) ...........40

**Cranberry juice** (*Ocean Spray* Premium 100%), 8 fl. oz..........140

**Cranberry juice blend,** 8 fl. oz., except as noted:

(*Mott's*), 11.5 fl. oz. .......................................................180

apple (*Juicy Juice*) .........................................................120

apple (*Ocean Spray* Granny Smith Premium 100%) ..............130

grape (*Ocean Spray* Concord Premium 100%) .....................150

lime (*Ocean Spray* Key Lime Premium 100%) .....................140

peach (*Ocean Spray* Georgia Premium 100%) .....................140

raspberry (*Ocean Spray* Pacific Premium 100%) ..................140

**Cranberry juice cocktail,** 8 fl. oz.:

(*Mott's*) ........................................................................150

(*Ocean Spray*) ................................................................140

(*Ocean Spray* Plus)......................................................160
(*Ocean Spray Lightstyle*)...........................................40
**Cranberry sauce,** canned, ¼ cup:
whole or jellied (*Ocean Spray*)...............................110
whole or jellied (*S&W*)..............................................100
**Cranberry-orange relish,** canned, ½ cup.................245
**Crayfish,** mixed species, meat only:
farmed, raw, 8 crayfish, 1 oz......................................20
farmed, boiled, poached, or steamed, 4 oz.............99
wild, raw, 8 crayfish, 1 oz...........................................21
wild, baked, broiled, or microwaved, 4 oz...............93
**Cream,** dairy pack:
half and half, 1 tbsp....................................................20
light, coffee or table, 1 tbsp.......................................29
medium (25% fat), 1 tbsp............................................37
whipped topping, see "Cream topping"
whipping, light, 1 tbsp., 2 tbsp. whipped.................44
whipping, heavy, 1 tbsp., 2 tbsp. whipped...............52
**Cream, double,** in jars (*Devon Cream Company English*
    *Double Devon*), 1 oz. ...........................................125
**Cream, sour,** 2 tbsp., except as noted:
(*Breakstone's* Reduced Fat)......................................45
(*Breakstone's/Knudsen Hampshire*)........................60
(*Breakstone's Free/Knudsen Free*)..........................35
(*Land O Lakes*)............................................................60
(*Land O Lakes* Light)..................................................35
(*Land O Lakes* No Fat)...............................................30
**"Cream," sour, nondairy** (*Tofutti Sour Supreme*), 2 tbsp.........50
**Cream topping,** 2 tbsp.:
(*Cool Whip/Cool Whip* Extra Creamy)......................25
(*Cool Whip Free/Kraft Free*)......................................15
(*Cool Whip Lite*)..........................................................20
(*Crowley*).......................................................................25
(*Kraft Dairy Whip*).......................................................15
(*Reddi Wip* Extra Creamy).........................................30
(*Reddi Wip* Fat Free)..................................................10
(*Reddi Wip* Original/Non Dairy)................................20
**Cream topping, mix** (*Dream Whip*), 2 tbsp.*............20
**Cream of tartar,** 1 tsp. ................................................2

**Creamer, nondairy:**
liquid (*Coffee-mate*), 1 tbsp..............................................20
liquid (*Coffee-mate* Fat Free/Low Fat), 1 tbsp. ...............10
liquid, flavored, all flavors (*Coffee-mate*), 1 tbsp. ...........40
liquid, flavored, all flavors (*Coffee-mate* Fat Free), 1 tbsp. .........25
powder (*Coffee-mate/Coffee-mate* Lite/Fat Free), 1 tsp. .............10
powder, flavored, all flavors (*Coffee-mate*), 4 tsp. .....................60
powder, flavored, all flavors (*Coffee-mate* Fat Free), 1 tsp. .........50
**Crème fraîche** (*Allouette*), 2 tbsp. ............................100
**Crepe** (*Frieda's*), 2 pcs. ...........................................50
**Croaker, Atlantic,** meat only:
raw, 4 oz. ..................................................................118
breaded, fried, 4 oz...................................................251
**Croissant:**
(*Sara Lee*), 1.5 oz. ..................................................170
butter (*Awrey's*), 3 oz. ............................................250
butter (*Awrey's*), 2 oz. ............................................170
margarine (*Awrey's*), 2.5 oz.....................................210
margarine (*Awrey's*), 2 oz.........................................170
mini (*Sara Lee* Petite), 2 pcs. ..................................230
**Crookneck squash,** fresh:
raw, baby (*Frieda's*), ⅔ cup, 3 oz..............................15
raw, sliced, 1 cup........................................................25
boiled, drained, sliced, 1 cup......................................36
**Crookneck squash, canned** (*Sunshine*), ½ cup .............25
**Crookneck squash, frozen:**
(*Birds Eye*), ½ cup......................................................50
sliced (*Birds Eye*), ⅔ cup...........................................15
**Croutons:**
Caesar (*Pepperidge Farm* Generous Cut), 6 pcs.............35
Caesar (*Pepperidge Farm* Generous Cut Fat Free), 6 pcs. .........30
cheese garlic (*Arnold* Classic), 2 tbsp...........................30
cheese and garlic (*Pepperidge Farm* Classic Cut), 9 pcs. .........35
Italian, zesty (*Pepperidge Farm* Generous Cut), 6 pcs. ...........35
seasoned (*Arnold* Classic), 2 tbsp.................................30
seasoned (*Pepperidge Farm* Classic Cut), 9 pcs.............35
**Cucumber,** fresh, raw:
(*Frieda's* Hothouse/Japanese), ⅔ cup, 3 oz.....................10
w/peel, 8¼" cucumber .................................................39

peeled, sliced, 1 cup ....................................................14
**Cumin seed,** ground, 1 tsp. ...................................8
**Currants,** fresh, raw:
black, European, 1 cup ............................................71
red or white, 1 cup ..................................................63
**Currants, dried,** zante, 1 cup ............................408
**Curry base,** 1 tsp.:
green (*A Taste of Thai*) ...........................................15
Mussaman or red (*A Taste of Thai*) .......................20
Panang (*A Taste of Thai*) .......................................25
yellow (*A Taste of Thai*) .........................................30
**Curry powder,** 1 tsp. ................................................7
**Curry paste,** 2 tbsp., except as noted:
(*Patak's* Balti) ........................................................115
(*Patak's* Biryani) ....................................................170
(*Patak's* Garam Masala), 2 tsp. ............................130
(*Patak's* Kashmiri Masala), 1 tsp. ...........................15
(*Patak's* Madras/Vindaloo) ....................................160
(*Patak's* Tikka Masala) ..........................................110
hot (*Patak's*) ..........................................................160
mild (*Patak's*) ........................................................170
**Curry sauce,** ½ cup, except as noted:
chili, hot, w/coriander (*Patak's* Vindaloo) ..............320
chili, hot, w/cumin (*Patak's* Madras 10 oz.) ...........280
coconut, rich, creamy, mild (*Patak's* Korma 10 oz.) .....210
coriander, tangy, and lemon (*Patak's* Tikka Masala 10 oz.) ......210
green or red (*A Taste of Thai* Dinner Kit Lite), 3.5 fl. oz. ..........90
Mussaman (*A Taste of Thai* Dinner Kit Lite), 3.5 fl. oz. ...........100
Panang or yellow (*A Taste of Thai* Dinner Kit Lite), 3.5 fl. oz. ..110
sweet peppers and coconut (*Patak's* Jalfrezi) ............140
tomato, rich, and onion (*Patak's* Dopiaza) ..............110
tomato, spicy, and cardamon (*Patak's* Rogan Josh 10 oz.) ......180
**Cusk,** meat only:
raw, 4 oz. ................................................................99
baked, broiled, or microwaved, 4 oz. ....................127
**Custard,** see "Pudding and pie filling mix"
**Cuttlefish,** meat only:
raw, 4 oz. ................................................................89
boiled, poached, or steamed, 4 oz. ........................179

# D

**Daikon,** see "Radish, Oriental"
**Daiquiri margarita mix,** strawberry (*Mr & Mrs T*),
   3.5 fl. oz. ............................................................150
*Dairy Queen/Brazier,* 1 serving:
*Basket,* chicken strip.....................................................1000
*Basket, The Great Steakmelt*..........................................750
burgers:
   *DQ Homestyle* bacon double cheeseburger........................610
   *DQ Homestyle* cheeseburger ..................................340
   *DQ Homestyle* double cheeseburger .........................540
   *DQ Homestyle* hamburger .....................................290
   *DQ Ultimate* burger ...........................................670
chicken sandwich, breast fillet...................................430
chicken sandwich, grilled .........................................310
hot dog .................................................................240
hot dog, chili 'n' cheese............................................330
fries, medium.........................................................440
fries, small ............................................................350
onion rings.............................................................320
*Blizzard* Flavor Treats:
   chocolate chip cookie dough, medium.............................950
   chocolate chip cookie dough, small................................660
   chocolate sandwich cookie, medium...............................640
   chocolate sandwich cookie, small .................................520
cones:
   chocolate, medium.................................................340
   chocolate, small.....................................................240
   dipped, medium ....................................................490
   dipped, small........................................................340
   *DQ* chocolate soft serve, ½ cup ...................................150
   *DQ* vanilla soft serve, ½ cup.......................................140
   vanilla, large .........................................................410
   vanilla, medium.....................................................330

vanilla, small .................................................................230
*DQ* cake, undecorated, frozen, 8" round, ⅛ cake .....................370
*DQ* cake, undecorated, layered, 8" round, ⅛ cake ...................330
*DQ Treatzza Pizza, Heath,* ⅛ pizza .............................................180
*DQ Treatzza Pizza, M&M's,* ⅛ pizza............................................190
malts, shakes, and smoothies:
   chocolate malt, medium..............................................880
   chocolate malt, small ................................................650
   chocolate shake, medium ...........................................770
   chocolate shake, small................................................560
   hot chocolate, frozen..................................................860
   strawberry banana *DQ Glacier Smoothy*............................670
*Misty* slush, medium ..............................................................290
*Misty* slush, small...................................................................220
novelties:
   *Buster Bar* .................................................................450
   chocolate *Dilly* bar......................................................210
   *DQ* fudge bar, no sugar added ......................................50
   *DQ* sandwich.............................................................150
   *DQ* vanilla orange bar, no sugar added...............................60
   lemon *DQ Freez'r,* ½ cup .............................................80
   *Starkiss* ....................................................................80
*Royal Treats:*
   banana split...............................................................510
   *Chocolate Rock* treat or *Peanut Buster* parfait .................730
   *Pecan Mudslide* treat .................................................650
   strawberry shortcake ...................................................430
sundae, chocolate, medium.......................................................400
sundae, chocolate, small ..........................................................280
yogurt, frozen:
   *Breeze, Heath,* medium ..............................................710
   *Breeze, Heath,* small...................................................470
   *Breeze,* strawberry, medium .........................................460
   *Breeze,* strawberry, small ............................................320
   cone, medium .............................................................260
   cup, medium ...............................................................230
   *DQ* nonfat, ½ cup.......................................................100
   strawberry sundae, medium ...........................................320
**Dandelion greens,** fresh, raw, chopped, 1 cup.........................25

**Danish,** 1 pc.:

all flavors (*Awrey's* Petite) ......................................................160
apple, cheese, or strawberry (*Awrey's*) ...............................290
apple, cheese, or strawberry (*Awrey's* Grande) ..................470
cinnamon (*Awrey's* Grande) ..................................................480
cinnamon swirl (*Awrey's* Grande) .........................................400
cinnamon swirl (*Awrey's*) ......................................................300
raspberry cheese swirl (*Awrey's* Grande)..............................360

**Date,** natural, dry:

pitted (*Dole*), 5–6 dates, 1.4 oz..........................................120
pitted, chopped (*Dole*), 1 oz...............................................120
domestic, 1 date, .3 oz. ..........................................................23

**Delicata squash** (*Frieda's*), ¾ cup, 3 oz. .........................30
**Dill dip mix,** dry (*Knorr*), ½ tsp........................................5
**Dill seed,** 1 tsp. ....................................................................6

**Dill weed,** fresh:

5 sprigs ...................................................................................<1
1 cup........................................................................................4

**Dill weed, dried,** 1 tsp..........................................................3
**Dock,** fresh, raw, chopped, 1 cup .......................................29

**Dolphin fish,** meat only:

raw, 4 oz. ...............................................................................96
baked, broiled, or microwaved, 4 oz. ...................................124

**Donut,** 1 piece, except as noted:

plain (*Awrey's*), 2 oz. ..........................................................210
plain (*Awrey's*), 1.5 oz. .......................................................150
chocolate, chocolate iced (*Awrey's*) ...................................190
chocolate iced (*Awrey's*)......................................................200
chocolate iced (*Hostess*) ....................................................170
chocolate iced (*Hostess Donettes*), 3 pcs. .........................230
coconut topped (*Awrey's*).....................................................210
crunch (*Awrey's*)...................................................................280
crunch topped (*Awrey's*) ......................................................160
custard filled, chocolate iced (*Awrey's* Bismarck) ...............330
devil's food, glazed (*Awrey's*) ..............................................300
jelly filled, powdered sugar (*Awrey's* Bismarck)...................250
jelly filled, vanilla iced (*Awrey's* Bismarck) .........................320
powdered sugar (*Awrey's*), 2 oz. .........................................240
powdered sugar (*Awrey's*), 1.5 oz........................................160

raised, glazed (*Hostess*) .............................................150
ring, chocolate iced (*Awrey's*), 2.7 oz. ....................300
ring, glazed (*Awrey's*), 2.5 oz. .................................270
sour cream (*Awrey's*) ...............................................370
sour cream, chocolate iced (*Awrey's*), 3.75 oz. .......430
sour cream, chocolate iced (*Awrey's*), 3 oz. ............310
sour cream, glazed (*Awrey's*), 3.75 oz. ....................420
sour cream, glazed (*Awrey's*), 3 oz. .........................300
sprinkle topped (*Awrey's*) .........................................160
white iced (*Awrey's*) .................................................200
**Drum,** freshwater, meat only:
raw, 4 oz. ..................................................................135
baked, broiled, or microwaved, 4 oz. .........................174
**Duck,** domesticated:
meat w/skin, 4 oz. .....................................................382
meat only, 4 oz. .........................................................228
meat only, chopped or diced, 1 cup ...........................281
duckling, breast, meat w/skin, 3 oz. ..........................172
duckling, leg, meat w/skin, 3.2 oz. ............................200
**Duck sauce,** see "Sweet and sour sauce"
**Dumpling entree,** frozen, Oriental style (*Lean Cuisine Everyday Favorites*), 9-oz. pkg. ...............................300
***Dunkin' Donuts:***
sandwich, *Omwich,* 1 piece:
    bagel, bacon/cheddar .............................................600
    bagel, Spanish/cheese............................................570
    bagel, 3 cheese .....................................................610
    croissant, bacon/cheddar or 3 cheese....................560
    croissant, Spanish/cheese .....................................530
    English muffin, bacon/cheddar or 3 cheese ............400
    English muffin, Spanish/cheese..............................370
sandwich, breakfast, ham/egg/cheese........................320
bagels, 1 piece:
    plain, blueberry, cinnamon raisin, onion or salt .......340
    egg or pumpernickel...............................................350
    everything, garlic or poppy seed.............................360
    sesame ...................................................................380
    wheat......................................................................330

**Dunkin' Donuts** *(cont.)*

cream cheese:

| | |
|---|---|
| plain, 1 pkt. | 200 |
| chive, 1 pkt. | 190 |
| lite, 1 pkt. | 130 |
| salmon or garden vegetable, 1 pkt. | 180 |

cookies, 1 pc.:

| | |
|---|---|
| chocolate chocolate chunk | 210 |
| chocolate chunk or oatmeal raisin pecan | 220 |
| chocolate chunk w/nuts or white chocolate chunk | 230 |
| peanut butter chocolate chunk w/nuts | 240 |
| peanut butter w/nuts | 240 |

croissant, 1 pc.:

| | |
|---|---|
| plain | 290 |
| almond | 350 |
| chocolate | 400 |

donuts, 1 piece:

| | |
|---|---|
| apple crumb | 230 |
| apple fritter | 300 |
| apple and spice | 200 |
| Bavarian kreme | 210 |
| black raspberry | 210 |
| blueberry cake | 290 |
| blueberry crumb | 240 |
| Boston kreme | 240 |
| bow tie | 300 |
| butternut cake | 300 |
| chocolate cake, double | 210 |
| chocolate cake, glazed | 290 |
| chocolate coconut cake | 300 |
| chocolate frosted | 200 |
| chocolate frosted cake | 300 |
| chocolate frosted coffee roll | 290 |
| chocolate iced, Bismarck | 340 |
| chocolate kreme filled | 270 |
| cinnamon bun | 510 |
| cinnamon cake | 270 |
| coconut cake | 290 |
| coconut cake, toasted | 300 |

coffee roll ...................................................................270
cruller, chocolate, glazed....................................280
cruller, glazed .................................................290
cruller, plain...................................................240
cruller, sugar .................................................250
*Dunkin' Donut* ...............................................240
éclair...........................................................270
glazed .........................................................180
glazed cake...................................................270
glazed fritter .................................................260
jelly filled ......................................................210
jelly stick .....................................................290
lemon ..........................................................200
maple frosted ................................................210
maple frosted coffee roll...................................290
old fashioned cake ..........................................250
powdered cake ...............................................270
powdered cruller .............................................270
strawberry .....................................................210
strawberry frosted............................................210
sugar raised ..................................................170
sugared cake .................................................250
vanilla frosted................................................210
vanilla frosted coffee roll....................................290
vanilla kreme .................................................270
whole wheat glazed..........................................310
*Munchkins,* cake:
  plain, 4 pcs....................................................220
  butternut or chocolate glazed, 3 pcs.....................200
  cinnamon or powdered, 4 pcs. ............................250
  coconut or toasted coconut, 3 pcs. .......................200
  glazed, 3 pcs. ...............................................200
  powdered, 4 pcs.............................................250
  sugared, 4 pcs...............................................240
*Munchkins,* yeast:
  glazed, 5 pcs. ...............................................200
  jelly filled, 5 pcs. ...........................................210
  lemon filled, 4 pcs...........................................170

**Dunkin' Donuts, Munchkins, yeast** (*cont.*)

sugar raised, 7 pcs.................................................................220

muffins, 1 pc.:

apple cinnamon.......................................................................510

apple and spice .....................................................................350

apple and spice, low fat ........................................................240

banana or blueberry, low fat .................................................250

banana nut .............................................................................360

blueberry, 6 oz. .....................................................................490

blueberry, 4 oz. .....................................................................320

blueberry, reduced fat ...........................................................450

bran........................................................................................390

bran, low fat ..........................................................................240

cherry ....................................................................................340

cherry or chocolate, low fat ..................................................250

chocolate chip, 6 oz. .............................................................590

chocolate chip, 4 oz. .............................................................400

chocolate hazelnut chunk......................................................610

corn, 6 oz. .............................................................................500

corn, 4 oz. .............................................................................390

corn, low fat ..........................................................................240

corn, reduced fat ...................................................................460

cranberry orange....................................................................470

cranberry orange, low fat ......................................................240

cranberry orange nut .............................................................350

honey bran raisin ...................................................................490

lemon poppy seed..................................................................360

oat bran..................................................................................370

beverages:

coffee *Coolatta,* w/cream, 16 oz.............................................410

coffee *Coolatta,* w/milk, 16 oz...............................................260

coffee *Coolatta,* w/milk, skim, 16 oz. ...................................230

*Dunkaccino,* 20 oz.................................................................510

*Dunkaccino,* 14 oz.................................................................360

*Dunkaccino,* 10 oz.................................................................250

hot cocoa, 14 oz.....................................................................330

hot cocoa, 10 oz.....................................................................230

orange mango fruit *Coolatta,* 16 oz. .....................................290

pink lemonade fruit *Coolatta,* 16 oz. .....................................350

raspberry lemonade or strawberry *Coolatta*, 16 oz. ............280
vanilla *Coolatta*, 16 oz. ...........................................450
**Durian:**
raw or frozen, 1.3 lb. .................................................885
chopped or diced, 1 cup.............................................357

# E

**FOOD AND MEASURE**                                     **CALORIES**

**Edamame,** raw (*Frieda's*), ½ cup ..............................................100
**Eel,** mixed species, meat only:
raw, 4 oz. ........................................................................209
baked, broiled, or microwaved, 4 oz. .........................................268
**Egg, chicken:**
raw, whole, 1 extra large .........................................................86
raw, whole, 1 large ................................................................75
raw, white only, 1 large...........................................................17
raw, yolk only (contains traces of white), 1 large .........................59
cooked, fried, 1 large..............................................................92
cooked, hard-boiled, chopped, 1 cup..........................................211
cooked, hard-boiled or poached, 1 large......................................75
cooked, omelet, 1 large ...........................................................93
**Egg, duck,** raw, whole, 1 egg.....................................................130
**Egg, quail,** raw, whole, 1 egg.....................................................14
**Egg, turkey,** raw, whole, 1 egg ...................................................135
**Egg pocket,** see "Breakfast sandwich/pocket"
**Egg roll,** frozen or refrigerated:
(*Empire Kosher*), 3-oz. pc........................................................190
chicken (*Chun King* Restaurant Style), 1 pc................................190
chicken (*La Choy* Restaurant Style), 1 pc. ................................210
chicken, mini (*Chun King/La Choy*), 6 pcs. ...............................210
chicken, sweet and sour (*La Choy* Restaurant Style), 1 pc. .....210
chicken, sweet and sour (*Yu Sing*), 6 pcs. ...............................190
chicken or shrimp (*Yu Sing*), 6 pcs. ........................................180
mini (*Empire Kosher*), 6 pcs., 4.9 oz.......................................280
pork (*La Choy* Restaurant Style), 1 pc......................................190
pork, sweet and sour (*Yu Sing*), 6 pcs......................................210
pork and shrimp (*Yu Sing*), 6 pcs............................................200
pork and shrimp, bite size (*La Choy*), 12 pcs.............................210
pork and shrimp, mini (*Chun King/La Choy*), 6 pcs.....................210
shrimp (*Chung's*), 1 pc. w/sauce pkt. .....................................140
shrimp (*Chun King/La Choy* Restaurant Style), 1 pc. ...............180

chicken or shrimp (*Yu Sing*), 6 pcs. ............................180
shrimp, mini (*Chun King/La Choy*), 6 pcs. ....................190
vegetable (*Chung's*), 1 pc. w/sauce pkt........................130
vegetable w/lobster, mini (*La Choy*), 6 pcs. ................190
**Egg roll entree,** frozen, vegetable (*Lean Cuisine Everyday
    Favorites*), 9-oz. pkg. ........................................300
**Egg roll wrapper,** refrigerated:
(*Frieda's*), 2 pcs., 1.7 oz. ........................................130
(*Nasoya*), 2 pcs., 1.6 oz..........................................120
**Egg substitute** (*Egg Beaters*), ¼ cup .......................30
**Eggnog,** canned (*Borden* Premium), ½ cup ..............160
**Eggplant,** fresh:
raw (*Frieda's* Chinese/Japanese), ⅔ cup, 3 oz............20
raw, peeled, 1 lb. (yield from 1¼-lb. eggplant) .............119
raw, cubed, 1 cup ....................................................21
boiled, drained, 1" cubes, 1 cup..................................28
**Eggplant, in jars:**
marinated (*Casa Visco*), 1 oz......................................15
sauteed (*Life in Provence*), ½ cup ............................270
strips, in sunflower oil (*Rienzi*), 1 oz..........................90
**Eggplant appetizer:**
(*Progresso* Caponata), 2 tbsp. ...................................25
(*Cedarlane* Caviar), 2 tbsp. .......................................30
**Eggplant dip,** 2 tbsp.
(*Victoria*) ................................................................30
roasted, w/red bell pepper (*Cedarlane*) .....................30
in jars (*Peloponnese* Babaganoush)............................40
**Eggplant entree,** Parmesan, frozen:
(*Cedarlane*), 5-oz. pkg. ...........................................160
(*Mrs. Paul's*), ½ cup...............................................190
w/linguine (*Michelina's*), 8-oz. pkg............................270
**Eggplant relish** (*Patak's* Brinjal), 1 tbsp. .................50
**Elderberry,** fresh, raw, 1 cup ..................................106
**Enchilada,** frozen, 1 pc., except as noted:
beef or cheese (*Patio* Family Pack), 2 pcs. w/sauce .................210
black bean vegetable (*Amy's*), 4.5 oz. .......................130
black bean vegetable (*Amy's* Family Size), ⅛ pkg. ......120
cheese (*Amy's*), 4.5 oz. ...........................................210
cheese (*Amy's* Family Size), ⅐ pkg. ..........................240

**Enchilada (*cont.*)**
chicken (*Stouffer's*), ¹⁄₁₂ of 57-oz. pkg....................220
vegetable (*Cedarlane*), 4.5 oz. ..................................135
**Enchilada dinner,** frozen, 1 pkg.:
beef, chili and beans (*Patio* Extra Large), 15.5 oz....................540
beef and cheese, chili and beans (*Patio* Extra Large), 15.5 oz. 670
black bean (*Amy's*), 10 oz. ...........................................250
cheese (*Amy's*), 9 oz. ..................................................330
suprema (*Healthy Choice* Meal), 11.3 oz. ..................300
**Enchilada entree,** frozen, 1 pkg., except as noted:
beef (*Banquet*), 11 oz.....................................................370
beef, and tamale, chili gravy w/ (*Morton*), 10 oz. ....................270
beef bake (*Ortega* Family Fiesta Meals), 9.25 oz., ¼ pkg. .......380
beef and tamale combo (*Banquet*), 11 oz....................450
beef or cheese (*Patio*), 12 oz.....................................370
cheese (*Banquet*), 11 oz. ..............................................360
chicken (*Banquet*), 11 oz. .............................................350
chicken (*Patio*), 12 oz...................................................400
chicken Suiza (*Healthy Choice* Entree), 10 oz. ..........280
chicken Suiza (*Lean Cuisine Everyday Favorites*), 9 oz.............280
Mexican style combo (*Banquet*), 11 oz. .....................380
Suiza, and Mexican style rice (*Lean Cuisine Everyday*
     *Favorites*), 9 oz.......................................................280
**Enchilada pie,** frozen (*Cedarlane*), 5.5-oz. pie ..............215
**Enchilada sauce,** ¼ cup:
green chili, fire roasted (*El Torito*) ...............................15
tomatillo (*El Torito*) .........................................................20
tomato, fire roasted (*El Torito*) ......................................45
**Enchilada sauce seasoning mix** (*Lawry's* Spices &
     Seasonings), 2 tsp. ...................................................20
**Endive,** fresh, raw:
1 head, 1.1 lbs. ................................................................87
chopped, ½ cup.................................................................4
**Endive, Belgian,** see "Chicory, witloof"
**Epazote,** fresh, raw, 1 sprig or 1 tbsp. .....................<1
**Eppaw,** fresh, raw, 1 cup..............................................150
**Escarole,** see "Endive"

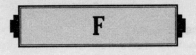

**FOOD AND MEASURE**                                    **CALORIES**

**Fajita dinner mix:**
(*Chi-Chi's* Dinner Kit), 2 shells and seasoning ........................300
chicken (*El Torito*), 3 oz. ...................................................................50
chicken (*Taco Bell Home Originals*), 2 fajitas* .......................340
**Fajita pocket** (*Mrs. Paterson's Aussie Pie*), 5.5-oz. pc............350
**Fajita seasoning mix:**
(*Chi-Chi's* Fiesta/*El Torito*), ¼ pkg. ...............................................35
(*Lawry's* Spices & Seasonings), 2 tsp. ......................................15
chicken (*Lawry's* Spices & Seasonings), 1 tsp. ..........................10
chicken (*Ortega*), 1½ tsp. ..............................................................15
chicken (*Taco Bell Home Originals*), 1 tbsp. ..............................20
**Fava beans,** see "Broad beans"
**Feijoa,** fresh, raw:
trimmed, 1 fruit, 1¾ oz. ....................................................................25
pureed, 1 cup.....................................................................................119
**Fennel,** bulb, raw:
1 bulb, 8.3 oz. .....................................................................................73
sliced, 1 cup.......................................................................................27
**Fennel seed,** 1 tsp. ...........................................................................7
**Fenugreek seed,** 1 tsp.....................................................................12
**Fettuccine:**
dry, see "Pasta"
refrigerated, plain (*Contadina Buitoni*), 1¼ cups......................240
refrigerated, plain or red bell pepper (*Di Giorno*), 2.5 oz. .........200
refrigerated, spinach (*Contadina Buitoni*), 1¼ cups .................260
**Fettuccine dishes, mix:**
Alfredo (*Knorr* TasteBreaks), 1 cont. .........................................230
Alfredo (*Pasta Roni*), approx. 1 cup* .........................................460
Alfredo (*Pasta Roni* Reduced Fat), approx. 1 cup* ..................310
Alfredo, classic (*Knorr*), ¾ cup...................................................280
w/creamy basil sauce (*Knorr* TasteBreaks), 1 cont. ..................220
**Fettuccine entree,** frozen, 1 pkg.:
Alfredo (*Banquet*), 9.5 oz. .............................................................350

**Fettuccine entree** (*cont.*)

Alfredo (*Freezer Queen*), 9 oz....................................................360
Alfredo (*Healthy Choice* Entree), 8 oz. .......................................240
Alfredo (*Lean Cuisine Everyday Favorites*), 9.25 oz. .................280
Alfredo (*Michelina's*), 9 oz........................................................380
Alfredo (*Stouffer's*), 11.5 oz. ....................................................540
Alfredo, w/broccoli and chicken (*Michelina's*), 8.5 oz...............310
Alfredo supreme (*Marie Callender's*), 13 oz. ............................450
Alfredo supreme, w/garlic bread (*Marie Callender's*), 14 oz. ....920
w/broccoli and chicken (*Marie Callender's*), 13 oz....................710
carbonara (*Michelina's*), 8 oz. ..................................................330
w/creamy pesto and vegetables (*Michelina's*), 8.5 oz..............250
primavera (*Lean Cuisine Everyday Favorites*), 10 oz. ...............270
primavera (*Michelina's*), 8 oz....................................................270
primavera (*Stouffer's*), 10 oz....................................................370
primavera, w/chicken (*Michelina's*), 8 oz. ................................280
primavera, w/tortellini (*Marie Callender's*), 14 oz.....................750

**Fig,** fresh:

1 large, 2.3 oz.............................................................................47
1 medium, 1.8 oz........................................................................37

**Fig, canned,** in light syrup, 1 fig w/liquid................................19

**Fig, dried:**

1 fig, ⅔ oz..................................................................................49
dried, calimyrna or mission (*Blue Ribbon Orchard
    Choice/Sun•Maid*), 1.5 oz., about 2 pcs.............................120

**Filbert, shelled:**

dried, 1 oz................................................................................179
dry roasted, 1 oz.......................................................................188

**Fish,** see specific listings

**Fish batter mix,** see "Fish seasoning and coating mix"

**Fish dinner,** frozen, 1 pkg.:

battered (*Swanson*), 10 oz. ......................................................490
herb baked (*Healthy Choice* Meal), 10.9 oz...............................340
lemon pepper (*Healthy Choice* Meal), 10.7 oz. .........................320
sticks (*Freezer Queen*), 6.5 oz.................................................290

**Fish entree,** frozen:

baked (*Lean Cuisine Cafe Classics*), 9-oz. pkg..........................290
breaded, w/macaroni and cheese (*Marie Callender's*),
    12-oz. pkg............................................................................550

cakes (*Mrs. Paul's*), 2 pcs., 3.7 oz. ............................................210
w/cheese and salsa (*Oven Poppers*), 4.5-oz. pc. ......................130
croquettes (*Dr. Praeger's*), 2.2-oz. pc. ...................................120
fillet (*Dr. Praeger's* Sandwich), 4-oz. pc. ................................210
fillet (*Stouffer's* Homestyle), 9-oz. pkg. .................................410
fillet, battered (*Mrs. Paul's* Hearty Size), 3.5-oz. pc. ................200
fillet, battered (*Mrs. Paul's*), 2.5-oz. pc. ..................................150
fillet, battered (*Van de Kamp's*), 2.6-oz. pc. ...........................170
fillet, breaded (*Dr. Praeger's*), 2.1-oz. pc. ..............................113
fillet, breaded (*Mrs. Paul's*), 2 pcs., 3.7 oz. ...........................280
fillet, breaded (*Van de Kamp's*), 2 pcs., 3.5 oz. .....................260
fillet, breaded (*Van de Kamp's* Hearty Size), 2-oz. pc. ..............150
fillet, breaded, baked, plain, garlic and herb, or lemon pepper:
   (*Mrs. Paul's* Healthy Selects), 2.9-oz. pc. ...........................130
   (*Van de Kamp's* Crisp & Healthy), 2 pcs., 3.7 oz. ...............170
fillet, grilled, garlic butter, lemon butter, or lemon pepper
   (*Van de Kamp's*), 1.7-oz. pc. ................................................120
fillet, grilled, Cajun, garlic butter, or lemon pepper
   (*Mrs. Paul's*), 4-oz. fillet ......................................................130
fillet sticks (*Dr. Praeger's*), 3 pcs., 2.9 oz. ..............................138
portion, battered (*Van de Kamp's*), 2.5-oz. pc. .........................160
portion, breaded (*Van de Kamp's*), 3 pcs., 4.5 oz. ...................360
w/shrimp, crab, vegetables (*Oven Poppers*), 4.5-oz. pc. ...........200
w/spinach and cheese (*Oven Poppers*), 4.5-oz. pc. ..................160
sticks (*Banquet*), 6.6 oz. ......................................................290
sticks, breaded:
   (*Mrs. Paul's*), 6 pcs., 3.35 oz. ............................................250
   (*Mrs. Paul's* Hearty Size), 5 pcs., 4 oz. ...............................300
   (*Van de Kamp's*), 6 pcs., 4 oz. ...........................................290
   (*Van de Kamp's* Club), 6 pcs., 3.4 oz. .................................240
   (*Van de Kamp's* Snack/Value), 6 pcs., 3.6 oz. .....................260
   baked (*Mrs. Paul's* Healthy Selects), 6 pcs., 4 oz. ..............190
   baked (*Van de Kamp's* Crisp & Healthy), 6 pcs., 3.7 oz. .....170
   minced (*Dr. Praeger's*), 1.7 oz. ...........................................90
   mini (*Van de Kamp's*), 13 pcs., 3.3 oz. ...............................250
strips, breaded (*Mrs. Paul's*), 4 pcs., 4 oz. .............................310
strips, breaded (*Van de Kamp's*), 4 pcs., 4 oz. .......................270
tenders, battered (*Mrs. Paul's/Van de Kamp's*), 4 pcs., 4 oz. ...290
**Fish sandwich,** frozen (*Hormel Quick Meal*), 5.2-oz. pc. ........420

**Fish seasoning and coating mix:**
(*Hodgson Mill Don's Chuck Wagon* Seafood Bake and Fry),
  ¼ cup .............................................................................95
(*Shake 'n Bake* Original Recipe), ¼ pkt. .....................................80
**Flan,** see "Pudding and pie filling mix"
**Flatfish,** meat only:
raw, 4 oz. ...................................................................103
baked, broiled, or microwaved, 4 oz. .........................................133
**Flax seed** (*Arrowhead Mills*), 3 tbsp.....................................140
**Flounder,** fresh, see "Flatfish"
**Flounder entree,** frozen:
(*Mrs. Paul's* Premium), 2.8-oz. fillet .......................................170
au gratin (*Oven Poppers*), 5-oz. pc. .........................................220
fillet, breaded (*Van de Kamp's* Premium), 4-oz. pc..........................230
stuffed w/broccoli and cheese (*Oven Poppers*), 5-oz. pc. ........150
stuffed w/crab (*Oven Poppers*), 5-oz. pc. ...................................250
stuffed w/garlic, shrimp, almonds (*Oven Poppers*), 5-oz. pc. ..250
**Flour,** see "Wheat flour" and other specific listings
**Focaccia, stuffed,** ½ piece, 5.5 oz.:
cheese and peppers (*Cedarlane* Italian) .....................................410
spinach and cheese (*Cedarlane* Mediterranean) .......................410
tomato and cheese (*Cedarlane* Roma) ......................................380
**Fondue,** ¼ cup:
(*Swiss Knight*) .............................................................120
(*SwissRose*) .................................................................140
**Frankfurter,** 1 link, except as noted:
(*Ball Park* Fat Free), 1.75 .................................................50
(*Ball Park* Lite), 1.75 oz. .................................................100
(*Ball Park Singles*), 1.6 oz. ...............................................150
(*Johnsonville*), 1.73 oz. ...................................................150
(*Louis Rich* Original 50% Less Fat), 1.6 oz................................90
(*Nathan's*), 2 oz. ..........................................................160
(*Oscar Mayer* Weiners), 1.6 oz. ..........................................140
(*Russer Light* Deli), 2 oz. .................................................120
beef (*Ball Park*), 2 oz. ....................................................180
beef (*Ball Park* Fat Free), 1.75 oz. ........................................55
beef (*Ball Park* Kosher), 1.5 oz. ..........................................140
beef (*Ball Park Singles*), 1.6 oz. ..........................................150
beef (*Boar's Head* Natural Casing), 2 oz....................................160

beef (*Boar's Head* Skinless), 1.6 oz.............................................120
beef (*Healthy Choice*), 1.75 oz. ...................................................80
beef (*Hebrew National*), 1.7 oz. .................................................150
beef (*Hebrew National* 97% Fat Free), 1.7 oz.............................45
beef (*Hebrew National* Cocktail), 5 links, 2 oz.........................180
beef (*Hebrew National* Dinner), 4 oz. .......................................350
beef (*Hebrew National* Family Pack/Party Pack), 2 oz. ............180
beef (*Hebrew National* Reduced Fat), 1.7 oz. ...........................120
beef (*Hormel* Fat Free Franks), 1.76 oz. .....................................45
beef (*Hormel* Natural Casing Franks), 2.4 oz. ...........................210
beef (*Hormel Light and Lean* Fat Free Hot Dogs), 1.76 oz.........45
beef (*Russer* Natural Casing), 2.6 oz. .......................................220
beef (*Wrangler's* Franks), 2 oz...................................................170
cheese (*Ball Park Singles*), 1.6 oz..............................................150
cheese or smoked (*Wrangler's* Franks), 2 oz. ...........................170
chicken (*Empire* Kosher), 2 oz. .................................................100
cocktail (*Johnsonville* Little Weiners), 6 links, 2 oz. .................180
pork and beef (*Boar's Head* Skinless), 2 oz. .............................150
smokie style (*Oscar Mayer Big & Juicy* Hot Dogs), 2.7 oz.......210
turkey (*Empire* Kosher), 2 oz......................................................90
turkey, pork and beef (*Healthy Choice* Low Fat), 1.75 oz............70
**Frankfurter sandwich,** frozen:
(*Ball Park Fun Franks*), 2 pcs. ...................................................340
(*Hebrew National* Franks in a Blanket), 5 pcs. ..........................290
beef (*Ball Park Fun Franks*), 2 pcs. ...........................................340
corn dog (*Ball Park Fun Franks*), 1 pc.......................................220
corn dog (*Hormel Quick Meal*), 3.5-oz. pc. ..............................272
corn dog (*Michelina's* Corn Dawgs), 5.5 oz. .............................320
corn dog, beef (*Ball Park Fun Franks*), 1 pc..............................220
corn dog, mini (*Hormel Quick Meal*), 10 pcs., 5.6 oz. .............490
**French beans,** mature, boiled, 1 cup......................................228
**French toast,** frozen:
(*Aunt Jemima* Homestyle/Cinnamon), 2 pcs. ............................240
sticks, cinnamon (*Aunt Jemima*), 4 pcs.....................................350
**Frosting,** ready-to-spread, 2 tbsp.:
all flavors:
    (*Betty Crocker* Soft Whipped)..............................................100
    except chocolate flavors (*Betty Crocker Creamy Deluxe*)....140

**Frosting, all flavors (*cont.*)**
    except chocolate and French vanilla (*Pillsbury Creamy*
      *Supreme*) ........................................................................150
all chocolate flavors:
    (*Pillsbury Creamy Supreme*) ...............................................140
    (*Sweet Rewards*) ...............................................................120
    w/frosting toppers (*Betty Crocker Creamy Deluxe*) .............140
    w/out frosting toppers (*Betty Crocker Creamy Deluxe*).......130
vanilla (*Sweet Rewards*) ...............................................................130
vanilla, French (*Pillsbury Creamy Supreme*) .............................160
**Frosting mix,** fudge or white (*"Jiffy"*), ⅙ pkg.........................150
**Fruit,** see specific listings
**Fruit, mixed, candied** (*S&W* Glacé Cake Mix), 2 tbsp..............90
**Fruit, mixed, canned** (see also "Fruit cocktail"), ½ cup,
    except as noted:
(*Del Monte Very Cherry*) ...............................................................90
in juice (*Del Monte Fruit Naturals* Chunky) .................................60
in juice (*Del Monte Fruit Cup Fruit Naturals*), 4 oz. ....................50
in juice (*Dole FruitBowls*), 4.6-oz. bowl .....................................90
in juice, chunky (*Libby's*) ..............................................................60
in juice, tropical (*Del Monte*) .......................................................60
in juice, tropical (*Dole FruitBowls*), 4-oz. bowl ..........................60
in light syrup, tropical (*Dole*)........................................................80
in light syrup, tropical, w/passion fruit juice (*Del Monte*)...........80
in lightly sweetened fruit juice (*S&W* Natural Style) ...................80
in extra light syrup (*Del Monte Lite* Chunky) ..............................60
in extra light syrup (*Del Monte Fruit Cup Lite*), 4 oz. .................50
in light syrup:
    (*Del Monte* Fruity Combo Fruit to Go Cup), 4 oz. .................70
    California (*Del Monte Orchard Select*) ................................80
    cherry flavored (*Del Monte Fruitrageous* Crazy Cherry
      Cup), 4 oz. .......................................................................90
    cherry flavored, natural (*Del Monte Fruit Pleasures*).............90
in heavy syrup (*Del Monte* Chunky) ...........................................100
in heavy syrup (*Del Monte Fruit Cup*), 4 oz.................................80
**Fruit, mixed, frozen** (*Birds Eye*), ½ cup .................................90
**Fruit bar,** frozen, 1 bar:
banana, creamy, chocolate dipped (*Edy's/Dreyer's*) .................210
banana cream (*Frozfruit*)............................................................150

cantaloupe (*Frozfruit*)................................................................60
cherry or watermelon (*Frozfruit*).............................................70
coconut cream (*Frozfruit*)......................................................200
lemon or pineapple (*Frozfruit*)................................................80
lemonade, lime, or strawberry (*Edy's/Dreyer's*).....................80
lime, strawberry, or tropical (*Frozfruit*)..................................90
mango (*Frozfruit*)....................................................................110
peach (*Edy's*)...........................................................................90
peach (*Frozfruit Smoothie. Yum Give Peach a Chance*)...........80
strawberry, creamy, chocolate dipped (*Edy's/Dreyer's*)........170
strawberry banana (*Frozfruit Smoothie. Yum Yumtonic*)........130
strawberry cream (*Frozfruit*)..................................................150
tangerine or wild berry (*Edy's*)................................................80
**Fruit cocktail,** canned, ½ cup:
in juice (*Del Monte Fruit Naturals*).........................................60
in lightly sweetened juice (*S&W* Natural Style).......................80
in extra light syrup (*Del Monte Lite*).......................................60
in heavy syrup (*Del Monte*)....................................................100
in heavy syrup (*S&W*)...............................................................90
**Fruit drink blend:**
(*Capri Sun All Natural Mountain Cooler*), 6.76 fl. oz. .............90
(*Capri Sun All Natural Pacific/Surfer Cooler*), 6.76 fl. oz........100
punch (*Capri Sun All Natural*), 6.76 fl. oz................................100
punch (*Hawaiian Punch Juicy Red*), 8 fl. oz............................120
punch (*Minute Maid*), 8 fl. oz.................................................110
tropical punch (*Kool-Aid Bursts*), 6.76 fl. oz..........................100
tropical punch (*Kool-Aid Splash*), 8 fl. oz. ............................120
**Fruit drink mix,** 8 fl. oz.*:
tropical punch (*Kool-Aid*) ......................................................100
tropical punch (*Kool-Aid* Sugar Sweetened)............................60
**Fruit glaze** (*Smucker's* Pie Glaze), 2 oz. ............................80
**Fruit juice,** see specific fruit listings
**Fruit juice blend,** 8 fl. oz.:
punch (*Florida's Natural Growers' Pride*)...............................130
punch (*Minute Maid* Calcium).................................................120
punch (*Mott's*)........................................................................120
punch (*Tropicana*)..................................................................130
punch, tropical (*Juicy Juice*)..................................................130
tropical (*Dole*)........................................................................110

**Fruit-nut mix,** see "Trail mix"
**Fruit pectin/protector** (*Sure-Jell*), ¼ tsp. .....................................5
**Fruit snack,** all fruits:
(*Fruit by the Foot*), .74-oz. roll.....................................80
(*Fruit Gushers*), .9-oz. pouch .....................................90
**Fruit spread,** all fruits:
(*Dickenson's*), 2 tbsp..................................................50
(*Polaner*), 1 tbsp. .........................................................40
(*Smucker's* Simply 100% Fruit), 1 tbsp. .....................50
**Fudge topping,** see "Chocolate topping"
**Fusilli dishes, mix:**
w/creamy pesto sauce (*Knorr*), ⅔ cup.....................250
and red beans (*Marrakesh Express*), 1 cup* ............210

# G

**Gai choy,** see "Cabbage, mustard"
**Gai lan,** see "Kale, Chinese"
**Garbanzo beans:**
dry (*Arrowhead Mills*), ¼ cup .................................................170
dry (*Frieda's*), ⅓ cup, 3 oz. ..................................................150
**Garbanzo beans, canned:**
(*Allens/East Texas Fair*), ½ cup .............................................120
(*Progresso*), ½ cup .............................................................120
(*Shari Ann's* Organic), ½ cup ................................................110
**Garlic,** fresh, raw:
1-oz. clove or 1 tsp. minced......................................................4
elephant (*Frieda's*), 1 tbsp. ....................................................5
**Garlic, pickled** (*Christopher Ranch*), 3 pcs. ...........................5
**Garlic paste** (*Italia In Tavola*), 1 tbsp.................................60
**Garlic powder:**
1 tsp...................................................................................10
w/parsley (*Lawry's*), ¼ tsp. ....................................................0
**Garlic relish,** in jars (*Patak's*), 1 tbsp.................................40
**Garlic salt** (*Lawry's*), ¼ tsp. ...............................................0
**Garlic spread:**
(*Lawry's* Ready-to-Spread), 1 tbsp. ........................................100
concentrate (*Lawry's*), 2 tsp. .................................................50
**Gefilte fish,** sweet, 1.5-oz. pc. ..............................................35
**Gelatin,** unflavored, dry (*Knox*), 1 pkt. ..................................25
**Gelatin dessert,** ready-to-eat, all flavors:
(*Jell-O*), 3.5-oz. cont. ...........................................................70
(*Jell-O* Sugar Free), 3¼-oz. cont. ...........................................10
(*Kozy Shack*), 4-oz. cont.......................................................100
(*Kozy Shack* Sugar Free), 4-oz. cont. .......................................10
(*Kraft Handi-Snacks*), 3.5-oz. cont. .........................................80
**Gelatin dessert mix,** ½ cup*, except as noted:
all flavors (*Jell-O*)................................................................80
all flavors (*Royal*) ................................................................70

**Gelatin dessert mix** (*cont.*)

all flavors (*Jell-O* Sugar Free)......................................................10
all flavors (*Royal* Sugar Free) ..................................................10
strawberry (*Jell-O 1–2–3*), ⅔ cup*...........................................130

**Gelato,** see "Ice cream"

**Gemelli dish, mix,** and white beans (*Marrakesh*
*Express*), 1 cup*....................................................................220

**Ginger,** root, fresh, raw:

(*Frieda's*), 1 tbsp........................................................................0
sliced, 1" diam., ¼ cup ................................................................17

**Ginger, crushed** (*Budarim*), 1 tsp..............................................2

**Ginger, crystallized** (*Frieda's*), 9 pcs., 1.1 oz. .......................100

**Ginger, ground,** 1 tsp.....................................................................6

**Ginger, pickled** (*Budarim* Sushi), 1 oz. .....................................20

**Ginger, Thai/Siamese** (*Frieda's* Galanga), ⅔ cup, 3 oz. ...........60

**Ginkgo nut,** shelled:

raw, 1 oz. ....................................................................................52
dried, 1 oz....................................................................................99

**Ginkgo nut, canned,** 1 cup........................................................172

**Glaze,** see "Fruit glaze" and "Ham glaze"

**Gluten,** see "Wheat gluten"

**Goa bean,** see "Winged bean"

**Goat,** roasted, 4 oz........................................................................162

**Golden nugget squash** (*Frieda's*), ¾ cup, 3 oz.........................30

**Goose,** domesticated, roasted:

meat w/skin, 4 oz......................................................................346
meat w/skin, chopped or diced, 1 cup .....................................427
meat only, 4 oz. .........................................................................270

**Goose fat,** 1 tbsp. .......................................................................115

**Gooseberry,** fresh, raw, 1 cup......................................................66

**Gooseberry, canned,** in light syrup, 1 cup..................................184

**Gourd strips,** see "Kanpyo"

**Grains,** see specific listings

**Granola,** see "Cereal, ready-to-eat"

**Granola and cereal bar,** 1 bar, except as noted:

(*Chex Milk 'n Cereal*), 1.4 oz...................................................160
(*Cinnamon Toast Crunch Milk 'n Cereal*), 1.6-oz. bar..............180
(*Honey Nut Cheerios Milk 'n Cereal*), 1.4 oz............................160
(*Kellogg's Rice Krispies Treats* Squares Original), .8 oz. ...........90

(*Kudos M&M's*), .8 oz. ...............................................................90
(*Kudos Snickers*), .8 oz. ...........................................................100
all varieties:
   (*Barbara's* Nature's Choice Cereal Fat Free), 1.3 oz. ............110
   (*Barbara's* Nature's Choice Granola), .75 oz. ......................80
   (*Golden Grahams Treats*), .8-oz. bar...............................90
   (*Nabisco* Fruit 'n Grain), 1.3 oz...................................130
   (*Nature Valley* Crunchy), 2 bars, 1.5 oz.............................180
   (*Nutri-Grain/Nutri-Grain Twists*), 1.3 oz............................140
apple or cinnamon raisin (*Nutri-Grain Fruit-full Squares*),
   1.7 oz. ...........................................................180
banana (*Nutri-Grain Fruit-full Squares*), 1.7 oz. ....................190
blueberry (*Little Debbie* Blastin'), 1.4 oz. ..........................140
chocolate chunk s'mores (*Golden Grahams Treats* King
   Size), 1.6-oz. bar.................................................190
chocolate fudge or chocolate chip (*Kudos*), 1 oz.....................120
cocoa (*Kellogg's Rice Krispies Treats* Squares), .8 oz. ............100
peanut butter (*Kudos*), 1 oz.........................................130
peanut butter, chocolate (*Kellogg's Rice Krispies Treats*
   Squares), .8 oz....................................................110
raspberry (*Little Debbie* Rappin'), 1.4 oz. ..........................140
**Grape,** fresh, raw:
(*Dole*), 1½ cups......................................................85
American type (slipskin), 10 medium ...................................15
American type (slipskin), 1 cup.......................................62
European type (adherent skin), w/seeds, 1 cup ........................109
European type (adherent skin), seedless, 10 medium ...................36
European type (adherent skin), seedless, 1 cup .......................114
**Grape, canned,** seedless, in heavy syrup, ½ cup .....................94
**Grape drink,** 8 fl. oz., except as noted:
(*Mott's*) ...........................................................130
(*Capri Sun All Natural*), 6.76 fl. oz................................100
(*Kool-Aid Bursts*), 6.76 fl. oz......................................100
white (*Welch's*) ....................................................140
white grape peach (*Welch's*) ........................................150
punch (*Hawaiian Punch Grape Geyser*) ................................120
punch (*Minute Maid*) ................................................120
punch, berry (*Kool-Aid Splash*)......................................120

**Grape drink mix,** 8 fl. oz.*:
(*Kool-Aid/Kool-Aid Grape Berry Splash*) ..................................100
(*Kool-Aid* Sugar Sweetened) ..............................................60
(*Kool-Aid Grape Berry Splash* Sugar Sweetened) ......................70
**Grape juice,** 8 fl. oz.:
(*Welch's*)....................................................................170
white (*Juicy Juice*) ......................................................150
**Grape juice blend:**
(*Mott's*), 8 fl. oz. ........................................................120
(*Mott's*), 11.5 fl. oz. ....................................................170
**Grape leaf,** in jars (*Krinos*), 1 leaf ......................................5
**Grape leaf, stuffed** (*Cedarlane*), 1 pc. ..............................50
**Grapefruit,** fresh:
(*Dole*), ½ grapefruit......................................................50
(*Ocean Spray*), ½ medium, 5.5 oz.....................................60
pink or red:
    ½ large, 4½" diam. ............................................53
    large sections w/juice, 1 cup..................................74
    medium sections w/juice, 1 cup ..............................69
    California or Arizona, ½ medium, 3¾" diam. ..............46
    California or Arizona, medium sections w/juice, 1 cup .........85
    Florida, ½ medium, 3¾" diam. ..............................37
    Florida, medium sections w/juice, 1 cup ..................69
white:
    ½ large, 4½" diameter ........................................53
    large sections w/juice, 1 cup..................................74
    medium sections w/juice, 1 cup ..............................76
    California, ½ medium, 3¾" diam. ............................44
    California, medium sections w/juice, 1 cup ..............85
    Florida, ½ medium, 3¾" diam. ..............................38
    Florida, sections w/juice, 1 cup..............................74
**Grapefruit, canned or chilled:**
in juice, 1 cup ..............................................................92
in light syrup, 1 cup......................................................152
**Grapefruit drink,** plain or blend (*Ocean Spray* Ruby Red),
    8 fl. oz. ............................................................130
**Grapefruit juice,** 8 fl. oz.:
(*Mott's*) ....................................................................110
(*Tropicana Pure Premium* Ruby Red w/Calcium) ..................90

fresh, raw, pink or white.................................................96
golden or ruby red (*Tropicana Pure Premium*)...........90
pink (*Ocean Spray* 100%)...........................................110
pink, blend (*Minute Maid*)...........................................125
ruby red (*Florida's Natural* Original/Calcium)............100
ruby red (*Florida's Natural Honey Sweetened Ruby Red*)........120
ruby red (*Tropicana Pure Premium* Grovestand/Calcium)..........90
white (*Ocean Spray* 100%).........................................100
frozen*, unsweetened.................................................101
**Grapefruit juice blend,** ruby red (*Minute Maid*), 8 fl. oz........110
**Gravy,** see specific listings
**Great northern bean,** mature:
dry, 1 cup................................................................620
boiled, 1 cup............................................................209
**Great northern bean,** canned, ½ cup:
(*Allens*)...................................................................100
w/sausage (*Trappey's*)..............................................100
**Green bean,** fresh:
raw (*Frieda's* Snap Beans), ⅔ cup, 3 oz....................25
raw, 10 beans, 4" long...............................................17
raw, 1 cup.................................................................34
boiled, drained, 1 cup.................................................44
**Green bean, canned,** ½ cup, except as noted:
(*Allens* Shell Out)......................................................30
(*Green Giant Kitchen Sliced*).......................................20
(*Walnut Acres Organic Farms*)....................................20
all styles, except Italian (*Del Monte*)...........................20
cut (*Allens/Sunshine/Alma/Crest Top/Stone Mountain*)..........30
cut (*Greene's Farm* Organic).......................................20
cut or French style (*Green Giant*)................................20
sliced, French style (*Greene's Farm* Organic)...............26
French style (*Allens*).................................................25
Italian (*Allens/Sunshine*)...........................................35
Italian (*Del Monte*)...................................................30
and potatoes (*Allens/Sunshine*).................................35
**Green bean, frozen:**
whole (*Birds Eye*), 21 pcs..........................................20
whole (*Birds Eye* Stir Fry), 1¾ cup............................100
whole (*Freshlike* Select), 1 cup..................................25

**Green bean, frozen** (*cont.*)

whole (*Freshlike* Stir Fry), 1 cup .................................................30
whole (*Seabrook Farms*), ¾ cup .............................................25
cut (*Birds Eye/Birds Eye* Deluxe), ½ cup ..........................25
cut (*Freshlike*), ⅔ cup.............................................................25
French (*Freshlike*), 1 cup........................................................25
Italian (*Birds Eye* Deluxe), ½ cup ........................................35
**Green bean, pickled,** spicy (*Hogue Farms*), ¼ cup .................15
**Green bean combination, frozen,** and baby carrots (*Birds Eye*
    Baby Blend), 1 cup...............................................................30
**Green bean dish,** frozen:
and almonds (*Green Giant*), ⅔ cup ......................................50
casserole (*Green Giant*), ⅔ cup.............................................90
casserole, mushroom (*Stouffer's*), ½ cup .........................130
and spaetzle (*Birds Eye* Bavarian Style), 1 cup ..............150
**Green peas,** see "Peas, green"
**Greens,** mixed (see also specific listings), canned
    (*Allens/Sunshine*), ½ cup .................................................30
**Green pepper,** see "Pepper, sweet"
**Grilling sauce** (see also specific listings):
(*San-J*), 2 tbsp. .......................................................................40
chipotle (*Chi-Chi's*), 2 tbsp...................................................60
ginger sesame, sweet (*House of Tsang* Hibachi), 1 tbsp. ..........40
salsa (*Chi-Chi's*), 2 tbsp........................................................50
Tex-Mex (*Chi-Chi's*), 2 tbsp..................................................35
**Grits,** see "Corn grits"
**Groundcherry,** fresh, raw, trimmed, 1 cup .............................74
**Grouper,** meat only:
raw, 4 oz. ................................................................................104
baked, broiled, or microwaved, 4 oz. ...................................134
**Guacamole,** refrigerated (*Calavo*), 2 tbsp. ...........................50
**Guacamole seasoning mix:**
(*El Torito*), 1/12 pkg..................................................................5
(*Lawry's* Spices & Seasonings), ½ tsp. .................................5
**Guava,** fresh, raw:
(*Frieda's*), 3-oz. fruit ..............................................................45
common, trimmed, 1 pc., 3.2 oz. ...........................................46
strawberry, trimmed, 1 pc., .2 oz. ...........................................4

**Guava nectar** (*Libby's*), 11.5-fl.-oz. can ...................................210
**Guava sauce,** cooked, 1 cup ......................................................86
**Guinea hen,** raw, 4 oz.:
meat w/skin ...............................................................................179
meat only ..................................................................................125

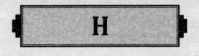

# H

**FOOD AND MEASURE**                                    **CALORIES**

**Haddock,** meat only:
raw, 4 oz. .................................................................99
baked, broiled, or microwaved, 4 oz. ........................127
smoked, 4 oz. ...........................................................132
**Haddock entree,** frozen:
fillet (*Mrs. Paul's* Premium), 4.2-oz. pc. ..................240
fillet, battered (*Van de Kamp's*), 2 pcs., 3.7 oz. .......220
fillet, breaded (*Van de Kamp's* Premium), 4-oz. pc...230
w/shrimp, crab, vegetables (*Oven Poppers*), 5-oz. pc. .............210
**Hake,** see "Whiting"
**Halibut, Atlantic or Pacific,** meat only:
raw, 4 oz. ...............................................................125
baked, broiled, or microwaved, 4 oz. ........................159
**Halibut, Greenland,** meat only:
raw, 4 oz. ...............................................................211
baked, broiled, or microwaved, 4 oz. ........................271
**Halibut entree,** frozen, fillet, battered (*Van de Kamp's*),
    3 pcs., 4 oz. ........................................................220
**Halvah,** 2 oz.:
chocolate covered (*Joyva*)........................................380
chocolate vanilla marble (*Joyva*) ..............................390
**Ham,** fresh, roasted:
whole leg, lean w/fat, 4 oz. .......................................310
whole leg, lean w/fat, chopped or diced, 1 cup..........369
whole leg, lean only, 4 oz. ........................................239
whole leg, lean only, chopped or diced, 1 cup ...........285
rump half, lean w/fat, 4 oz. .......................................286
rump half, lean w/fat, chopped or diced, 1 cup ..........340
rump half, lean only, 4 oz. ........................................234
rump half, lean only, chopped or diced, 1 cup............278
shank half, lean w/fat, 4 oz. ......................................328
shank half, lean w/fat, chopped or diced, 1 cup .........390
shank half, lean only, 4 oz. .......................................244

shank half, lean only, chopped or diced, 1 cup...........................290
**Ham, cured,** 4 oz., except as noted:
whole leg, lean w/fat, unheated.................................................279
whole leg, lean w/fat, roasted..................................................276
whole leg, lean w/fat, roasted, chopped or diced, 1 cup...........341
whole leg, lean only, unheated.................................................167
whole leg, lean only, roasted ...................................................178
whole leg, lean only, roasted, chopped or diced, 1 cup............219
boneless (11% fat), unheated ..................................................206
boneless (11% fat), roasted.....................................................202
boneless (11% fat), roasted, chopped or diced, 1 cup..............249
boneless, extra lean (5% fat), unheated...................................149
boneless, extra lean (5% fat), roasted .....................................164
**Ham, refrigerated or canned,** 3 oz., except as noted:
(*Black Label* Canned)...............................................................109
(*Black Label* Cured) ................................................................111
(*Cure 81*).................................................................................100
(*Curemaster*).............................................................................80
(*Hormel Always Tender*), 4 oz..................................................270
(*Jones Dairy Farm* Country Club)..............................................100
(*Jones Dairy Farm* Fully Cooked) .............................................240
(*Jones Dairy Farm* Homestead).................................................140
(*Jones Dairy Farm* Old Fashioned).............................................220
(*Jones Dairy Farm* Semi-Boneless)............................................180
(*Jones Dairy Farm* Skinless Shankless/Spiral Sliced)...............160
(*Spiral Cure 81* Half)................................................................150
all varieties (*Jones Dairy Farm Country Carved*) .....................100
steak (*Jones Dairy Farm Lean Choice*) ....................................100
**Ham entree,** frozen, honey smoked steak, w/macaroni and
    cheese (*Marie Callender's*), 14 oz.......................................490
**Ham-cheese loaf** (*Russer*), 2 oz.............................................120
**Ham-cheese pocket,** frozen, 1 piece:
(*Deli Stuffs*), 4.5 oz................................................................340
(*Hot Pockets*), 4.5 oz..............................................................310
(*Toaster Breaks* Melts), 2.2 oz................................................180
w/broccoli (*Healthy Choice Meals To Go*), 6.1 oz. .................320
cheddar (*Lean Pockets*), 4.5 oz...............................................280
cheddar (*Croissant Pockets*), 4.5 oz. ......................................330

**Ham glaze,** in jars:
(*Boar's Head* Brown Sugar and Spice), 2 tbsp......................120
(*Reese's*), 1 tbsp.....................................................................20
**Ham lunch meat,** 2 oz., except as noted:
(*Boar's Head* Cappy/Deluxe) ..................................................60
(*Boar's Head* Deluxe Low Sodium)...........................................50
(*Boar's Head* Sweet Slice) ...................................................100
(*Carl Buddig*), 2.5-oz. pkg. ..................................................120
(*Carl Buddig*), 9 slices, 2 oz. ................................................85
(*Hansel 'n Gretel* 95% Fat Free) .............................................50
(*Healthy Deli* Deluxe/Less Sodium)..........................................60
(*Healthy Deli* Old Tyme Taverne 97% Fat Free) ..........................60
(*Hormel Light and Lean* 97 Half), 3 slices, 3 oz............................90
(*Hormel Light and Lean* 97 Sliced), 1-oz. slice .............................25
(*Jones Dairy Farm* Lean Choice), 2 slices, 1.6 oz..........................50
(*Oscar Mayer* Lower Sodium), 3 slices, 2.2 oz. ...........................70
(*Sara Lee* Bavarian) ............................................................70
(*Sara Lee* Homestyle/Smokehouse) .........................................60
(*Sara Lee* Old Fashioned Cooked) ...........................................50
all varieties (*Russer* Fat Free) .................................................45
baked (*Healthy Choice*), 1-oz. slice .........................................30
baked (*Russer*)...................................................................70
baked or cooked (*Healthy Choice Deli Thin Deli Traditions*),
   6 slices, 1.9 oz. ..............................................................60
Black Forest (*Russer*)...........................................................60
Black Forest, smoked (*Healthy Deli* 97% Fat Free) .....................60
boiled (*Sara Lee* Deli), 2 slices, 1.6 oz. ...................................40
brown sugar (*Carl Buddig* Premium Lean Slices), 2.5-oz. pkg...90
brown sugar or maple cured (*Sara Lee*) .....................................70
cappicola (*Healthy Deli* Cappi).................................................60
chopped (*Black Label*) .........................................................140
cinnamon apple (*Healthy Deli* Grove)........................................70
cooked (*Healthy Choice*)........................................................60
cooked (*Hormel* Deli)............................................................60
cooked (*Russer/Russer Light*) .................................................60
glazed (*Healthy Deli* Deluxe)..................................................60
honey (*Carl Buddig*), 2.5-oz. pkg. ..........................................120
honey (*Carl Budding*), 9 slices, 2 oz. .......................................90
honey (*Healthy Choice*), 1-oz. slice .........................................30

honey (*Healthy Deli* Honey Valley) .............................................60
honey (*Oscar Mayer*), 3 slices, 2.2 oz. ......................................70
honey baked (*Carl Buddig* Premium Lean), 2.5-oz. pkg. ............80
honey baked or brown sugar cured (*Healthy Choice Hearty
    Deli Flavor*), 3 slices, 2 oz. ....................................................70
honey cured (*Russer*) ..............................................................60
honey cured (*Sara Lee*), 2 oz. ...................................................60
honey maple cured (*Russer*) .....................................................70
honey mustard or honey and maple (*Healthy Choice*)................60
honey, honey maple, or honey mustard (*Healthy Choice Deli
    Thin Savory Selections*), 6 slices, 1.9 oz. ..............................60
hot (*Healthy Deli* Rodeo) ...........................................................60
hot (*Russer*)...........................................................................70
jalapeno (*Healthy Deli*) ............................................................60
maple (*Boar's Head Maple Glazed Honey Coat*) .........................60
maple (*Healthy Deli* Vermont) ...................................................60
maple (*Russer* Canadian) .........................................................70
maple, flame seared (*Healthy Deli*) ...........................................70
pepper (*Boar's Head*) ...............................................................60
pepper (*Healthy Deli* Tutta Bella) ..............................................70
rosemary and sun-dried tomato (*Boar's Head*) ..........................60
smoked (*Healthy Choice*) ..........................................................60
smoked (*Oscar Mayer*), 3 slices, 2.2 oz. ...................................60
smoked (*Russer* Old Fashioned) ................................................70
smoked, double (*Healthy Deli* 97% Fat Free) ..............................60
spiced (*Boar's Head*) ..............................................................120
spiced (*Russer*)......................................................................160
Virginia (*Healthy Choice*) ..........................................................60
Virginia (*Healthy Deli* Less Sodium)...........................................70
Virginia (*Healthy Deli*)..............................................................60
Virginia (*Sara Lee* Deli), 3 slices, 1.8 oz....................................60
Virginia, baked (*Healthy Deli*)....................................................70
Virginia, pineapple topped or smoked (*Boar's Head*) .................60
Virginia, smoked (*Russer*) ........................................................70
**Ham patty,** plain or w/cheese (*Hormel*), 2-oz. patty ...............180
**Ham salad spread,** 1 tbsp. .......................................................32
**Ham spread,** deviled:
(*Hormel Cure 81*), 4 tbsp. .......................................................150
(*Underwood*), ¼ cup...............................................................140

**Hamburger,** see "Beef sandwich/pocket" and specific restaurant
   listings
**"Hamburger," vegetarian,** see "Burger, vegetarian"
**Hamburger entree mix** (*Hamburger Helper*), 1 cup\*, except
   as noted:

| | |
|---|---|
| bacon cheeseburger | 380 |
| barbecue beef | 320 |
| beef pasta | 270 |
| beef Romanoff | 300 |
| beef stew | 260 |
| beef taco | 280 |
| beef teriyaki | 290 |
| cheddar 'n bacon | 330 |
| cheddar and broccoli | 350 |
| cheddar cheese melt | 310 |
| cheddar spirals, reduced sodium | 300 |
| cheeseburger macaroni | 360 |
| cheese, nacho | 320 |
| cheese, 3 | 340 |
| cheesy Italian | 320 |
| cheesy shells | 330 |
| chili macaroni | 290 |
| fettuccine Alfredo | 300 |
| hash browns, cheesy | 400 |
| Italian, zesty | 300 |
| Italian herb, reduced sodium | 270 |
| Italian Parmesan | 300 |
| lasagne | 270 |
| lasagne, 4 cheese | 330 |
| meat loaf, 1/6 loaf\* | 270 |
| Mexican, zesty | 280 |
| mushroom and wild rice | 310 |
| Philly cheesesteak or double cheese pizza | 330 |
| pizza, pepperoni | 310 |
| pizza pasta, w/cheese topping | 280 |
| potatoes au gratin or rice Oriental | 280 |
| potatoes Stroganoff | 260 |
| ravioli, w/white cheese topping | 310 |
| Salisbury or spaghetti | 270 |

Southwestern beef.................................................................300
Stroganoff...............................................................................320
**Hard sauce,** brandied (*Crosse & Blackwell*), 2 tbsp. ..............180
**Hazelnut,** see "Filbert"
**Head cheese** (*Boar's Head*), 2 oz.........................................90
**Heart,** beef, simmered, 4 oz..................................................199
**Hearts of palm,** see "Palm"
**Herb seasoning blend** (*Lawry's* Pinch of Herbs), ¼ tsp. ............0
**Herbs,** see specific listings
**Herring,** fresh, meat only:
Atlantic, raw, 4 oz. ..............................................................179
Atlantic, baked, broiled, or microwaved, 4 oz. ......................230
Atlantic, kippered, 4 oz. .......................................................246
Pacific, raw, 4 oz..................................................................221
Pacific, baked, broiled, or microwaved, 4 oz..........................284
**Herring, canned,** see "Sardine"
**Herring, in jars:**
(*Vita* Party Snacks), 2 oz., about ¼ cup................................120
in sour cream (*Nathan's*), ¼ cup..........................................120
in sour cream (*Vita*), ¼ cup .................................................120
in wine sauce (*Skansen* Tidbits), 5 pcs., 1.9 oz. .....................85
**Herring salad,** chopped (*Blue Ridge Farms*), ⅓ cup ...............150
**Hickory nut,** dried, shelled, ¼ cup.........................................197
**Hoisin sauce,** 1 tbsp...............................................................36
**Hollandaise sauce,** in jars:
(*Concord Foods*), 1½ tbsp. .....................................................60
(*Melba*), 2 tbsp. ......................................................................90
(*Reese's*), 2 tbsp. ....................................................................90
**Hollandaise sauce mix,** dry (*Knorr* Classic), 1 tsp...................10
**Hominy,** canned:
golden (*Allens/Uncle William*), ½ cup....................................120
white (*Allens/Uncle William*), ½ cup .....................................100
white, 1 cup..........................................................................119
yellow, 1 cup.........................................................................205
**Hominy grits,** dry, see "Corn grits"
**Honey** (*Aunt Sue's/Grandma's/Sue Bee*), 1 tbsp........................60
**Honey bun,** see "Bun, sweet"
**Honey loaf,** see "Lunch meat"
**Honey mustard,** see "Mustard blends"

**Honey spread,** flavored, all flavors (*Bigelow*), 1 tbsp................70
**Honeydew melon,** fresh, raw:
(*Dole*), ¹⁄₁₀ melon......................................................50
cubed, 1 cup, approx. 20 pcs.......................................56
**Horned melon** (*Frieda's*), 3.5-oz. fruit..............................25
**Horseradish,** fresh:
(*Frieda's*), 1 tbsp.......................................................0
leafy tips, raw, chopped, 1 cup.....................................13
leafy tips, boiled, drained, chopped, 1 cup....................25
**Horseradish, prepared,** 1 tsp.:
(*Boar's Head*) ...........................................................5
(*Kraft/Kraft* Cream Style) ...........................................0
all styles (*Gold's*) ......................................................0
**Horseradish sauce** (*Kraft*), 1 tsp..................................20
**Horseradish tree:**
leafy tips, boiled, drained, chopped, 1 cup....................25
pods, boiled, drained, sliced, 1 cup..............................43
**Hot dog,** see "Frankfurter"
**Hot fudge sauce,** see "Chocolate topping"
**Hot sauce** (see also "Pepper sauce" and specific listings):
(*Frank's RedHot*), 1 tsp..............................................0
(*Lottie's* Traditional Barbados Recipe), 1 tsp................5
(*Tabasco*), 1 tsp.......................................................0
(*Taco Bell Home Originals* Restaurant Hot Sauce) 1 tsp........<1
all varieties (*Trappey's*), 1 tsp....................................0
chili, sweet, green or red (*A Taste of Thai*), 1 tsp.........10
garlic (*A Taste of Thai*), 1 tsp....................................10
habanero (*Shotgun Willie's/Sontava* XXX), 2 tbsp.........10
jalapeno (*Buffalo*), 1 tbsp..........................................0
**Hubbard squash,** fresh:
raw (*Frieda's*), ¾ cup, 3 oz.......................................35
raw, cubed, 1 cup ....................................................46
baked, cubed, 1 cup ...............................................103
**Hummus,** 2 tbsp., except as noted:
(*Cedar's*) ................................................................50
basil and sun-dried tomato (*Cedarlane*) ......................50
garlic, roasted (*Cedarlane*), 1 oz...............................45
red pepper, roasted (*Cedarlane*) ...............................50
**Hunter gravy mix** (*Knorr* Gravy Classics), ¼ cup*...........25

**Hyacinth bean,** immature:
raw, 1 cup ...................................................................................37
boiled, drained, 1 cup ................................................................44
**Hyacinth bean, mature:**
dry, 1 cup .................................................................................722
boiled, 1 cup ............................................................................227

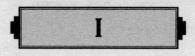

**FOOD AND MEASURE**                                       **CALORIES**

**Ice:**

| | |
|---|---:|
| all flavors, except lemon (*Luigi's*), 6 fl. oz. | 110 |
| cherry (*Mama Tish's*), 4 fl. oz. | 90 |
| lemon (*Luigi's*), 6 fl. oz. | 100 |
| lemon or strawberry (*Mama Tish's*), 4 fl. oz. | 80 |
| lemon or strawberry (*Mama Tish's* No Sugar), 4 fl. oz. | 70 |
| orange (*Frozfruit Orange Overload*), 4.5 oz. | 100 |
| raspberry (*Mama Tish's*), 4 fl. oz. | 100 |
| raspberry, blue (*Frozfruit Blue Raspberry Blast Chill*), 4.5 oz. | 100 |
| strawberry (*Frozfruit Verry Strawberry Chill*), 4.5 oz. | 90 |
| watermelon (*Frozfruit Wild Watermelon Wipeout*), 4.5 oz. | 80 |

**Ice bar** (see also "Fruit bar" and "Sherbet bar"), 1 bar:

| | |
|---|---:|
| all flavors (*Popsicle* 12 Pack), 1.75 fl. oz. | 45 |
| all flavors (*Popsicle* Sugar Free 12 Pack), 1.75 fl. oz. | 15 |

**Ice cream,** ½ cup, except as noted:

| | |
|---|---:|
| all flavors, except hazelnut (*Häagen-Dazs* Gelato) | 240 |
| almond, toasted (*Dreyer's* Grand) | 150 |
| apple pie à la mode (*Edy's/Dreyer's Homemade*) | 140 |
| *Banana Boogie* (*Edy's/Dreyer's Dreamery*) | 290 |
| (*Ben & Jerry's Blondes are a Swirl's Best Friend* Low Fat) | 200 |
| (*Ben & Jerry's Bovinity Divinity*) | 290 |
| (*Ben & Jerry's Cherry Garcia*) | 260 |
| (*Ben & Jerry's Chubby Hubby*) | 350 |
| (*Ben & Jerry's Chunky Monkey*) | 310 |
| (*Ben & Jerry's Dilbert's World Totally Nuts*) | 310 |
| (*Ben & Jerry's Phish Food*) | 300 |
| (*Ben & Jerry's 2-Twisted Everything But The . . .*) | 320 |
| (*Ben & Jerry's 2-Twisted From Russia With Buzz*) | 280 |
| (*Ben & Jerry's 2-Twisted Half Baked*) | 290 |
| (*Ben & Jerry's 2-Twisted Jerry's Jubilee*) | 260 |
| (*Ben & Jerry's 2-Twisted Monkey Wrench*) | 310 |
| (*Ben & Jerry's 2-Twisted Pulp Addiction*) | 240 |

(*Ben & Jerry's 2-Twisted Urban Jumble*) ....................310
(*Ben & Jerry's Wavy Gravy*)....................................340
berry pie (*Edy's/Dreyer's Dreamery* Blue Ribbon)....................260
blueberry cobbler (*Edy's/Dreyer's* Fat Free/No Sugar) ...........100
blueberry hill (*Healthy Choice* Old Fashioned) ...............120
brownies à la mode (*Edy's/Dreyer's Homemade*) ...............150
butter almond (*Breyers* All Natural)........................160
butter pecan (*Breyers* All Natural)........................170
butter pecan (*Breyers* Homemade) .........................170
butter pecan (*Edy's/Dreyer's* Grand).......................160
butter pecan (*Edy's/Dreyer's* No Sugar) ....................110
butter pecan (*Edy's/Dreyer's* Grand Light) .................120
butter pecan (*Edy's/Dreyer's Homemade* Old Fashioned) .........160
butter pecan (*Häagen-Dazs*)................................310
butter pecan crunch (*Healthy Choice*).......................120
butterscotch blondie (*Healthy Choice* Old Fashioned) ......140
cappuccino chocolate chunk (*Healthy Choice*) ..............120
*Cappuccino Commotion* (*Häagen-Dazs*) ....................310
cappuccino mocha chunk (*Healthy Choice*)...................120
caramel (*Ben & Jerry's Triple Caramel Chunk*)..............290
caramel (*Edy's Grand Light* Crazy for Caramel) ............120
caramel crème (*Edy's/Dreyer's Dreamery*) .................260
caramel peanut brittle (*Edy's/Dreyer's Homemade*) .........160
caramel pecan, creme (*Häagen-Dazs*)........................320
caramel praline crunch (*Breyers* All Natural) .............170
caramel praline crunch (*Edy's/Dreyer's* Fat Free) .........110
caramel toffee bar (*Edy's/Dreyer's Dreamery* Heaven).........270
*Cashew Praline Parfait* (*Edy's/Dreyer's Dreamery*).........260
cherry, black, vanilla (*Edy's/Dreyer's* Grand) ............160
cherry chocolate chip (*Edy's* Grand) ......................150
cherry chocolate chunk (*Healthy Choice*)...................110
cherry vanilla (*Breyers* All Natural)......................140
cherry vanilla (*Häagen-Dazs*)..............................240
cherry vanilla (*Healthy Choice* Old Fashioned).............120
chocolate (*Breyers* All Natural)...........................160
chocolate (*Edy's/Dreyer's* Grand) .........................150
chocolate (*Häagen-Dazs*)...................................270
chocolate (*Starbucks Double Shot*) ........................290
chocolate, dark, Belgian (*Godiva*).........................280

**Ice cream** (*cont.*)

chocolate, French (*Breyers* All Natural Light)............................150
chocolate, triple (*Edy's/Dreyer's* No Sugar)............................100
chocolate chip (*Breyers* All Natural).....................................170
chocolate chip (*Edy's/Dreyer's* Grand) .................................170
chocolate chip (*Edy's/Dreyer's* Homemade Cookie Jar)............170
chocolate chunk, double (*Edy's/Dreyer's* Homemade)...............170
chocolate chocolate chip (*Häagen-Dazs*) ...............................300
chocolate chocolate chunk (*Healthy Choice*) ..........................120
chocolate chocolate fudge (*Häagen-Dazs*) .............................290
chocolate cream pie (*Edy's/Dreyer's* Homemade).....................170
chocolate fudge (*Edy's/Dreyer's* Fat Free) .............................110
chocolate fudge (*Edy's/Dreyer's* Fat Free/No Sugar) ................100
chocolate fudge mousse (*Edy's/Dreyer's* Grand Light) .............120
chocolate fudge, double (*Breyers* Homemade) .........................170
chocolate fudge brownie (*Ben & Jerry's*)................................280
chocolate fudge brownie (*Häagen-Dazs* Low Fat).....................190
chocolate fudge mousse (*Edy's* Grand)...................................160
chocolate fudge sundae (*Edy's* Grand)...................................170
chocolate hazelnut truffle (*Godiva*).......................................340
chocolate peanut butter chunk (*Edy's* Fat Free) ......................120
chocolate peanut butter chunk (*Edy's/Dreyer's* Dreamery) ......310
chocolate rainbow (*Breyers* Rainbow)....................................140
*Chocolate Raspberry Escape* (*Edy's/Dreyer's* Grand Light)......120
chocolate raspberry truffle (*Godiva*)......................................280
*Chocolate Swirl* (*Edy's/Dreyer's* Dreamery Galactic) ................280
chocolate Swiss almond (*Häagen-Dazs*) .................................300
chocolate truffle (*Edy's/Dreyer's* Dreamery Explosion) .............280
cinnamon (*Häagen-Dazs*) ...................................................270
coconut cream pie (*Ben & Jerry's* Low Fat)..............................160
coconut cream pie (*Healthy Choice*) .....................................120
coffee (*Ben & Jerry's* Coffee Hazelnut Swirl)............................280
coffee (*Breyers* All Natural).................................................140
coffee (*Edy's/Dreyer's* Grand) .............................................140
coffee (*Edy's/Dreyer's* Dreamery Cuppa Joe)...........................230
coffee (*Häagen-Dazs*) .......................................................270
coffee (*Starbucks* Italian Roast) ..........................................230
coffee (*Starbucks* Java Chip)...............................................250
coffee (*Starbucks* Latte Low Fat)..........................................170

coffee almond fudge (*Starbucks*) ................................250
coffee w/cinnamon and coffee cake (*Starbucks Coffee
   Cake Streusel*) ................................................250
coffee crunch (*Ben & Jerry's Heath Bar*) ...................310
coffee fudge (*Edy's* Fat Free/No Sugar) ....................100
coffee fudge (*Häagen-Dazs* Low Fat) .........................170
coffee mocha (*Starbucks Frappuccino* Low Fat) ........170
coffee mocha chip (*Häagen-Dazs*) .............................290
coffee mousse crunch (*Edy's/Dreyer's Grand Light*) ...120
coffee toffee (*Starbucks* Java Toffee) ........................260
cookie chunk (*Edy's/Dreyer's* Fat Free) .....................110
cookie creme de mint (*Healthy Choice*) .....................130
cookie dough (*Dreyer's* Grand) ..................................180
cookie dough (*Edy's* Grand) .......................................170
cookie dough (*Edy's/Dreyer's Grand Light*) ...............120
cookie dough, chocolate chip (*Ben & Jerry's*) ............300
cookie dough, chocolate chip (*Breyers* All Natural) ....180
cookie dough chip (*Häagen-Dazs*) .............................310
cookies and cream (*Häagen-Dazs*) ............................270
cookies and cream (*Edy's/Dreyer's* Grand) ................160
cookies and cream (*Edy's/Dreyer's Grand Light*) .......120
cookies and cream (*Healthy Choice*) .........................120
cookies and fudge (*Häagen-Dazs* Low Fat) ...............180
cookies in cream (*Breyers* All Natural) ......................170
(*Dreyer's* Grand Gold Miner's Dream) .......................170
(*Dreyer's* Grand Ice Cream Sandwich) ......................150
dulce de leche (*Breyers* All Natural) ..........................160
dulce de leche (*Edy's/Dreyer's* Grand) ......................150
dulce de leche (*Häagen-Dazs*) ..................................290
dulce de leche (*Starbucks*) ........................................260
(*Edy's* Grand Ice Cream Sandwich) ...........................160
(*Edy's/Dreyer's* Chips 'N Swirls No Sugar) ................100
(*Edy's/Dreyer's* Dreamery Sticky Bun) .......................270
(*Edy's/Dreyer's* Dreamery Hit Chilly Chili) .................260
(*Edy's/Dreyer's* Dreamery Grandma's Cookie Jar*) ....270
(*Edy's/Dreyer's* Dreamery Nuts About Malt*) .............280
(*Edy's/Dreyer's* Grand Light French Silk*) .................120
eggnog and cream (*Edy's/Dreyer's* Homemade) .........140
espresso chip (*Edy's* Grand) ......................................150

**Ice cream (*cont.*)**

espresso fudge chip (*Edy's/Dreyer's* Grand Light) ....................120
fruit rainbow (*Breyers Rainbow*) ................................................140
fudge brownie (*Breyers* Homemade) .......................................180
fudge brownie (*Healthy Choice*) ..............................................120
fudge brownie, double (*Edy's/Dreyer's* Grand) .........................170
fudge brownie, double (*Edy's* No Sugar) .................................100
fudge chunk (*Ben & Jerry's* New York Super) .........................320
hazelnut (*Häagen-Dazs* Gelato) ..............................................260
macadamia brittle (*Häagen-Dazs*) ...........................................300
mango (*Häagen-Dazs*) ..............................................................250
mint (*Ben & Jerry's 2-Twisted Entangled Mints*) .....................290
mint (*Edy's/Dreyer's Dreamery*) ...............................................280
mint chocolate chip (*Breyers* All Natural) ................................170
mint chocolate chip (*Breyers* All Natural Light) .......................140
mint chocolate chip (*Edy's/Dreyer's* Grand) .............................170
mint chocolate chip (*Edy's/Dreyer's* Grand Light) ....................120
mint chocolate chip (*Healthy Choice*) ......................................120
mint chocolate cookie (*Ben & Jerry's*) ....................................280
mint chip (*Häagen-Dazs*) ..........................................................290
mocha almond fudge (*Dreyer's* Grand) ....................................160
*Mocha Latte* (*Ben & Jerry's* Low Fat) .....................................150
Neapolitan (*Breyers* Homemade) .............................................150
Neapolitan (*Dreyer's* Grand) ....................................................140
*Nutty Waffle Cone* (*Ben & Jerry's*) ........................................310
orange and cream (*Ben & Jerry's*) ...........................................230
peach (*Breyers* All Natural) ......................................................130
peach (*Edy's/Dreyer's Dreamery* Harvest) ...............................220
peach (*Edy's/Dreyer's* Homemade Grovestand) ......................110
peanut butter (*Edy's/Dreyer's All About PB* No Sugar) ............130
peanut butter cup (*Ben & Jerry's*) ...........................................380
peanut butter cup (*Edy's/Dreyer's* Grand Light) ......................130
peanut butter cup (*Healthy Choice*) .........................................110
pecan caramel truffle (*Godiva*) ................................................320
pecan pie (*Ben & Jerry's Southern Pecan Pie*) ........................290
pineapple coconut (*Häagen-Dazs*) ...........................................230
pistachio (*Häagen-Dazs*) ..........................................................280
*Pistachio Pistachio* (*Ben & Jerry's*) .......................................240
pralines and caramel (*Breyers* All Natural Light) .....................140

praline and caramel or caramel cluster (*Healthy Choice*) .........130
pralines and cream (*Häagen-Dazs*) ...........................................290
raspberry, black (*Edy's/Dreyer's Dreamery* Avalanche).............250
raspberry marble chunk (*Edy's/Dreyer's* Fat Free) ....................110
raspberry truffle, wild (*Healthy Choice*)....................................120
raspberry vanilla swirl (*Edy's/Dreyer's* Fat Free/No Sugar) ........90
rocky road (*Breyers* All Natural)................................................180
rocky road (*Breyers* All Natural Light).......................................140
rocky road (*Edy's/Dreyer's* Grand)............................................170
rocky road (*Edy's/Dreyer's* Grand Light) ...................................120
rocky road (*Healthy Choice*) .....................................................140
rum raisin (*Häagen-Dazs*)..........................................................270
s'mores (*Ben & Jerry's* Low Fat)...............................................190
strawberries and cream (*Edy's/Dreyer's Homemade*) ...............120
strawberry (*Breyers* All Natural)................................................130
strawberry (*Breyers* All Natural Light).......................................110
strawberry (*Edy's* No Sugar Added) ............................................90
strawberry (*Edy's/Dreyer's* Grand) ............................................130
strawberry (*Häagen-Dazs*).........................................................250
strawberry (*Healthy Choice* Old Fashioned) ..............................110
strawberry cheesecake (*Edy's/Dreyer's Dreamery* New York)...250
turtle fudge cake (*Healthy Choice*) ...........................................130
vanilla (*Ben & Jerry's World's Best*) ..........................................250
vanilla (*Breyers* All Natural) ......................................................150
vanilla (*Breyers* All Natural Calcium Rich).................................130
vanilla (*Breyers* Fat Free/No Sugar)............................................90
vanilla (*Breyers* Homemade) .....................................................140
vanilla (*Breyers* Light)................................................................130
vanilla (*Edy's* Grand).................................................................140
vanilla (*Edy's/Dreyer's* Fat Free)...............................................100
vanilla (*Edy's/Dreyer's* Fat Free/No Sugar) .................................90
vanilla (*Edy's/Dreyer's Dreamery*) .............................................260
vanilla (*Edy's/Dreyer's* Grand Light) .........................................100
vanilla (*Edy's/Dreyer's Homemade* All Natural) .........................130
vanilla (*Häagen-Dazs*)...............................................................270
vanilla (*Häagen-Dazs* Low Fat) .................................................170
vanilla (*Healthy Choice*).............................................................100
vanilla bean (*Edy's/Dreyer's* Grand)..........................................140
vanilla bean (*Healthy Choice*)....................................................110

**Ice cream (*cont.*)**

vanilla or French vanilla (*Breyers* All Natural Light) .................120
vanilla, French (*Breyers* All Natural) ........................................160
vanilla, French (*Edy's/Dreyer's* Grand) ....................................160
vanilla almond (*Starbucks* Bliss) .............................................260
vanilla caramel (*Häagen-Dazs* Low Fat) ..................................180
vanilla and caramel (*Edy's* Fat Free/No Sugar) ........................100
vanilla caramel fudge (*Ben & Jerry's*) ......................................300
vanilla cashew crunch (*Starbucks*) ...........................................280
vanilla and chocolate (*Breyers Take Two* All Natural) .................150
vanilla chocolate swirl (*Edy's/Dreyer's* Fat Free/No Sugar) .......100
vanilla/chocolate (*Edy's* Grand) ...............................................150
vanilla/chocolate/strawberry (*Breyers* All Natural) .....................140
vanilla/chocolate/strawberry (*Breyers* All Natural Light) ...........120
vanilla/chocolate/strawberry (*Breyers* No Sugar) ........................90
vanilla/chocolate/strawberry (*Edy's* Grand) ..............................140
vanilla custard (*Edy's* Homemade) ..........................................140
vanilla fudge twirl (*Breyers* All Natural) ...................................150
vanilla fudge twirl (*Breyers* No Sugar) .....................................100
vanilla and orange sherbet (*Breyers Take Two* All Natural) .......130
vanilla Swiss almond (*Häagen-Dazs*) .......................................310
white chocolate macadamia toffee (*Godiva*) .............................250
white chocolate raspberry (*Godiva*) ..........................................250
**"Ice cream," nondairy,** ½ cup:
all flavors, soft-serve (*Tofutti*) .................................................190
all flavors, soft-serve (*Tofutti* Lite) ............................................90
*Better Pecan* (*Tofutti* Premium) .............................................220
chocolate or vanilla fudge sundae (*Tofutti* Fat/Sugar Free) .........80
chocolate cookie crunch (*Tofutti* Premium) ..............................210
chocolate supreme (*Tofutti* Premium) .......................................180
chocolate or vanilla fudge (*Tofutti* Low Fat Supreme) ...............120
coffee marshmallow (*Tofutti* Low Fat Supreme) ........................100
honey vanilla chamomile (*Tofutti*) .............................................190
peach mango or strawberry banana (*Tofutti* Low Fat
    Supreme) .............................................................................100
vanilla (*Tofutti/Tofutti* Premium) ...............................................190
*Vanilla Almond Bark* (*Tofutti* Premium) ..................................210
vanilla strawberry sundae (*Tofutti* Fat/Sugar Free) .....................80
wildberry supreme (*Tofutti* Premium) ........................................190

**Ice cream bar,** (see also "Sherbet bar"), 1 bar:
almond, toasted (*Good Humor*), 3 fl. oz. ................................180
(*Ben & Jerry's Phish Stick*) ................................................290
(*Ben & Jerry's Totally Nuts*) .............................................370
candy bar swirl (*Klondike*), 5 fl. oz. ....................................320
cappuccino (*Klondike*), 5 fl. oz. ..........................................290
caramel or strawberry, soft (*Breyers* Magnum), 3.75 fl. oz. .....360
caramel crunch (*Klondike*), 5 fl. oz. .....................................290
chocolate:
    chocolate coated (*Klondike*), 5 fl. oz. ...........................280
    dark chocolate coated (*Häagen-Dazs*) ...........................350
    milk chocolate and almond coated (*Häagen-Dazs*) .............310
    eclair (*Good Humor* 6 Pack), 3 fl. oz. .............................150
    peanut butter, milk chocolate coated (*Häagen-Dazs*
      Swirl*) ......................................................................320
coconut pineapple, w/white chocolate (*Häagen-Dazs*
    Tropical) ....................................................................340
coffee, w/milk chocolate (*Häagen-Dazs* Almond Crunch) .........360
coffee caramel (*Starbucks Frappuccino*) ...............................110
coffee mocha (*Starbucks Frappuccino*) .................................120
cookie dough (*Ben & Jerry's*) ..............................................410
cookies and cream (*Good Humor*), 3 fl. oz. ...........................190
cookies and cream crunch (*Häagen-Dazs*) ............................380
dulce de leche, w/caramel (*Häagen-Dazs*) ............................300
mint, w/dark chocolate (*Häagen-Dazs*) .................................340
Neapolitan (*Klondike*), 5 fl. oz. ...........................................280
peanut butter (*Good Humor Reese's Peanut Butter Cup*),
    3 fl. oz. ....................................................................250
*S'mores Pop* (*Ben & Jerry's*) ..............................................330
strawberry, w/white chocolate (*Häagen-Dazs*) ......................270
strawberry shortcake (*Good Humor*), 3 fl. oz. ........................180
strawberry swirl (*Klondike*), 5 fl. oz. ....................................290
vanilla (*Ben & Jerry's*) .......................................................330
vanilla, almond coated (*Klondike*), 5 fl. oz. ...........................310
vanilla, chocolate coated:
    (*Klondike* Original), 5 fl. oz. .........................................290
    (*Klondike* Reduced Fat/No Sugar Added), 4 fl. oz. ...........190
    (*Popsicle* Rainbow Choc Pops 8 Pack), 2.1 fl. oz. ...........130
    w/crisps (*Klondike* Krispy Krunch), 5 fl. oz. ...................300

**Ice cream bar, vanilla, chocolate coated** (*cont.*)
    w/sprinkles (*Popsicle* Sprinklers 8 Pack), 2.1 fl. oz. ...........130
    dark chocolate (*Klondike*), 5 fl. oz. ......................................290
    dark or milk chocolate (*Good Humor*), 3 fl. oz. .................180
    milk chocolate (*Häagen-Dazs*) ..............................................330
    milk chocolate and almonds (*Häagen-Dazs*) ......................370
  vanilla, sherbet coated, see "Sherbet bar"
  vanilla, toffee coated (*Klondike Heath*), 5 fl. oz. ......................300
  *Vanilla Heath Bar Crunch* (*Ben & Jerry's*) ...............................320
**"Ice cream" bar, nondairy,** 1 bar:
  chocolate fudge (*Tofutti* Treats).................................................30
  fruit, mixed, chocolate coated (*Tofutti Frutti*) ........................120
  fudge (*Tofutti Teddy Fudge*).......................................................70
  peanut butter (*Tofutti* Monkey Bars) ......................................220
  strawberry, crumb coated (*Tofutti* Crumb Cakes) ..................220
  vanilla fudge, crumb coated (*Tofutti* Crumb Cakes)................230
**Ice cream cake:**
  cappuccino or vanilla (*Viennetta*), 2.4-oz. pc. .......................190
  chocolate, triple (*Viennetta*), 2.4-oz. pc...............................180
  vanilla (*Viennetta* Snack Size), 2.6-oz. pc. ............................240
**Ice cream cone or cup,** plain, unfilled, 1 pc.:
  bowl, waffle (*Keebler*) ..............................................................50
  cone, all varieties, except fudge-dipped (*Keebler*).....................50
  cone, chocolate (*Oreo*) .............................................................50
  cone, fudge-dipped (*Keebler*) ...................................................35
  cone, sugar (*Comet*) .................................................................60
  cup (*Comet/Comet* Rainbow) ....................................................20
  cup (*Keebler*)............................................................................15
**Ice cream cone, filled:**
  (*Good Humor*), 4 fl. oz.............................................................270
  caramel or fudge (*Klondike Big Bear*), 5 fl. oz.......................370
  vanilla (*Klondike Big Bear*), 5 fl. oz.......................................350
**Ice cream sandwich,** 1 pc.:
  (*Good Humor*), 3 fl. oz.............................................................160
  (*Klondike Choco Taco*), 3.9 fl. oz............................................240
  Neapolitan or vanilla (*Klondike Big Bear*), 4.23 fl. oz. ..............200
  chocolate chip cookie (*Klondike Big Bear*), 4 fl. oz. ................290
**Italian sausage,** see "Sausage"
**Italian seasoning,** zesty (*Wyler's Shakers*), 1 tsp......................10

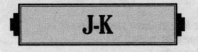

**J-K**

| FOOD AND MEASURE | CALORIES |
|---|---|

*Jack in the Box,* 1 serving:

breakfast items:

| | |
|---|---|
| bacon | 20 |
| biscuit | 190 |
| biscuit, sausage | 380 |
| biscuit, sausage, egg, cheese | 510 |
| *Breakfast Jack* | 280 |
| *Country Crock Spread* | 25 |
| croissant, sausage | 660 |
| croissant, supreme | 530 |
| French toast sticks | 420 |
| grape jelly | 40 |
| hash browns | 170 |
| sandwich, sourdough | 450 |
| sandwich, ultimate | 600 |
| syrup | 130 |

burgers:

| | |
|---|---|
| cheeseburger, bacon | 760 |
| cheeseburger, double | 440 |
| cheeseburger, ultimate | 950 |
| cheeseburger, ultimate, w/bacon | 1050 |
| hamburger | 250 |
| hamburger w/cheese | 300 |
| *Jumbo Jack* | 550 |
| *Jumbo Jack* w/cheese | 640 |
| *Sourdough Jack* | 690 |

chicken and more:

| | |
|---|---|
| cheese, American, 1 slice | 40 |
| Swiss style, 1 slice | 45 |
| chicken breast, 5 pcs. | 360 |

chicken sandwiches:

| | |
|---|---|
| chicken | 400 |
| chicken fajita pita | 320 |

**Jack in the Box, chicken sandwiches (cont.)**

| | |
|---|---|
| chicken fillet, grilled | 480 |
| chicken supreme | 830 |
| *Jack's Spicy Chicken* | 570 |

dipping sauces, 1 oz.:

| | |
|---|---|
| barbecue | 45 |
| buttermilk house | 130 |
| *Frank's Red Hot Buffalo* | 10 |
| sweet and sour | 45 |
| fish and chips | 780 |
| taco | 170 |
| taco, monster | 270 |
| salsa | 10 |
| tartar sauce | 210 |

salads and teriyaki bowl:

| | |
|---|---|
| chicken teriyaki bowl | 670 |
| garden chicken salad | 200 |
| side salad | 50 |
| croutons | 50 |
| soy sauce | 5 |

salad dressings:

| | |
|---|---|
| blue cheese | 210 |
| buttermilk house | 290 |
| Italian, low calorie | 25 |
| Thousand Island | 250 |

sides:

| | |
|---|---|
| fries, curly, chili cheese | 650 |
| fries, curly, seasoned | 410 |
| fries, jumbo | 430 |
| fries, regular | 350 |
| fries, super scoop | 610 |
| onion rings | 450 |
| potato wedges, bacon cheddar | 750 |

snacks:

| | |
|---|---|
| egg roll, 1 pc. | 150 |
| egg rolls, 3 pcs. | 440 |
| jalapenos, stuffed, 3 pcs. | 230 |
| jalapenos, stuffed, 7 pcs. | 530 |
| sour cream | 60 |

shakes, regular:

cappuccino or chocolate ............................................630

*Oreo* cookie ...............................................................740

strawberry .................................................................640

vanilla .......................................................................610

desserts:

apple turnover, hot ...................................................340

cheesecake ...............................................................320

double fudge cake .....................................................300

**Jackfruit,** fresh, sliced (*Frieda's*), 1 cup .....................120

**Jackfruit, dried** (*Frieda's*), ½ cup ...............................80

**Jalapeno,** see "Pepper, jalapeno"

**Jalapeno dip** (see also "Cheese dip"), (*Kraft*), 2 tbsp. .............60

**Jam and preserves** (see also "Fruit spread" and "Jelly, fruit"):

all fruits (*Smucker's* Preserves/Marmalade), 1 tbsp. ............50

all fruits (*Smucker's* Low Sugar Preserves), 1 tbsp. ............25

all fruits (*Smucker's* Light Sugar Free Preserves), 1 tbsp. .........10

amaretto, peach and pecan (*D. L. Jardine's*), 2 tbsp. .................80

marmalade, orange (*Crosse & Blackwell*), 1 tbsp. .....................60

**Java plum,** fresh, raw, 3 pcs., .3 oz. .................................5

**Jelly, fruit,** 1 tbsp.:

all fruits (*Smucker's* Jelly), 1 tbsp. ...............................50

apple (*Musselman's*) ...................................................50

apple, mint flavored (*Crosse & Blackwell*) ...........................50

guava or red currant (*Crosse & Blackwell*) ...........................60

**Jelly, hot,** 2 tbsp., except as noted:

hot pepper (*Reese's*), 1 tbsp. .......................................50

jalapeno (*D. L. Jardine's* Hotter) ....................................80

jalapeno cherry or habanero (*D. L. Jardine's* Hotter) .................70

**Jerusalem artichoke,** fresh, raw, sliced, 1 cup .............114

**Jicama,** see "Yam bean tuber"

**Jute,** potherb, boiled, drained, 1 cup .............................32

**Kabocha squash** (*Frieda's*), ¾ cup, 3 oz. ...................30

**Kale,** fresh:

raw, chopped, 1 cup ....................................................34

boiled, drained, chopped, 1 cup .....................................36

**Kale, canned** (*Allens/Sunshine*), ½ cup ........................30

**Kale, Chinese,** fresh (*Frieda's* Gai Lan), 1 cup, 3 oz. ...............15

**Kale, frozen,** chopped, boiled, drained, ½ cup .....................20

**Kale, Scotch,** fresh, boiled, drained, chopped, 1 cup ................36
**Kamut flour** (*Arrowhead Mills*), ¼ cup ...................................110
**Kanpyo,** .2-oz. strip .................................................................16
**Kasha,** see "Buckwheat groats"
**Kelp,** see "Seaweed"
**Ketchup,** 1 tbsp., except as noted:
(*Del Monte*) ..............................................................................15
(*Heinz*) .....................................................................................15
(*Muir Glen* Organic/*Muir Glen* Organic Spicy) .....................15
*KFC,* 1 serving:
chicken, *Original Recipe:*
    breast .................................................................................400
    drumstick or whole wing ....................................................140
    thigh ..................................................................................250
chicken, *Extra Crispy:*
    breast .................................................................................470
    drumstick ...........................................................................195
    thigh ..................................................................................380
    wing, whole ........................................................................220
chicken, Hot & Spicy:
    breast .................................................................................505
    drumstick ...........................................................................175
    thigh ..................................................................................355
    wing, whole ........................................................................210
chicken, popcorn, large ...........................................................620
chicken, popcorn, small ...........................................................362
chicken pot pie, chunky ...........................................................770
chicken sandwiches, w/sauce:
    honey BBQ flavored ..........................................................310
    *Original Recipe* ...............................................................450
    *Tender Roast* ..................................................................350
    *Triple Crunch* ..................................................................490
    *Triple Crunch Zinger* .......................................................550
chicken wings, honey BBQ, 6 pcs. ...........................................607
chicken wings, *Hot Wings,* 6 pcs. ...........................................471
*Crispy Strips, Colonel's,* 3 pcs. ..............................................300
*Crispy Strips,* spicy, 3 pcs. .....................................................335
salads and sides:
    BBQ baked beans ..............................................................190

biscuit, 2-oz. pc.................................................................180
coleslaw.........................................................................232
corn on the cob...............................................................150
macaroni and cheese .......................................................180
mashed potatoes w/gravy .................................................120
potato salad...................................................................230
potato wedges................................................................280
desserts, 1 slice or serving:
  chocolate chip cake, double................................................320
  *Colonel's* pie, apple .........................................................310
  *Colonel's* pie, pecan ........................................................490
  *Colonel's* pie, strawberry creme.........................................280
  *Little Bucket* parfait, chocolate cream...............................290
  *Little Bucket* parfait, fudge brownie ..................................280
  *Little Bucket* parfait, lemon creme .....................................410
  strawberry shortcake .....................................................200
**Kidney,** beef, simmered, 4 oz. ...........................................163
**Kidney bean,** mature:
dry (*Arrowhead Mills*), ¼ cup .............................................160
boiled, 1 cup ..................................................................225
**Kidney bean, canned,** ½ cup:
red (*S&W*)....................................................................100
red or dark red (*Progresso*) ...............................................110
red, Creole style (*Trappey's*)..............................................100
red, dark (*Allens/Trappey's*)..............................................130
red, light (*Allens/Trappey's*)..............................................120
red, light, w/jalapeno (*Trappey's*) ......................................110
red, light, New Orleans style, w/bacon (*Trappey's*) ..............110
red, w/chili gravy (*Trappey's*) ............................................110
white (*Progresso* Cannellini) ...............................................100
white, whole (*Shari Ann's* Organic Cannellini) .........................100
**Kidney beans, sprouted,** raw, 1 cup .....................................53
**Kielbasa** (see also "Polish sausage"):
(*Boar's Head*), 2 oz. .......................................................120
pork and beef, .9-oz. slice .................................................81
turkey (*Louis Rich* Polska), 2 oz. .........................................90
turkey, pork, and beef (*Healthy Choice*), 2 oz. ..........................70
**Kielbasa loaf** (*Russer*), 2 oz. ..........................................120
**Kim chee** (*Frieda's*), ¼ cup, 2 oz. .....................................15

**Kiwi,** fresh:
| | |
|---|---|
| (*Dole*), 2 medium | 90 |
| (*Frieda's*), 5 oz. | 90 |
| w/out skin, 1 large, 3.2 oz. | 56 |
| w/out skin, 1 medium, 2.7 oz. | 46 |
| baby or gold (*Frieda's*), 5 oz. | 90 |

**Kiwi drink blend,** 8 fl. oz., except as noted:
| | |
|---|---|
| lime (*Kool-Aid Bursts Kickin'*), 6.76 fl. oz. | 100 |
| strawberry (*Kool-Aid Splash*) | 110 |
| mix*, lime (*Kool-Aid Kickin'*) | 100 |
| mix*, lime (*Kool-Aid Kickin' Sugar Sweetened*) | 60 |

**Knockwurst:**
| | |
|---|---|
| (*Ball Park*), 4 oz. | 360 |
| (*Karl Ehmer*), 4-oz. link | 250 |
| beef (*Ball Park*), 4 oz. | 340 |
| beef (*Boar's Head*), 4-oz. link | 310 |
| beef (*Hebrew National*), 3 oz. | 260 |

**Kohlrabi,** fresh:
| | |
|---|---|
| raw (*Frieda's*), ⅔ cup, 3 oz. | 25 |
| raw, .6-oz. slice | 4 |
| boiled, drained, sliced, 1 cup | 48 |

**Kumquat,** fresh, raw, trimmed, ⅔-oz. pc. ..................12
**Kumquat, pickled,** sweet, in jars (*Haddon House*), 1 pc. ..........10

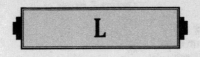

**L**

**FOOD AND MEASURE** **CALORIES**

**Lamb,** domestic, choice, meat only, trimmed to ¼" fat,
   4 oz., except as noted:

cubed, leg and shoulder, braised, lean only ...............................253
cubed, leg and shoulder, broiled, lean only................................211
ground, raw .................................................................................320
ground, broiled ...........................................................................321
ground, broiled, 1 cup ................................................................328
foreshank, braised, lean w/fat.....................................................276
foreshank, braised, lean only......................................................212
leg, whole, roasted, lean w/fat....................................................293
leg, whole, roasted, lean w/fat, 1 slice, 3 diam. by ¼"...............73
leg, whole, roasted, lean only .....................................................217
leg, whole, roasted, lean only, 1 slice, 3" diam. by ¼" ...............54
leg, shank half, roasted, lean w/fat.............................................255
leg, shank half, roasted, lean only ..............................................204
leg, sirloin half, roasted, lean w/fat ............................................331
leg, sirloin half, roasted, lean only..............................................231
loin, roasted, lean w/fat ..............................................................350
loin, roasted, lean only ...............................................................229
loin chop, broiled, lean w/fat ......................................................358
loin chop, broiled, lean w/fat, 2.25 oz. (4.2 oz. raw w/bone)....201
loin chop, broiled, lean only, 1.6 oz. (4.2 oz. raw w/bone) .......100
rib, broiled, lean w/fat.................................................................409
rib, broiled, lean only ..................................................................266
rib, roasted, lean w/fat.................................................................407
rib, roasted, lean only ..................................................................263
shoulder, whole, braised, lean w/fat ...........................................390
shoulder, whole, braised, lean only .............................................321
shoulder, whole, broiled, lean w/fat.............................................315
shoulder, whole, broiled, lean only ..............................................238
shoulder, whole, roasted, lean w/fat............................................313
shoulder, whole, roasted, lean only .............................................231

**Lamb (*cont.*)**
shoulder arm chop:
    braised, lean w/fat................................................................393
    braised, lean only ..............................................................316
    broiled, lean w/fat..............................................................319
    broiled, lean w/fat, 3.2 oz. (5.6 oz. raw w/bone) ................261
    broiled, lean only................................................................227
    broiled, lean only, 2.6 oz. (5.6 oz. raw w/bone)..................148
    roasted, lean w/fat.............................................................316
    roasted, lean only ..............................................................218
shoulder, blade, braised, lean w/fat.......................................391
shoulder, blade, braised, lean only ........................................327
shoulder, blade, broiled, lean w/fat........................................315
shoulder, blade, broiled, lean only.........................................239
shoulder, blade, roasted, lean w/fat.......................................319
shoulder, blade, roasted, lean only ........................................237
**Lamb's-quarter,** boiled, drained, chopped, 1 cup......................58
**Lasagna entree, canned or packaged:**
(*Dinty Moore American Classics*), 1 bowl................................340
w/meat sauce (*Hormel* Microcup Meals), 1 cup .....................210
**Lasagna entree, frozen,** 1 pkg., except as noted:
Alfredo (*Michelina's*), 9 oz.....................................................360
bake (*Stouffer's*), 11.5 oz......................................................450
cheese (*Amy's*), 10.25 oz......................................................310
cheese (*Lean Cuisine Everyday Favorites* Classic), 11.5 oz......290
cheese, casserole (*Lean Cuisine Everyday Favorites*), 10 oz. ...270
cheese, chicken scallopini (*Lean Cuisine Cafe Classics*),
    10 oz. ...............................................................................270
cheese, extra (*Marie Callender's*), 15 oz...............................590
cheese, 5 (*Lean Cuisine Everyday Favorites*), 8 oz. ................210
cheese, 5 (*Lean Cuisine* Family Style Favorites), 1 cup ...........210
cheese, 5 (*Stouffer's*), 10.75 oz............................................360
cheese, 4 (*Michelina's*), 8 oz. ...............................................290
chicken (*Lean Cuisine Everyday Favorites*), 10 oz. .................280
chicken (*Lean Cuisine* Family Style Favorites), 1 cup .............200
chicken (*Stouffer's*), 1 cup ...................................................310
w/meat sauce (*Banquet*), 9.5 oz. ..........................................260
w/meat sauce (*Banquet* Family), 1 cup .................................270
w/meat sauce (*Freezer Queen*), 10 oz. .................................290

w/meat sauce (*Lean Cuisine Everyday Favorites*), 10.5 oz. ......300
w/meat sauce (*Marie Callender's*), 15 oz. ...............................630
w/meat sauce (*Marie Callender's* Family), 1 cup.......................350
w/meat sauce (*Michelina's*), 8 oz. ........................................240
w/meat sauce (*Michelina's*), 9 oz. ........................................290
w/meat sauce (*Michelina's*), 10 oz. ......................................400
w/meat sauce (*Stouffer's*), 10.5 oz.......................................370
pollo (*Michelina's*), 8 oz. ....................................................280
pomodoro (*Michelina's*), 8 oz...............................................260
primavera (*Michelina's*), 8 oz. ..............................................270
Roma (*Healthy Choice* Entree), 13.5 oz. ...............................420
w/tomato sauce, Italian sausage (*Stouffer's*), 10⅞ oz. ............420
vegetable (*Amy's* Family), ⅙ pkg. .........................................200
vegetable (*Cedarlane* Low Fat), 10 oz. ..................................280
vegetable (*Lean Cuisine Everyday Favorites*), 10.5 oz. .............260
vegetable (*Michelina's*), 8 oz. ..............................................210
vegetable (*Michelina's*), 8.5 oz. ...........................................240
vegetable (*Stouffer's*), 10.5 oz.............................................400
vegetable or tofu vegetable (*Amy's*), 9.5 oz. ..........................300
w/white sauce (*Michelina's*), 10 oz.......................................540
**Leek,** fresh, lower leaf and bulb portion:
raw (*Frieda's*), ⅓ cup, 3 oz......................................................50
raw, 3.1-oz. leek or 1 cup chopped .........................................54
boiled, drained, 1 leek, 4.4 oz.................................................38
boiled, drained, chopped or diced, ½ cup.................................16
**Leek, freeze-dried,** lower leaf and bulb portion, ¼ cup.............3
**Lemon,** fresh, raw:
(*Dole*), 1 lemon.....................................................................18
w/peel, seeded, 3.8-oz. lemon.................................................22
**Lemon curd** (*Crosse & Blackwell*), 1 tbsp.............................50
**Lemon grass,** fresh:
(*Frieda's*), 1 tbsp...................................................................0
1 cup.....................................................................................66
1 tbsp......................................................................................5
**Lemon grass hearts,** in jars (*A Taste of Thai*), 1 pc. ...............0
**Lemon herb sauce mix,** dry (*Knorr* Classic), 1 tbsp..................30
**Lemon juice:**
fresh, 2 tbsp............................................................................8
bottled, from concentrate (*ReaLemon*), 1 tsp. ............................0

**Lemon-lime drink mix** (*Kool-Aid*), 8 fl. oz.*.............................100
**Lemon peel,** fresh, raw, 1 tbsp...............................................3
**Lemonade,** 8 fl. oz.:
(*Country Time*)........................................................................90
(*Minute Maid*)........................................................................110
(*Sunkist*)...............................................................................120
(*Tropicana*)...........................................................................120
(*Welch's*)..............................................................................110
pink (*Country Time*).............................................................90
raspberry (*Minute Maid*).......................................................120
**Lemonade mix,** 8 fl. oz.*:
(*Kool-Aid* Sugar Free)............................................................5
(*Kool-Aid* Sugar Sweetened)...............................................70
all flavors (*Country Time Lem'N Berry Sippers*)...................90
regular or pink (*Country Time*)..............................................70
regular or pink (*Country Time* Sugar Free)............................5
regular or pink (*Kool-Aid*).....................................................100
strawberry (*Country Time Lem'N Berry Sippers* Sugar Free).......5
strawberry (*Kool-Aid Soarin'*)..............................................100
(*Kool-Aid Soarin'* Sugar Free)...............................................5
strawberry (*Kool-Aid Soarin'* Sugar Sweetened)...................70
**Lentil:**
dry, green or red (*Arrowhead Mills*), ¼ cup.........................150
cooked, ½ cup........................................................................115
**Lentil, sprouted,** raw, 1 cup..................................................82
**Lettuce,** fresh:
Bibb or Boston, 5"-diam. head................................................21
Bibb or Boston, chopped or shredded, 1 cup...........................7
iceberg (*Andy Boy*), ⅙ medium head....................................16
iceberg (*Dole*), ⅙ medium head, 3.2 oz. ..............................15
iceberg, 1 large head, 1⅔ lb. .................................................91
iceberg, chopped or shredded, 1 cup.......................................7
limestone (*Frieda's*), ⅔ cup, 3 oz..........................................10
looseleaf, shredded (*Andy Boy*), 1½ cups.............................15
looseleaf, shredded (*Dole*), 1½ cups ....................................15
looseleaf, shredded, ½ cup.......................................................5
romaine (*Andy Boy*), 6 leaves...............................................20
romaine (*Dole*), 6 leaves, 3 oz. ............................................20
romaine or cos, shredded, ½ cup..............................................1

**Lima beans, immature,** fresh:
raw, 1 cup ...................................................................176
boiled, drained, 1 cup ...............................................209
**Lima beans, mature:**
baby, dry, 1 cup ........................................................677
baby, boiled, 1 cup ...................................................229
large, dry, 1 cup .......................................................602
large, boiled, 1 cup ..................................................216
**Lima beans, canned:**
(*Allens/East Texas Fair* Green Limas) ....................120
(*Del Monte*)...............................................................80
(*Sunshine* Green Butterbeans) ...............................120
baby or large (*Allens* Butterbeans).........................120
green and white (*Allens* Limas)...............................110
w/bacon, baby white (*Trappey's* Lima) ...................130
w/bacon, green (*Trappey's* Lima) ............................120
w/sausage, large white (*Trappey's* Butterbeans) ......110
**Lima beans, frozen:**
(*Birds Eye* Butter Beans/Speckled Butter Beans) ......100
(*Seabrook Farms* Petite)...........................................110
baby (*Birds Eye/Birds Eye* Deluxe) .........................130
baby (*Freshlike*) ......................................................110
baby (*Green Giant*)....................................................80
Fordhook (*Birds Eye/Birds Eye* Deluxe)...................100
Fordhook (*Freshlike*)..................................................90
**Lime,** fresh:
(*Frieda's* Key Lime), 3 oz. ........................................25
2" diam., 2.4 oz..........................................................20
**Lime juice:**
fresh, 2 tbsp................................................................8
bottled, from concentrate (*ReaLime*), 1 tsp. ................0
**Lime relish,** Indian, hot or mild (*Patak's*), 1 tbsp. ......30
**Ling,** meat only:
raw, 4 oz. ...................................................................99
baked, broiled, or microwaved, 4 oz. .......................126
**Ling cod,** meat only:
raw, 4 oz. ...................................................................96
baked, broiled, or microwaved, 4 oz. .......................124

**Linguine:**

dry, see "Pasta"

refrigerated, plain (*Contadina Buitoni*), 1¼ cups......................240

refrigerated, plain or herb (*Di Giorno*), 2.5 oz...........................200

refrigerated, spinach (*Di Giorno*), 2.5 oz..................................190

**Linguine entree, frozen,** w/clams (*Michelina's*), 8.5 oz...........290

**Linguine entree, mix,** about 1 cup*:

chicken and broccoli (*Pasta Roni*)............................................370

chicken Parmesan, creamy (*Pasta Roni*)..................................410

**Litchee,** see "Lychee"

**Liquor,**[1] 1 fl. oz.:

80 proof...................................................................................65

100 proof.................................................................................83

**Liver,** 4 oz., except as noted:

beef, pan fried.......................................................................246

chicken, simmered, chopped or diced, 1 cup .........................219

lamb, pan-fried ......................................................................270

turkey, simmered, chopped, 1 cup.........................................237

veal (calves'), pan-fried .........................................................278

**Liver cheese,** 1.3-oz. slice..................................................116

**Liverwurst** (see also "Braunschweiger"):

(*Boar's Head* Strassburger), 2 oz. .........................................170

1 oz..........................................................................................92

**Lo bok,** see "Radish, Oriental"

**Lobster** (see also "Spiny lobster"), northern, meat only:

raw, 1 lobster, 5.3 oz.............................................................135

raw, 4 oz. ..............................................................................102

boiled, poached, or steamed, 4 oz. ........................................111

boiled, poached, or steamed, 1 cup, 5.1 oz. ..........................142

**Lobster sauce,** canned (*Progresso*), ½ cup.........................100

**Loganberry,** fresh, 1 cup....................................................89

**Long beans,** see "Yard-long beans"

**Loquat,** fresh:

(*Frieda's*), 5 oz......................................................................70

1 large, .7 oz. ...........................................................................9

cubed, 1 cup ...........................................................................70

---

[1]*Includes all pure distilled liquors: bourbon, brandy, gin, rum, scotch, tequila, vodka, etc.*

**Lotus root,** fresh:
raw (*Frieda's*), 1 cup, 3 oz. ........................................................50
raw, 9½"-long root ............................................................85
raw, sliced, 2½" diam., 10 slices .................................60
boiled, drained, ½ cup ....................................................40
**Lotus seed:**
raw, 1 oz. ......................................................................24
dried, 1 oz., 42 medium ..................................................94
**Lox,** see "Salmon, smoked"
**Lunch meat,** loaf (see also specific listings):
barbecue, .8-oz. slice ......................................................40
Dutch or Italian (*Russer*), 2 oz. ..................................130
honey, 1-oz. slice ............................................................36
jalapeno, w/Monterey jack cheese (*Russer*), 2 oz. ..............160
luxury, pork, 1-oz. slice ..................................................40
mother's, pork, ¾-oz. slice ..............................................60
old fashioned (*Russer* Light), 2 oz. ................................90
olive (*Boar's Head*), 2 oz. ............................................130
olive (*Russer*), 2 oz. ..................................................160
pepper (*Russer*), 2 oz. ..................................................90
pickle and pimento (*Russer*), 2 oz. ................................160
pickle and pimento (*Russer* Light), 2 oz. ......................100
Polish (*Russer*), 2 oz. ..................................................140
**Lunch meat, canned,** 2 oz.:
(*Spam* Lite) ..................................................................110
(*Spam/Spam* Less Salt/Smoked) ..................................170
**Lupin,** mature:
dry, 1 cup ....................................................................668
boiled, 1 cup ................................................................198
**Lychee:**
(*Frieda's*), 1 fruit ..........................................................60
fresh, raw, shelled and seeded, 1 cup ..........................125
dried, 1 oz. ....................................................................78

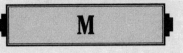

## FOOD AND MEASURE                                      CALORIES

**Macadamia nut,** shelled:
(*Frieda's*), 5 pcs., 1.1 oz. ...........................................................210
raw or dry roasted, 1 oz., 10–12 kernels ...................................204
raw or dry roasted, whole or halves, ¼ cup ............................241
**Macaroni, dry** (see also "Pasta, dry"), 2 oz.:
elbow or spiral.............................................................................210
protein fortified ...........................................................................213
vegetable (tricolor) ....................................................................208
whole wheat..................................................................................197
**Macaroni, dry, cooked** (see also "Pasta, dry, cooked"), 1 cup:
elbow .............................................................................................197
small shells, protein fortified, or spirals.....................................189
vegetable (tricolor) ....................................................................172
whole wheat..................................................................................174
**Macaroni entree, canned or packaged:**
w/beef, tomato sauce (*Chef Boyardee Beefaroni*), 1 cup .........260
w/beef, tomato sauce (*Chef Boyardee Beefaroni* Microwave
    Bowl), 1 bowl ...........................................................................200
beefy (*Kid's Kitchen*), 1 cup........................................................190
and cheese (*Chef Boyardee*), 1 cup.............................................230
and cheese (*Franco-American*), 1 cup .......................................210
and cheese (*Hormel* Mac & Cheese), 7.5-oz. can.....................270
and cheese (*Hormel* Microcup Meals), 1 cup ............................270
and cheese/and cheesy beef (*Kid's Kitchen*), 1 cup .................260
and cheese, w/*Cure 81* ham (*Dinty Moore American*
    *Classics*), 1 bowl....................................................................330
**Macaroni entree, frozen,** 1 pkg., except as noted:
and beef (*Freezer Queen*), 9 oz. ................................................230
and beef (*Healthy Choice* Entree), 8.5 oz. ...............................220
and beef (*Lean Cuisine Everyday Favorites*), 10 oz..................270
and beef (*Michelina's*), 8 oz.......................................................250
and beef (*Stouffer's*), 11.5 oz. ...................................................380
and cheese (*Amy's*), 9 oz. ..........................................................410

and cheese (*Banquet*), 12 oz. ...................................................420
and cheese (*Boston Market* Home Style Meals), 10 oz. ...........430
and cheese (*Freezer Queen*), 8 oz. ......................................350
and cheese (*Healthy Choice* Entree), 9 oz. ..........................240
and cheese (*Howard Johnson's*), 10 oz. ................................410
and cheese (*Lean Cuisine Everyday Favorites*), 10 oz. .............290
and cheese (*Marie Callender's*), 12 oz. .................................540
and cheese (*Michelina's*), 8 oz. ............................................270
and cheese (*Morton*), 1 cup .................................................240
and cheese (*Stouffer's*), ½ of 12-oz. pkg. ............................320
and cheese, w/broccoli (*Stouffer's*), 10.5 oz. .......................400
and cheese, cheddar, sharp (*Michelina's*), 10 oz. ..................430
and cheese, w/ham (*Michelina's*), 8 oz. ................................340
and cheese, pot pie (*Banquet*), 7 oz. ....................................210
and "cheese," nondairy (*Amy's* Soy Cheeze), 9 oz. ................360
**Macaroni entree mix,** and cheese:
(*Creamette*), 2.5 oz. ...........................................................250
(*Kraft* Light Deluxe Dinner), about 1 cup* ............................290
(*Kraft Thick 'N Creamy* Premium Dinner), about 1 cup* ..........420
(*Land O Lakes*), 1 cup* ......................................................400
(*Land O Lakes* Deluxe Plus), 1 cup* ...................................360
all varieties, (*Kraft* Deluxe Dinner), about 1 cup* ..................320
all varieties, (*Kraft* Dinner), about 1 cup* ............................410
**Macaroni salad,** refrigerated:
(*Blue Ridge Farms*), ½ cup .................................................240
(*Chef's Express*), 4 oz. .......................................................210
**Macchiato pasta,** frozen, stuffed w/gorgonzola walnut
    agnolotti (*Cafferata*), ½ of 9-oz. pkg. .............................330
**Mace,** ground, 1 tsp. ............................................................8
**Mackerel,** meat only:
Atlantic, raw, 4 oz. ..............................................................230
Atlantic, baked, broiled, or microwaved, 4 oz. .....................297
king, raw, 4 oz. ..................................................................119
king, baked, broiled, or microwaved, 4 oz. ..........................152
Pacific and jack, raw, 4 oz. .................................................179
Pacific and jack, baked, broiled, or microwaved, 4 oz. ..........228
Spanish, raw, 4 oz. .............................................................158
Spanish, baked, broiled, or microwaved, 4 oz. ......................179
**Mackerel, canned,** in oil, drained (*Reese*), 4.375-oz. can .......240

**Mackerel, smoked,** fillet, 2 oz.:
herb (*Ducktrap River*) ..................................................................110
peppered (*Ducktrap River*) ........................................................120
**Madras sauce,** see "Curry sauce"
**Mahi mahi,** see "Dolphin fish"
**Mai tai drink mix,** bottled (*Mr & Mrs T*), 4.5 fl. oz. .............140
**Malanga** (*Frieda's*), ⅔ cup, 3 oz. ...........................................90
**Malt syrup,** 1 tbsp. ..................................................................76
**Malted milk powder,** natural or chocolate flavor (*Carnation*),
    3 tbsp. ...............................................................................90
**Mammy apple,** fresh, raw, untrimmed, 1 fruit, 1.9 lb. ...........432
**Manicotti entree,** frozen, 1 pkg.:
cheese (*Stouffer's*), 9 oz. .........................................................360
cheese, 3 (*Healthy Choice* Entree), 11 oz. ..............................300
cheese-spinach (*Lean Cuisine Hearty Portions*), 15½ oz. ........370
**Mango,** fresh:
(*Frieda's* Pango), 5-oz. fruit ......................................................90
trimmed, 1 fruit, 7.3 oz. ...........................................................135
sliced, 1 cup .............................................................................107
sliced, peeled (*Dole*), ½ cup ....................................................54
**Mango, canned or in jars:**
sliced, in light syrup (*Ka•Me*), 4 pcs. .....................................102
sliced, in syrup (*Haddon House*), ¼ cup ...................................90
**Mango, dried** (*Frieda's*), 4 pcs., 1.4 oz. ...............................130
**Mango drink mix,** 8 fl. oz.:
(*Kool-Aid Man-O-Mango-Berry*) ...............................................100
(*Kool-Aid Man-O-Mango-Berry* Sugar Sweetened) .....................60
(*Tang*) .....................................................................................100
**Mango nectar** (*Libby's*), 8 fl. oz. ...........................................140
**Mango relish,** hot or mild (*Patak's*), 1 tbsp. ............................40
**Mangosteen,** canned, in syrup, 1 cup ....................................158
**Maple syrup,** 1 tbsp. ................................................................52
**Margarine,** salted or unsalted, 1 tbsp.:
(*Earth Balance* Vegan) .............................................................100
(*Land O Lakes* Country Morning Blend Stick/Tub) .....................100
(*Land O Lakes* Stick/Tub) .........................................................100
(*Land O Lakes* Stick/Tub Light) ..................................................50
(*Land O Lakes* Spread w/Sweet Cream Stick) ............................90
(*Land O Lakes* Spread w/Sweet Cream Tub) ..............................80

(*Smart Balance*) ........................................................80
(*Smart Balance* Light) ..............................................45
(*Smart Beat* Trans Fat Free) ...................................20
**Margarita mix,** bottled:
(*D. L. Jardine's*), 1 fl. oz. .......................................90
(*Mr & Mrs T*), 4 fl. oz. ...........................................130
strawberry (*Mr & Mrs T*), 3.5 fl. oz. ......................150
**Marinade** (see also "Stir-fry sauce" and specific listings),
   1 tbsp., except as noted:
(*House of Tsang Mandarin*) ....................................25
Caribbean jerk (*Lawry's*) .........................................25
citrus grill or tequila lime (*Lawry's*) .......................15
coriander ginger (*Patak's* Tikka Marinade/Grill), 2 tbsp. ....40
Dijon and honey, Hawaiian, or hickory (*Lawry's*) ..........20
fajitas meat (*D. L. Jardine's*) ....................................5
garlic, lemon pepper, Mediterranean, or Thai ginger
   (*Lawry's*) ...........................................................10
ginger and garlic (*Patak's* Tandoori Marinade/Grill), 2 tbsp. ....35
lemon grass herb (*Annie Chun's*), 2 tbsp. ...............60
London broil (*Lawry's* Weekday Gourmet) ...............10
mesquite (*Lawry's*) ..................................................5
**Marinade seasoning mix,** all flavors (*Adolph's Marinade in*
   *Minutes* Tenderizing), ¾ tsp. ...............................5
**Marjoram,** dried, 1 tsp. .............................................2
**Marmalade,** see "Jam and preserves"
**Marrow squash,** raw, trimmed, 1 oz. ......................4
**Marshmallow topping** (*Smucker's* Spoonable), 2 tbsp. ....120
**Matzo balls** (*Mrs. Adler's*), 3 pcs. w/liquid ............190
**Mayonnaise,** 1 tbsp.:
(*Hellmann's/Best Foods*) .........................................100
(*Hellmann's/Best Foods* Light) .................................50
(*Kraft*) ....................................................................100
(*Kraft* Fat Free) .......................................................10
(*Kraft* Light) .............................................................50
(*Smart Balance* Light) ..............................................50
dressing (*Miracle Whip*) ..........................................70
dressing (*Miracle Whip* Light) .................................35
dressing (*Miracle Whip Free*) ..................................15
dressing (*Smart Beat*) .............................................10

***McDonald's,*** 1 serving:

breakfast:

    bagel, ham, egg, and cheese ...............................................550

    bagel, Spanish omelet....................................................690

    bagel, steak, egg, and cheese .........................................700

    biscuit, plain...............................................................290

    biscuit, bacon, egg, and cheese......................................540

    biscuit, sausage ..........................................................470

    biscuit, sausage and egg ...............................................550

    breakfast burrito..........................................................320

    *Egg McMuffin*.............................................................290

    eggs, scrambled, 2.......................................................160

    English muffin, plain ....................................................140

    hash browns ...............................................................130

    hot cakes, plain ...........................................................340

    hot cakes, w/syrup, margarine.........................................600

    sausage ....................................................................170

    *Sausage McMuffin* ......................................................360

    *Sausage McMuffin,* w/egg .............................................440

danish and muffin:

    apple bran muffin, low fat ..............................................300

    apple danish...............................................................340

    cheese danish ............................................................400

    cinnamon roll .............................................................390

sandwiches:

    *Big Mac*....................................................................590

    *Big Xtra!*...................................................................710

    *Big Xtra!* w/cheese .....................................................810

    cheeseburger..............................................................330

    *Chicken McGrill* .........................................................450

    *Chicken McGrill* w/out mayo .........................................340

    *Crispy Chicken* ..........................................................550

    *Filet-O-Fish* ...............................................................470

    hamburger..................................................................280

    *Quarter Pounder*.........................................................430

    *Quarter Pounder* w/cheese............................................530

*Chicken McNuggets:*

    4 pcs. .......................................................................190

   6 pcs. ....................................................................290
   9 pcs. ....................................................................430
*McNuggets* sauce pkt.:
   barbeque or honey ...............................................45
   honey mustard or sweet and sour ........................50
   hot mustard............................................................60
   mayonnaise, light...................................................40
fries:
   large ....................................................................540
   medium .................................................................450
   *Super Size* ............................................................610
   small.....................................................................210
salads, w/out dressing:
   chef salad .............................................................150
   garden salad..........................................................100
   grilled chicken Caesar salad..................................100
   croutons, 1 pkg. .....................................................50
salad dressing, 1 pkg.:
   Caesar or honey mustard......................................150
   ranch ....................................................................170
   red French, reduced calorie, or Thousand Island ......130
   vinaigrette, fat free herb .........................................30
desserts and shakes:
   baked apple pie .....................................................260
   chocolate chip cookie............................................170
   fruit'n yogurt parfait ...............................................380
   fruit'n yogurt parfait, w/out granola.......................280
   *McDonaldland Cookies,* 1 pkg. ..............................180
   *McFlurry, Butterfinger* ...........................................620
   *McFlurry, M&M's or Nestlé Crunch* .......................630
   *McFlurry, Oreo* .....................................................570
   shake, chocolate, strawberry or vanilla, small....................360
   sundae, hot caramel...............................................360
   sundae, hot fudge .................................................340
   sundae, strawberry ...............................................290
   sundae nuts.............................................................40
   vanilla cone, reduced fat .......................................150
**Meat, lunch,** see "Lunch meat" and specific listings

**Meat, potted:**
(*Armour*), ¼ cup ...................................................................80
(*Hormel*), 4 tbsp. .............................................................100
**Meat loaf dinner,** frozen, 1 pkg.:
(*Banquet Extra Helping*), 16 oz. .....................................610
(*Freezer Queen*), 9.5 oz. .................................................310
(*Swanson*), 10.75 oz. .......................................................380
(*Swanson Hungry-Man*), 16.5 oz. ...................................630
traditional (*Healthy Choice* Meal), 12 oz. .......................330
**Meat loaf entree,** frozen:
(*Banquet*), 9.5 oz. ...........................................................280
(*Freezer Queen*), 1 patty and sauce ...............................200
(*Hormel Always Tender*), 5 oz. .......................................240
(*Stouffer's* Homestyle), 9⅞ oz. .......................................390
and gravy, w/mashed potato (*Marie Callender's*), 14 oz. .........540
and gravy, w/mashed potato (*Michelina's*), 8 oz. .............340
and gravy, w/sour cream mashed potato (*Michelina's*),
    10.5 oz. .....................................................................390
gravy, savory, and (*Banquet* Family), 1 patty w/gravy ..............190
in gravy (*Stouffer's*), ⅙ of 59-oz. pkg. ...........................220
w/gravy (*Boston Market*), 9 oz. ......................................400
w/mashed potato (*Stouffer's Hearty Portions*), 17 oz. .............590
w/mashed potato and gravy (*Boston Market*), 16 oz. .............740
tomato sauce w/ (*Morton*), 9 oz. .....................................250
w/whipped potato (*Lean Cuisine Cafe Classics*), 9⅜ oz. ..........260
**Meat loaf mix** (*Adolph's Meal Makers*), 1 tbsp. .........................25
**Meat tenderizer,** all varieties (*Adolph's*), ¼ tsp. ...........................0
**Meatball entree, canned,** 1 cup:
pasta and, in tomato sauce (*Franco-American Garfield*) ..........260
stew (*Dinty Moore*) ...........................................................250
**Meatball entree, frozen,** 1 pkg.:
Italian, in wine sauce (*Michelina's*), 8 oz. ......................210
mashed potatoes and (*Michelina's*), 8.5 oz. ...................270
Swedish (*Lean Cuisine Everyday Favorites*), 9⅛ oz. ..............290
Swedish (*Marie Callender's*), 12.5 oz. ............................520
Swedish (*Stouffer's*), 11.5 oz. ........................................520
Swedish, and gravy (*Michelina's*), 10 oz. .......................400
**Meatball sandwich/pocket,** frozen, 1 pc.:
Italian style (*Healthy Choice Meals To Go*), 6.1 oz. .................330

and mozzarella (*Hot Pockets*), 4.5 oz.................................320
and mozzarella (*Lean Pockets*), 4.5 oz.............................300
**Melon,** see specific listings
**Melon, mixed,** balls, frozen, unthawed, 1 cup .....................57
**Menudo,** canned (*Juanita's* Menudito), 1 cup .....................170
**Mexican entree,** frozen, 1 pkg.:
fiesta (*Patio*), 12 oz. ...........................................................350
Mexican style (*Patio*), 13.5 oz. .........................................470
ranchero (*Patio*), 13 oz.......................................................470
**Mexican squash** (*Frieda's*), ½ cup, 3 oz................................35
**Milk,** dairy pack or packaged, 1 cup:
buttermilk, cultured ..............................................................99
whole, 3.3% fat....................................................................150
reduced/low fat, 2% fat .......................................................121
reduced/low fat, 2%, protein fortified.................................137
reduced/low fat, 1% fat .......................................................102
1%, protein fortified.............................................................119
skim/fat free...........................................................................86
**Milk, canned:**
condensed, sweetened (*Carnation*), 2 tbsp..........................130
evaporated (*Carnation*), 2 tbsp............................................40
evaporated (*Carnation* Lowfat/*Carnation* Fat Free), 2 tbsp..........25
**Milk, chocolate,** see "Chocolate milk"
**Milk, dry:**
buttermilk, 1 tbsp. ................................................................25
whole, 1 tbsp. .......................................................................40
nonfat (*Carnation*), ⅓ cup ...................................................80
nonfat, regular, 1 tbsp. .........................................................27
nonfat, instant, 1 tbsp...........................................................15
**Milk, goat,** 1 cup ...................................................................168
**Milk, human,** 1 cup ...............................................................171
**Milkfish,** meat only:
raw, 4 oz. ..............................................................................167
baked, broiled, or microwaved, 4 oz. ..................................216
**Millet:**
dry, 1 cup..............................................................................756
cooked, 1 cup .......................................................................207
**Millet flour** (*Arrowhead Mills*), ¼ cup ..................................110
**Mincemeat,** see "Pie filling"

**Mint sauce** (*Crosse & Blackwell*), 1 tsp. ......................................5
**Miso,** soy:
1 oz. ..............................................................................................58
1 cup ..........................................................................................567
**Molasses:**
all varieties (*Brer Rabbit*), 1 tbsp. ............................................60
regular, mild or robust (*Grandma's*), 1 tbsp. ............................50
**Monkfish,** meat only:
raw, 4 oz. ....................................................................................86
baked, broiled, or microwaved, 4 oz. ........................................110
**Mortadella** (*Russer*), 2 oz. ..................................................170
**Mothbean,** mature:
dry, 1 cup ..................................................................................672
boiled, 1 cup ............................................................................207
**Muffin,** 1 pc., except as noted:
apple (*Awrey's*) ........................................................................230
apple, blueberry, or banana nut (*Awrey's*) ..............................130
banana nut (*Awrey's* Grande) ..................................................410
banana nut or lemon poppy (*Awrey's* Petite) ..........................160
banana walnut (*Hostess* Mini), 3 pcs. ....................................160
blueberry (*Awrey's*) ..................................................................210
blueberry (*Awrey's* Grande) ....................................................380
blueberry (*Awrey's* Petite) ......................................................150
blueberry (*Entenmann's* Light Fat Free) ................................120
blueberry (*Hostess* Mini), 3 pcs. ............................................150
cheese streusel (*Awrey's*) ......................................................380
chocolate chip (*Hostess* Mini), 3 pcs. ....................................160
chocolate chocolate chip (*Awrey's* Grande) ............................480
corn (*Awrey's*), 4 oz. ..............................................................410
corn (*Awrey's*), 1.25 oz. ..........................................................130
corn (*Entenmann's*) ................................................................210
cranberry nut (*Awrey's*) ..........................................................150
English (*Awrey's*) ....................................................................140
English (*Thomas'* Original) ......................................................120
English (*Thomas'* Original Super Size) ....................................190
English, blueberry, cinnamon raisin, or cranberry (*Thomas'*) ..140
English, cinnamon or maple French toast (*Thomas'*) ..............150
English, honey wheat (*Thomas'*) ..............................................130
lemon poppy seed (*Awrey's*) ..................................................420

raisin bran (*Awrey's*), 4 oz............................................................350
raisin bran (*Awrey's*), 2.5 oz.........................................................200
raisin bran (*Awrey's*), 1.5 oz.........................................................110
sourdough (*Thomas'*) .................................................................120
sourdough (*Thomas' Super Size*)..................................................200
**Muffin mix,** 1 pc.\*, except as noted:
apple cinnamon (*Betty Crocker Smart Size Pouch*) .................170
apple cinnamon (*Betty Crocker Sweet Rewards*).....................140
apple cinnamon (*"Jiffy"*) .............................................................190
apple streudel (*Betty Crocker*) ....................................................210
banana (*Pillsbury Quick Bread & Muffin Mix*)............................180
banana nut (*Betty Crocker/Betty Crocker Smart Size Pouch*)...170
banana nut (*"Jiffy"*).....................................................................180
blueberry (*Betty Crocker Smart Size Pouch*) ............................160
blueberry (*"Jiffy"*) .......................................................................190
blueberry, twice the (*Betty Crocker*) ..........................................140
blueberry, wild (*Betty Crocker*) ..................................................170
blueberry, wild (*Betty Crocker Sweet Rewards*).......................130
bran, w/dates (*"Jiffy"*)..................................................................170
bran, corn, or whole wheat (*Hodgson Mill*), ⅙ pkg. ................130
chocolate, double (*Betty Crocker*) ..............................................200
chocolate chip (*Betty Crocker Smart Size Pouch*) ...................170
corn (*"Jiffy"*) ...............................................................................180
corn, golden (*Betty Crocker Smart Size Pouch*) .......................160
cranberry (*Pillsbury Quick Bread & Muffin Mix*)........................160
cranberry orange (*Betty Crocker*) ...............................................150
lemon poppy seed (*Betty Crocker*) .............................................190
lemon poppy seed (*Betty Crocker Smart Size Pouch*).............180
lemon poppy seed (*Pillsbury Quick Bread & Muffin Mix*).........180
nut (*Pillsbury Quick Bread & Muffin Mix*)...................................170
oat bran, wheat free (*Arrowhead Mills*), ⅓ cup .......................160
raspberry (*"Jiffy"*) .......................................................................180
**Mulberry,** fresh, raw, 10 berries, .5 oz.............................................7
**Mullet,** striped, meat only:
raw, 4 oz. .....................................................................................133
baked, broiled, or microwaved, 4 oz. .........................................170
**Mung bean,** mature:
dry, 1 cup......................................................................................718
boiled, 1 cup.................................................................................212

**Mung bean sprout,** fresh:

raw, 1 cup ....................................................................31

boiled, drained, 1 cup ..................................................26

stir-fried, 1 cup ............................................................62

**Mung bean sprout, canned,** drained, 1 cup .............15

**Mungo bean,** mature:

dry, 1 cup ..................................................................706

boiled, 1 cup ..............................................................189

**Mushroom,** fresh:

raw, whole, 1 cup .........................................................24

raw, pieces or slices, 1 cup ........................................18

boiled, drained, pieces, 1 cup .....................................42

brown, Italian or crimini, raw, .5-oz. pc. .......................3

enoki (*Frieda's*), ¼ pkg., .9 oz. .................................10

oyster, raw, 1 large, 5.2 oz. ........................................55

oyster, raw, 1 small, .5 oz. ............................................6

portobello, caps or sliced, raw (*Phillips*), 2 oz. ...........4

enoki, 1 large, .2 oz. .....................................................2

enoki, 1 medium, .1 oz. ..................................................1

shiitake, cooked, 4 mushrooms, 2.5 oz. .....................40

shiitake, cooked, 1 cup ................................................80

**Mushroom, canned or in jars:**

whole or sliced (*BinB*), 3-oz. jar ................................40

whole or sliced (*Green Giant*), ½ cup .......................30

drained, 1 cup .............................................................37

straw, drained, 1 cup ..................................................58

**Mushroom, dried:**

chanterelle (*Frieda's*), 2 pcs. ....................................15

cloud ear, .2-oz. pc. ....................................................13

cloud ear, 1 cup ..........................................................80

morel, oyster, or wood ear (*Frieda's*), 3 pcs. ............15

oyster or porcini (*Epicurean Specialty*), ⅓ oz. .......131

padi straw (*Frieda's*), 6 pcs. .....................................15

porcini (*Frieda's*), 5 pcs. ...........................................15

portobello, thin sliced (*Frieda's*), 7 pcs. ......................5

shiitake (*Frieda's*), ¼ cup ..........................................10

shiitake, 4 mushrooms, ½ oz. .....................................44

**Mushroom batter mix** (*Hodgson Mill Don's Chuck Wagon*),

¼ cup ..........................................................................95

**Mushroom gravy,** ¼ cup:
(*Heinz* Home Style)..................................................25
(*Franco-American/Franco-American* Creamy).............20
**Mushroom sauce:**
(*Pasta Gusto*), ⅓ cup ..........................................160
carciofi or porcini (*Italia In Tavola*), 2 tbsp..............110
shiitake (*Annie Chun's/Annie Chun's* Spicy), 1 tbsp...............15
**Mussel,** blue, meat only:
raw, 4 oz. ..............................................................90
raw, 1 cup ...........................................................119
boiled, poached, or steamed, 4 oz. ......................194
**Mussel, canned,** in red sauce, drained (*Reese*), 4-oz. can......120
**Mussel, smoked** (*Ducktrap River*), ¼ cup.................140
**Mustard,** prepared, 1 tsp.:
all varieties except honey (*Grey Poupon*).....................5
brown (*Gulden's*) .....................................................5
yellow (*Boar's Head* Delicatessen Style).......................0
yellow (*Hebrew National* Deli) .................................4
yellow (*Kraft*)...........................................................0
**Mustard blends:**
honey (*Boar's Head*), 1 tsp. ....................................10
honey (*Grey Poupon*), 1 tsp. ..................................10
horseradish (*Kraft*), 1 tsp..........................................0
mayonnaise (*Hellmann's Dijonnaise*), 1 tbsp. ..........20
**Mustard greens,** fresh:
raw, chopped, 1 cup ................................................15
boiled, drained, chopped, 1 cup .............................21
**Mustard greens, canned** (*Allens/Sunshine*), ½ cup ..........30
**Mustard greens, frozen:**
chopped (*Birds Eye*), 1 cup.....................................30
chopped, boiled, drained, 1 cup .............................29
**Mustard seed,** yellow, 1 tsp....................................16
**Mustard spinach,** see "Spinach, mustard"

| FOOD AND MEASURE | CALORIES |
|---|---|

**Nacho mix** (*Taco Bell Home Originals*), 12 nachos* ..............240
**Natto:**
1 oz. ..........................................................................................60
1 cup .......................................................................................371
**Navy bean,** mature, boiled, 1 cup.........................................258
**Navy bean, canned,** ½ cup:
(*Allens*) ...................................................................................110
Creole style (*Trappey's*).........................................................110
w/bacon or bacon and jalapeno (*Trappey's*)...........................110
**Navy bean sprout,** from mature seeds, raw, 1 cup ................70
**Nectarine,** fresh, raw:
(*Dole*), 5 oz.............................................................................70
2½" diam., 4.8 oz......................................................................67
sliced, 1 cup.............................................................................68
**New Zealand spinach,** see "Spinach, New Zealand"
**Newburg sauce mix,** dry (*Knorr* Classic), 1 tbsp....................35
**Noodle, Chinese,** uncooked:
(*Nasoya*), 1 cup .....................................................................210
cellophane or long rice, 2 oz. ................................................200
chow mein, fresh (*Frieda's*), 4 oz. ........................................270
chow mein, regular or spinach (*Annie Chun's*), 2 oz. ............200
crispy (*Frieda's*), ½ cup........................................................160
**Noodle, egg,** dry, 2 oz.:
(*Hodgson Mill*).......................................................................200
(*Kluski*) ..................................................................................210
all widths (*Mueller's*)..............................................................220
whole wheat, plain or spinach (*Hodgson Mill*).......................190
yolk free (*Borden*)...................................................................210
**Noodle, egg,** cooked, 1 cup.................................................213
**Noodle, egg, refrigerated,** spinach (*Nasoya*), 1 cup...........210
**Noodle, Japanese,** uncooked, except as noted:
soba (*Annie Chun's*), 2 oz. ...................................................200
soba, 2 oz. .............................................................................191

soba, cooked, 1 cup ...................................................113
somen, 2 oz. ...............................................................202
somen, cooked, 1 cup .................................................231
refrigerated (*Nasoya*), 1 cup......................................210
**Noodle, rice,** uncooked, except as noted:
(*A Taste of Thai*), 2 oz..............................................200
2 oz. ...........................................................................206
cooked, 1 cup ............................................................192
all styles and flavors (*Annie Chun's*), 2 oz. ...............210
**Noodle dish, mix:**
Alfredo (*Lipton* Noodles & Sauce), 1 cup* .................330
beef flavor (*Lipton* Noodles & Sauce), 1 cup* ............280
butter and herb (*Lipton* Noodles & Sauce), 1 cup* .....300
cheddar cheese (*Kraft Noodle Classics*), approx. 1 cup* .........400
chicken, savory (*Kraft Noodle Classics*), approx. 1 cup* .........340
chicken broccoli (*Lipton* Noodles & Sauce), 1 cup*.....310
chicken flavor (*Lipton* Noodles & Sauce), 1 cup* .......290
Stroganoff (*Lipton* Noodles & Sauce), 1 cup* ............300
**Noodle entree, canned or packaged,** 1 cup:
and beef, in Stroganoff (*Dinty Moore* Microwave)....................240
and chicken (*Hormel* Microcup Meals) ......................200
rings, and chicken (*Kid's Kitchen*)..............................150
**Noodle entree, frozen,** 1 pkg., except as noted:
Alfredo (*Michelina's*), 8 oz......................................330
Alfredo, w/pepperoni (*Michelina's*), 8 oz...................370
Alfredo, and vegetables (*Michelina's*), 8 oz. ............320
with beef (*Freezer Queen* Family), 1 cup ..................200
and cheese, w/pepperoni (*Michelina's*), 8 oz............280
and chicken (*Michelina's*), 8 oz.................................290
and chicken, homestyle (*Banquet*), 12 oz. ................390
w/chicken, peas and carrots (*Michelina's*), 8 oz. .......227
escalloped, and chicken (*Marie Callender's*), 13 oz. .............740
escalloped, and chicken (*Marie Callender's* Family), 1 cup........280
marinara (*Michelina's*), 8 oz.....................................230
Romanoff (*Stouffer's*), ½ of 12-oz. pkg....................240
Romanoff, w/meatballs (*Michelina's*), 10 oz. ............300
w/beef and brown gravy (*Banquet* Family), 1 cup .....150
stir-fry, Asian (*Amy's*), 10 oz. ..................................240
Stroganoff (*Michelina's*), 8 oz. .................................350

**Noodle entree, frozen (*cont.*)**

and tomatoes, red and green (*Michelina's*), 8 oz. ....................240

and vegetables, w/beef (*Michelina's*), 8 oz. ...............................220

**Nopale:**

raw, sliced, 1 cup...............................................................................14

cooked, 1 pad ......................................................................................4

cooked, 1 cup .....................................................................................22

(*Doña Maria* Nopalitos), 2 tbsp. .......................................................5

**Nutmeg,** ground, 1 tsp. ....................................................................12

**Nut,** see specific listings

**Nuts, mixed,** 1 oz., except as noted:

(*Planters/Planters* Lightly Salted/Unsalted/Deluxe)..................170

(*Sweet Roasts* Cinnamon/Honey/Vanilla)...................................160

dry roasted, w/peanuts....................................................................168

dry roasted, w/peanuts, ¼ cup.......................................................203

honey roasted or sesame (*Planters*) ...........................................160

oil roasted, w/peanuts .....................................................................175

oil roasted, w/peanuts, ¼ cup.........................................................219

oil roasted, w/out peanuts...............................................................174

oil roasted, w/out peanuts, ¼ cup...................................................221

**Oat** (see also "Cereal, cooking/hot" and "Cereal, ready-to-eat"):

steel cut (*Arrowhead Mills*), ¼ cup ..............................................170

whole grain, 1 cup.............................................................................607

**Oat bran** (see also "Cereal, ready-to-eat"):

dry (*Arrowhead Mills*), ⅓ cup .......................................................150

raw, 1 cup..........................................................................................231

cooked, 1 cup .....................................................................................88

**Oat flakes,** rolled (*Arrowhead Mills*), ⅓ cup ............................130

**Oat flour:**

(*Arrowhead Mills*), ⅓ cup..............................................................120

bran (*Hodgson Mill* Blend/Organic), scant ¼ cup.....................110

bran (*Hodgson Mill*), ¼ cup ..........................................................160

**Oat groats** (*Arrowhead Mills*), ¼ cup .......................................160

**Oatmeal,** see "Cereal, cooking/hot"

**Oca** (*Frieda's*), ½ cup, 3 oz. .........................................................70

**Ocean perch,** meat only:

Atlantic, raw, 4 oz. ...........................................................................107

baked, broiled, or microwaved, 4 oz. .............................................137

**Ocean perch entree,** frozen, fillet, battered (*Van de Kamp's*),
2 pcs., 3.7 oz.........................................................................220
**Octopus,** meat only:
raw, 4 oz. .............................................................................93
boiled, poached or steamed, 4 oz. .............................................186
**Oheloberry,** fresh, raw, 10 berries, .4 oz. .....................................3
**Oil,** 1 tbsp., except as noted:
(*Arrowhead Mills* Essential Balance) .............................................130
(*House of Tsang Mongolian Fire*), 1 tsp. .........................................45
almond, apricot kernal, babassu, corn, cottonseed, cupu
    assu, grapeseed, hazelnut, oat, palm, poppy seed, rice bran,
    safflower, sesame, shea nut, soybean, sunflower, tea seed,
    walnut, or wheat germ ......................................................120
avocado, canola, or mustard .....................................................124
butter ................................................................................112
coconut or palm ....................................................................117
cod liver, herring, menhaden, salmon, or sardine........................123
flax seed (*Arrowhead Mills*).....................................................130
menhaden, fully hydrogenized....................................................113
peanut or olive......................................................................119
sesame (*Sun Luck*), 1 tsp.........................................................45
sesame, pure or hot chili (*House of Tsang*), 1 tsp. ....................45
wok (*House of Tsang*) .............................................................130
**Okra,** fresh:
raw, 8 pods, 3" long, 3.4 oz.......................................................31
raw, 1 cup ..............................................................................33
boiled, drained, 8 pods, 3" long.................................................27
boiled drained, sliced, ½ cup......................................................26
**Okra, canned,** ½ cup:
cut (*Allens/Trappey's*) ..............................................................30
w/tomatoes or tomatoes and corn (*Allens/Trappey's*)................30
gumbo, Creole (*Trappey's*) .......................................................30
**Okra, frozen:**
whole (*Birds Eye/Freshlike*), 9 pods .............................................25
cut (*Birds Eye/Freshlike*), ¾ cup .................................................25
boiled, drained, sliced, ½ cup......................................................26
and tomatoes (*Birds Eye*), ¾ cup................................................25
**Okra, pickled,** in jars:
(*Talk o' Texas*), 2 pcs., .8 oz. ......................................................10

**Okra, pickled (*cont.*)**
hot (*Trappey's* Cocktail), 1.1 oz. ...................................................10
**Olive,** pickled:
(*Peloponnese* Mixed), 4 pcs. .......................................................30
Atalanti (*Peloponnese*), 3 pcs. ....................................................25
black, see "ripe," below
green, cracked (*Krinos*), 2 pcs. ....................................................20
green, Italian (*Rienzi*), 2 pcs. ......................................................25
green, pitted, queen, stuffed w/garlic or capers (*Roland*),
   2 pcs. ......................................................................................20
green, pitted, Spanish, salad (*Early California*), 1 tbsp. ..............25
green, pitted, Spanish, stuffed (*Early California*), 4 pcs. ..............25
green, pitted, stuffed w/anchovy (*Reese's*), 4 pcs. .....................20
Ionian (*Peloponnese*), 3 pcs. .......................................................15
Kalamata (*Krinos*), 3 pcs. ...........................................................45
Kalamata, unpitted or pitted (*Peloponnese*), 5 pcs. ....................40
Nafplion (*Peloponnese*), 4 pcs. ...................................................15
ripe, Greek (*Krinos* Black), 2 pcs. ...............................................35
ripe, pitted (*Early California*), 6 small, 5 medium or 4 large .......25
ripe, pitted (*Lindsay*), 6 small, 5 medium, 4 large or 3
   extra large .............................................................................25
ripe, pitted (*Orbetti*), 5 medium or 3 extra large ......................25
ripe, pitted (*Orbetti*), 2 colossal ...............................................20
and jalapeno (*D. L. Jardine's* Texas Caviar), 2 pcs. ....................15
**Olive spread,** Kalamata, in jars (*Peloponnese*), 1 tsp. ...............15
**Onion,** fresh:
raw (*Frieda's* Boiler/Cipolline), 3 onions, 3 oz. ...........................30
raw (*Frieda's* Maui), 1/3 cup, 1.1 oz. ...........................................10
raw (*Frieda's* Pearl), 2/3 cup, 3 oz. .............................................30
raw, sliced, 1 cup ........................................................................44
raw, chopped (*Dole* Vidalia), 1/2 cup ...........................................30
raw, chopped, 1 cup ....................................................................61
boiled, drained, chopped, 1 cup ..................................................92
boiled, drained, chopped, 1 tbsp. ..................................................7
**Onion, canned or in jars:**
2.2-oz. onion................................................................................12
whole (*Hanover* O&C), 1/2 cup ....................................................25
whole, small (*S&W*), 1/2 cup .......................................................40
chopped or diced, 1/2 cup .............................................................21

white, boiled (*Twin Tree Gardens*), 1 oz. ...............5
in sauce (*Boar's Head Sweet Vidalia*) 1 tbsp. ...............10
**Onion, dehydrated,** flakes, 1 tbsp. ...............18
**Onion, dried,** minced, w/green onion (*Lawry's*), ¼ tsp. ...............0
**Onion, frozen** (see also "Onion rings"):
whole, small (*Birds Eye*), 7 pcs. ...............30
chopped (*Ore-Ida*), ¾ cup ...............25
boiled, drained, whole, 1 cup ...............59
boiled, drained, chopped, ½ cup ...............29
boiled, drained, chopped, 1 tbsp. ...............4
diced (*Birds Eye*), ⅔ cup ...............30
pearl, in cream sauce (*Birds Eye*), ½ cup ...............60
**Onion, green** (scallion), fresh:
chopped (*Andy Boy*), ¼ cup ...............10
chopped (*Dole*), ¼ cup, .9 oz. ...............10
chopped, 1 tbsp. ...............2
**Onion dip,** 2 tbsp.:
creamy or French (*Kraft* Premium) ...............45
French (*Breakstone's Free/Knudsen Free/Kraft Free*) ...............25
French (*Dean's Dips for One*) ...............60
French (*Dean's Dips for One* Lite) ...............35
French (*Frito-Lay*) ...............60
French or green (*Kraft*) ...............60
French or toasted (*Breakstone's*) ...............50
**Onion dip mix,** dry, chive (*Knorr*), ½ tsp. ...............5
**Onion gravy** (*Heinz* Home Style), ¼ cup ...............25
**Onion powder,** 1 tsp. ...............7
**Onion relish,** Vidalia, in jars, 1 tbsp.:
sweet (*Best of the South*) ...............15
zesty (*Braswell's*) ...............25
**Onion rings,** breaded, frozen:
(*Mrs. Paul's*), 4 pcs. ...............190
(*Ore-Ida Onion Ringers*), 3.2 oz., 6 pcs. ...............220
(*Ore-Ida Vidalia O's*), 3.2 oz., 5 pcs. ...............240
partially fried, oven heated, 10 large rings, 3–4" diam. ...............289
**Onion ring mix,** regular or sweet Vidalia (*Hodgson Mill*
    *Don's Chuck Wagon*), ¼ cup ...............100
**Opo squash** (*Frieda's*), ⅔ cup, 3 oz. ...............10

**Orange,** fresh:
(*Frieda's* Blood), 5 oz.................................................70
(*Frieda's* Seville), 3-oz. fruit......................................40
all common varieties:
    3¹⁄₁₆" diam..............................................................87
    sections, 1 cup....................................................85
California:
    navel, 2⁷⁄₈" diam.................................................65
    navel, sections w/out membrane, 1 cup...............76
    Valencia, 2⁵⁄₈" diam. .........................................59
    Valencia, sections w/out membrane, 1 cup..........88
Florida:
    2⁵⁄₈" diam............................................................65
    sections w/out membrane, 1 cup ......................85
w/peel, seeded, 5.6 oz. ............................................64
w/peel, sections, 1 cup.............................................68
**Orange, mandarin,** see "Tangerine"
**Orange drink:**
(*Capri Sun All Natural*), 6.76 fl. oz. ........................100
punch (*Hawaiian Punch Orange Ocean*), 8 fl. oz......120
**Orange drink blend,** 8 fl. oz., except as noted:
pineapple (*Kool-Aid Bursts Oh Yeah*), 6.76 fl. oz. ...100
pineapple apple (*Welch's*).......................................140
strawberry banana (*Chiquita*) ..................................120
**Orange drink mix,** 8 fl. oz.*:
(*Kool-Aid*)..............................................................100
(*Kool-Aid* Sugar Sweetened) ....................................60
(*Tang*)....................................................................90
pineapple (*Kool-Aid Oh Yeah*) ................................100
pineapple (*Kool-Aid Oh Yeah* Sugar Sweetened) ......60
pineapple (*Tang*)....................................................100
**Orange juice,** 8 fl. oz., except as noted:
(*Minute Maid* Original/Pulp Free) ............................110
(*Mott's*), 10-fl.-oz. bottle........................................130
(*Mott's* 16 oz.) ......................................................100
(*Mott's* 64 oz.) ......................................................130
all styles (*Florida's Natural/Florida's Natural Growers'*
    *Pride*)................................................................120
all styles (*Tropicana Pure Premium*) .......................110

fresh.....................................................................................112
canned, unsweetened .......................................................105
chilled, including from concentrate ................................110
frozen*, unsweetened........................................................112
**Orange juice blend,** 8 fl. oz.:
banana (*Tropicana Pure Premium* Calcium)..........................140
grapefruit, ruby red (*Tropicana Pure Premium* Calcium) .........100
grapefruit, unsweetened ...................................................106
kiwi passion fruit (*Tropicana Pure Tropics*)...............................100
mango peach (*Tropicana Pure Tropics*) ....................................110
pineapple (*Tropicana Pure Premium* Calcium).........................130
pineapple (*Tropicana Pure Tropics*).........................................120
punch (*Juicy Juice*) ...............................................................120
strawberry (*Tropicana Pure Premium* Calcium)........................130
strawberry banana (*Tropicana Pure Tropics*) ...........................110
tangerine (*Minute Maid/Minute Maid* Calcium)........................120
tangerine (*Tropicana Pure Premium* Calcium) .........................110
**Orange peel,** fresh, raw, 1 tbsp.............................................6
**Orange roughy,** see "Roughy"
**Oregano,** dried, ground, 1 tsp. ..............................................5
**Oriental sauce,** see "Stir-fry sauce" and specific listings
**Oyster,** meat only:
Eastern:
    farmed, raw, 6 medium, 3 oz...............................................50
    farmed, raw, 4 oz. ..............................................................67
    farmed, baked, broiled, or microwaved, 4 oz. ......................90
    wild, raw, 6 medium, 3 oz....................................................57
    wild, raw, 4 oz......................................................................77
    wild, raw, 1 cup..................................................................169
    wild, baked, broiled, or microwaved, 4 oz. ..........................82
    wild, boiled, poached, or steamed, 4 oz. ...........................155
    wild, breaded, fried, 6 medium, 3.1 oz. .............................173
Pacific, raw, 1 medium, 1¾ oz. ..........................................41
Pacific, raw, 4 oz..................................................................92
Pacific, boiled, poached or steamed, 1 medium, .9 oz. .......41
Pacific, baked, broiled, or microwaved, 4 oz........................185
**Oyster, canned:**
whole, drained (*Bumble Bee* Fancy), ⅓ of 8-oz. can .................70
Eastern, drained, 1 cup......................................................112

smoked (*Reese's*), 2 oz. ...........................................................110
smoked (*Bumble Bee* Fancy), ½ of 3.75-oz. can ......................120
**Oyster plant,** see "Salsify"
**Oyster sauce,** 1 tbsp. ...................................................................2
**Oyster stew,** see "Soup, canned, condensed"

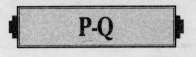

**FOOD AND MEASURE**                                    **CALORIES**

**Pad Thai sauce** (*A Taste of Thai*), 2 tbsp. .............................90
**Palm,** hearts of, canned, 1.2-oz. pc. ..........................9
**Pancake, frozen,** 3 pcs., except as noted:
(*Aunt Jemima* Homestyle) ...............................................210
(*Aunt Jemima* Low Fat) ...................................................170
(*Hungry Jack* Original) ....................................................270
blueberry or buttermilk (*Aunt Jemima*) ...........................210
buttermilk (*Eggo*), 2 pcs. ................................................190
mini (*Aunt Jemima*), 13 pcs. ...........................................240
**Pancake batter,** frozen, ½ cup:
(*Aunt Jemima* Homestyle) ...............................................260
blueberry (*Aunt Jemima*) .................................................290
buttermilk (*Aunt Jemima*) ...............................................270
**Pancake mix,** dry, ⅓ cup, except as noted:
(*Betty Crocker* Complete Original) ...................................200
(*Betty Crocker* Original Smart Size Pouch), ½ cup ............190
(*Bisquick Shake 'n Pour* Original), ½ cup .........................220
(*Hungry Jack* Extra Light and Fluffy) ...............................160
(*Hungry Jack* Original/Extra Light and Fluffy Complete) ...........150
blueberry (*Bisquick Shake 'n Pour*), ½ cup.........................240
buckwheat, oat bran, or wild rice (*Arrowhead Mills*) .............140
buttermilk:
(*Arrowhead Mills*) ......................................................120
(*Betty Crocker* Complete) .........................................200
(*Betty Crocker* Complete Smart Size Pouch), ½ cup .........210
(*Bisquick Shake 'n Pour*), ½ cup ...............................220
(*"Jiffy"* Complete) .....................................................160
corn, blue (*Arrowhead Mills*) ...........................................150
kamut (*Arrowhead Mills*), ¼ cup ......................................130
multi-grain or whole grain (*Arrowhead Mills*), ¼ cup..............120
**Pancake syrup,** ¼ cup:
(*Log Cabin* Lite) .............................................................100
(*Log Cabin* Original/*Mrs. Butterworth's* Original) .....................210

**Pancake syrup (*cont.*)**
(*Vermont Maid*)......................................................210
(*Vermont Maid* Light)..........................................100
cinnamon apple (*Mrs. Butterworth's*).................210
strawberry (*Mrs. Butterworth's*).........................220
**Pancreas,** 4 oz.:
beef, braised.........................................................307
veal, braised.........................................................290
***Papa John's Pizza:***
original crust pizza, 1 slice of 14" pie:
    *All the Meats*...............................................390
    cheese.........................................................270
    garden special............................................290
    pepperoni....................................................305
    sausage.......................................................335
    *The Works*...................................................345
thin crust pizza, 1 slice of 14" pie:
    *All the Meats*...............................................345
    cheese.........................................................225
    garden special............................................240
    pepperoni....................................................260
    sausage.......................................................285
    *The Works*...................................................295
sides:
    breadstick, 1 pc...........................................140
    cheese sticks, 2 pcs....................................180
    garlic sauce, 1 tbsp.......................................30
    nacho cheese sauce, 1 tbsp...........................14
    pizza sauce, 1 tbsp........................................10
**Papaya,** fresh:
(*Frieda's*), 1 cup, 5 oz.........................................50
cubed, peeled (*Dole*), ½ cup...............................27
mashed, 1 cup.......................................................90
**Papaya, dried** (*Frieda's*), ⅓ cup.....................140
**Papaya nectar** (*Libby's*), 11.5-fl.-oz. can.......210
**Paprika,** 1 tsp........................................................6
**Parsley,** fresh, ½ cup...........................................11
**Parsley, dried:**
1 tbsp.......................................................................4

freeze-dried, ¼ cup.............................................................................4
freeze-dried, 1 tbsp............................................................................1
**Parsley root,** raw (*Frieda's*), ⅔ cup, 3 oz.................................10
**Parsnip,** fresh:
raw, sliced, 1 cup...........................................................................100
boiled, drained, sliced, ½ cup ......................................................63
**Passion fruit,** fresh, raw:
(*Frieda's*), 5 oz. ............................................................................140
purple, 1 cup...................................................................................229
purple, trimmed, 1 fruit, .6 oz. ....................................................18
**Passion fruit drink mix** (*Crystal Light*), 8 fl. oz.* .....................5
**Passion fruit juice,** fresh, 8 fl. oz.:
purple...............................................................................................126
yellow................................................................................................148
**Pasta, dry** (see also "Macaroni" and "Noodles"), uncooked,
    2 oz., dry, except as noted:
all styles (*Delverde*) .....................................................................200
all styles (*Mueller's* Classic/Italian Style/*Savory Collection*) .....210
corn...................................................................................................202
spaghetti, plain ..............................................................................210
spaghetti, protein fortified ...........................................................213
spaghetti, spinach..........................................................................211
spaghetti, whole wheat..................................................................197
rice, brown (*Lundberg* Organic).................................................210
**Pasta, dry, cooked,** 1 cup:
corn...................................................................................................375
spaghetti, plain ..............................................................................197
spaghetti, protein fortified ...........................................................230
spaghetti, whole wheat..................................................................174
spinach .............................................................................................182
**Pasta, refrigerated,** see specific pasta listings
**Pasta dish, frozen** (see also specific pasta listings):
(*Birds Eye* Italian Style), 1 cup .................................................150
(*Birds Eye* New England Style), 9-oz. pkg................................260
cheddar (*Freshlike Pasta Combo's* Classic), 2 cups.................200
cheddar (*Stouffer's*), 11-oz. pkg................................................500
cheddar, white (*Birds Eye Pasta Secrets*), 2 cups....................240
cheese, 3 (*Birds Eye Pasta Secrets*), 2 cups............................230
cheese, 3, and broccoli (*Cedarlane*), 9-oz. pkg. .......................430

**Pasta dish, frozen (*cont.*)**

garlic, herb (*Freshlike Pasta Combo's*), 2 cups.........................260
garlic, zesty (*Birds Eye Pasta Secrets*), 2 cups ........................240
herb, Italian (*Freshlike Pasta Combo's*), 2⅓ cups....................240
pepper, roasted (*Freshlike Pasta Combo's*), 1 cup...................310
peppercorn (*Freshlike Pasta Combo's*), 2¼ cups .....................320
peppercorn, creamy (*Birds Eye Pasta Secrets*), 2⅓ cups.........300
pesto, Italian (*Birds Eye Pasta Secrets*), 2⅓ cups ...................240
primavera (*Birds Eye Pasta Secrets*), 2⅓ cups.........................230
primavera (*Green Giant*), 9-oz. pkg. .........................................300
primavera, creamy (*Freshlike Pasta Combo's*), 2¼ cups..........230
Stroganoff sauce, w/meatballs (*Freezer Queen*), 1 cup ............240
**Pasta dish, mix** (see also specific pasta listings):
Alfredo (*Bowl Appetite!*), 1 bowl ...............................................360
Alfredo, garlic (*Pasta Roni*), about 1 cup* ................................360
broccoli (*Pasta Roni*), about 1 cup*..........................................340
broccoli au gratin (*Pasta Roni*), about 1 cup*...........................280
cheddar, mild (*Pasta Roni*), about 1 cup* .................................290
cheddar, zesty (*Lipton* Pasta & Sauce), 1 cup* ........................320
cheddar broccoli (*Lipton* Pasta & Sauce), 1 cup* ....................340
chicken (*Pasta Roni*), about 1 cup*...........................................310
chicken (*Pasta Roni* Homestyle), about 1 cup* ........................230
chicken and garlic (*Pasta Roni* Low Fat), about 1 cup*............210
garlic, creamy (*Lipton* Pasta & Sauce), 1 cup* ........................350
garlic, roasted, chicken flavor (*Lipton* Pasta & Sauce),
   1 cup*.................................................................................290
herb and butter (*Pasta Roni*), about 1 cup* ..............................380
mushroom, creamy (*Lipton* Pasta & Sauce), 1 cup*................320
Parmesano (*Pasta Roni*), about 1 cup*......................................390
Romanoff (*Pasta Roni*), about 1 cup* ........................................400
salad, Caesar (*Suddenly Salad*), ¾ cup*...................................230
salad, Caesar, creamy (*Kraft*), approx. ¾ cup ..........................340
salad, classic (*Suddenly Salad*), ¾ cup* ..................................250
salad, garden Italian (*Suddenly Salad*), ¾ cup* .......................140
salad, garden primavera (*Kraft*), approx. ¾ cup........................240
salad, garlic, roasted, Parmesan (*Suddenly Salad*), ¾ cup* ....260
salad, herb and garlic (*Kraft*), approx. ¾ cup............................280
salad, Italian (*Kraft* 97% Fat Free), approx. ¾ cup ..................190
salad, Parmesan, creamy (*Suddenly Salad*), 1 cup* ................360

salad, Parmesan peppercorn (*Kraft*), approx. ¾ cup ...............360
salad, ranch and bacon (*Kraft*), approx. ¾ cup .......................350
salad, ranch and bacon (*Suddenly Salad*), ¾ cup\* .................330
**Pasta entree, canned** (see also specific listings):
**Pasta entree, frozen** (see also "Pasta dish, frozen" and specific
    pasta listings), 1 pkg., except as noted:
Alfredo primavera (*Lean Cuisine Everyday Favorites*), 10 oz. ...290
cheddar, country (*Amy's*), 1 cup .........................................250
pizza (*Michelina's*), 8.5 oz. ................................................350
primavera (*Amy's* Skillet Meals), 9.5 oz. .............................320
stuffed trio (*Marie Callender's*), 10.5 oz. .............................380
w/tomato Parmesan sauce (*Michelina's*), 8 oz .....................250
and vegetables Alfredo (*Amy's* Skillet Meals), 1 cup ..............220
**Pasta flour,** see "Semolina flour"
**Pasta salad,** see "Pasta dish, mix"
**Pasta sauce, canned or in jars** (see also "Tomato sauce" and
    specific listings), tomato, ½ cup, except as noted:
(*Del Monte* Traditional) ...........................................................60
(*Healthy Choice* Traditional) ..................................................50
(*Prego* No Salt) ...................................................................110
(*Prego* Traditional) ..............................................................140
(*Ragú Old World Style* Traditional) .........................................80
basil (*Amy's*) .........................................................................80
basil (*Classico* Di Napoli) .......................................................50
basil (*Del Monte*) ...................................................................70
basil (*Muir Glen* Organic) .......................................................50
beef, onion and garlic, sauteed (*Ragú Robusto!*) ...................100
cheese, 4 (*Classico* Di Parma) ...............................................80
cheese, 4 (*Del Monte*) ...........................................................70
cheese, 6 (*Ragú Robusto!*) .....................................................90
cheese, 3 (*Prego*) ................................................................100
cheese, Romano (*Muir Glen* Organic) ......................................90
garden combination (*Prego* Extra Chunky) .............................100
garden combination (*Ragú* Chunky Gardenstyle) .....................110
garlic:
    (*Prego* Extra Chunky Supreme) ........................................140
    and herb (*Del Monte* Chunky) ...........................................60
    and herb (*Healthy Choice*) .................................................50
    mushroom (*Amy's*) ..........................................................120

**Pasta sauce, canned or in jars, garlic (*cont.*)**

mushroom (*Healthy Choice* Garlic Lovers)............................45

and onion (*Del Monte*)................................................60

and onion (*Healthy Choice* Garlic Lovers) ........................40

and onion (*Muir Glen* Organic) ....................................55

roasted (*Classico* Di Sorrento)......................................60

roasted (*Healthy Choice* Garlic Lovers) ..........................50

roasted (*Muir Glen* Organic) .......................................50

roasted (*Ragú Robusto!*)............................................80

roasted, and herb (*Prego*)..........................................110

roasted, Parmesan (*Prego* Extra Chunky) .......................120

roasted, primavera (*Ragú* Light)...................................60

roasted, and sun-dried tomato (*Healthy Choice* Garlic

    Lovers) ...............................................................50

and Romano (*Healthy Choice* Mediterranean Harvest) .........60

super (*Ragú* Chunky Gardenstyle)..................................100

hamburger (*Prego*) ....................................................120

herb, chunky (*Muir Glen* Organic)....................................50

herb, Italian (*Del Monte* Chunky) ....................................60

herb, Italian (*Muir Glen* Organic)....................................55

marinara (*Amy's*) .......................................................50

marinara (*Prego*) .......................................................110

marinara (*Ragú Old World Style*) .....................................80

marinara, cabernet (*Muir Glen* Organic).............................50

marinara, mushroom (*Muir Glen* Organic)............................45

marinara, w/pizza sauce (*Aunt Millie's*) .............................70

marinara, sweet basil (*Classico* Di Campania) ......................70

marinara, w/wine (*Healthy Choice* Mediterranean Harvest) ........50

meat (*Del Monte*)........................................................60

meat (*Prego*)...........................................................140

meat (*Ragú Old World Style*) ..........................................80

mushroom:

    (*Del Monte*) .......................................................60

    (*Healthy Choice* Super Chunky) ................................40

    (*Prego* Extra Chunky Supreme) ................................130

    (*Prego* Made with Mushrooms)..................................150

    (*Ragú* Super Chunky Gardenstyle) .............................120

    (*Ragú Old World Style*)...........................................80

    garlic (*Healthy Choice* Super Chunky) .........................45

garlic (*Prego*) ..................................................................110
garlic (*Ragú* Light Chunky) ...........................................70
green pepper (*Prego* Extra Chunky) ............................110
green pepper (*Ragú* Chunky Gardenstyle).....................110
Parmesan (*Prego*) ........................................................130
portobello (*Classico* Di Toscana) ..................................70
portobello (*Muir Glen* Organic) .....................................50
and ripe olive (*Classico* Di Sicilia)................................70
and roasted garlic (*Ragú* Chunky Gardenstyle) ..................110
and sweet pepper, chunky (*Healthy Choice* Super) ..............45
and tomato, diced (*Prego* Extra Chunky).......................110
onion, balsamic roasted (*Muir Glen* Organic) ............................50
onion, diced, and garlic (*Prego*) ..................................120
onion and garlic, sauteed (*Ragú Robusto!*)..................90
onion and mushroom, sauteed (*Ragú Robusto!*)...............80
olive (*Pasta Gusto*), ⅓ cup........................................150
olive, green (*Muir Glen* Organic) ..................................60
Parmesan and Romano (*Ragú Robusto!*) ......................90
pepper (*Pasta Gusto*), ⅓ cup......................................100
pepper, green, and mushroom (*Del Monte*).....................60
pepper, green, and mushroom (*Muir Glen* Organic) ..................70
pepper, red, roasted, and garlic (*Prego*)......................110
pepper, red, spicy (*Classico* Di Roma Arrabbiata)...................60
pepper, red, spicy (*Ragú Robusto!*)...............................90
pepper, red, roasted (*Muir Glen* Organic)......................60
pepper, red, roasted, and onion (*Ragú* Chunky Gardenstyle) ...120
pepper, roasted, and onion (*Classico* Di Salerno) ......................60
pepper, sweet, and onion (*Muir Glen* Organic) ............................40
pepperoni (*Prego*) ......................................................120
red wine and herbs (*Ragú Robusto!*) ..............................80
Romano, peccorino, and herb (*Classico* Di Palermo)................80
sausage, Italian, and garlic (*Prego*)..............................120
sausage, Italian, w/green peppers, onions (*Classico*
    D'Abruzzi)......................................................................70
sausage, sweet, and cheese (*Ragú Robusto!*) ............................100
spinach and cheese Florentine (*Classico* Di Firenze) ..................80
tomato:
    (*Prego* Extra Chunky Supreme) ............................130
    Alfredo (*Classico* Di Liguria).................................60

**Pasta sauce, canned or in jars, tomato (*cont.*)**

basil (*Prego*)............................................................110
basil (*Ragú* Light) ...................................................50
basil (*Ragú* Light No Sugar Added) .......................60
basil and Italian cheese (*Ragú* Chunky Gardenstyle)...........110
fire roasted, and garlic (*Classico* Di Siena)...........60
garlic and onion (*Ragú* Chunky Gardenstyle) .....................120
olive oil and garlic (*Ragú* Robusto! ) ...................100
onion and garlic (*Prego* Extra Chunky)................................110
Parmesan (*Prego*) .................................................140
7 herb (*Ragú* Robusto! ) ........................................80
spicy, and pesto (*Classico* Di Genoa) ...................90
spinach and cheese (*Ragú* Chunky Gardenstyle) .................120
sun-dried (*Classico* Capri) .....................................80
sun-dried (*Muir Glen* Organic) ...............................55
sun-dried, and herb (*Healthy Choice* Mediterranean
   Harvest) ..............................................................60
vegetable (*Prego* Extra Chunky Supreme) ....................120
vegetable, garden (*Muir Glen* Organic) .........................50
vegetables, Italian style (*Healthy Choice*)....................40
vegetable primavera (*Ragú* Chunky Gardenstyle Super)...........110
vegetable primavera, chunky (*Healthy Choice* Super)................45
**Pasta sauce, refrigerated** (see also specific listings),
   tomato, ½ cup:
cheese, 4 (*Di Giorno*) .............................................160
marinara (*Contadina Buitoni*).................................80
marinara (*Di Giorno*)...............................................70
marinara, mushroom (*Contadina Buitoni*) ...............70
marinara, roasted garlic (*Contadina Buitoni*).............60
tomato cream (*Di Giorno*) .....................................160
tomato herb Parmesan (*Contadina Buitoni*) .............140
tomato and mushroom (*Di Giorno*)........................60
red pepper, roasted, cream (*Di Giorno*) ...................140
vegetable, garden (*Contadina Buitoni*)....................40
**Pasta sauce mix,** dry, 2 tbsp.:
Alfredo, carbonara, cheddar, or Parma rosa (*Knorr*)................60
4 cheese or garlic herb (*Knorr*) ...............................70

**Pasta sauce seasoning mix:**
(*Lawry's* Extra Rich and Thick Spaghetti Sauce Spices &
  Seasonings), 1 tbsp. ................................................................35
(*Lawry's* Original Style Spaghetti Sauce Spices &
  Seasonings), 1½ tbsp. .............................................................30
spatini (*Lawry's* Spaghetti Sauce Spices & Seasonings), 2 tsp. 20
**Pastrami** (see also "Turkey pastrami"):
(*Carl Buddig*), 2.5-oz. pkg. ..........................................................100
(*Boar's Head* Red Round), 2 oz. ....................................................80
(*Boar's Head* Round), 2 oz. ...........................................................70
(*Boar's Head* First Cut/Red First Cut), 2 oz. ................................90
(*Healthy Choice*), 2 oz. .................................................................60
(*Healthy Choice Deli Thin Savory Selections*), 6 slices,
  1.9 oz. .....................................................................................70
(*Healthy Deli* 95% Fat Free), 2 oz. ...............................................80
(*Hebrew National*), 4 slices, 2 oz. ................................................90
(*Russer*), 2 oz. ..............................................................................80
**Pastry flour,** see "Wheat flour"
**Pastry mix,** see "Baking mix"
**Pastry shell,** see "Puff pastry"
**Pâté** (see also specific listings):
chicken liver, 1 tbsp. .....................................................................26
duck and pork mousse w/truffles (*Marcel & Henri*), 2 oz. .......240
glazed, w/truffles (*Tour Eiffel Campagnard Française*), 2 oz. ....210
goose liver, smoked, 1 oz. ............................................................131
goose liver, smoked, 1 tbsp. ..........................................................60
**Pea pod, Chinese,** see "Peas, edible pod"
**Peach,** fresh, raw:
(*Dole*), 2 peaches ..........................................................................70
(*Frieda's* Donut/*Frieda's* Late Season), 5 oz. ..............................60
2¾" diam., approx. 2½ per lb .........................................................68
sliced, 1 cup ...................................................................................73
**Peach, canned,** ½ cup, except as noted:
in juice, halves or slices, 1 cup ....................................................109
in juice, slices (*Del Monte Fruit Naturals* Cling) ...........................80
in juice, diced (*Del Monte Fruit Cup Fruit Naturals*), 4 oz. ...........50
in juice, diced (*Dole FruitBowls*), 4.6-oz. bowl .............................80
in lightly sweetened juice, slices (*S&W* Natural Style Cling) ......80
in extra light syrup, halves or slices (*Del Monte* Lite) .................60

**Peach, canned (*cont.*)**

in extra light syrup, diced (*Del Monte Fruit Cup* Lite), 4 oz. .......50
in light syrup, slices (*Del Monte Orchard Select* Cling) .............80
in light syrup, peach flavor (*Del Monte Fruit To-Go*), 4 oz. ..........70
in heavy syrup:
    halves (*Del Monte* Cling Melba)............................................100
    halves (*S&W* Cling)...............................................................100
    halves or slices (*Del Monte* Cling/Freestone) ......................100
    diced (*Del Monte Fruit Cup*), 4 oz. ........................................80
cinnamon, in light syrup (*Del Monte* Chunky Cut Cling).............80
raspberry flavor, in light syrup (*Del Monte* Cling) ......................80
raspberry flavor, natural, in light syrup (*Del Monte Fruit*
    *Pleasures*) ..............................................................................80
raspberry flavor, wild (*Del Monte Fruitrageous* Cup), 4 oz. .......80
spiced, whole, in heavy syrup, 1 cup .........................................182
spiced, whole, in heavy syrup (*Del Monte* Cling).......................100
spiced, slices, in light syrup (*Del Monte* Cling)...........................80
in sauce (*Del Monte Fruitrageous Peachy Pie* Cup), 4 oz. ..........80
**Peach, dehydrated,** sulfured, uncooked, 1 cup ......................377
**Peach, dried,** sulfured:
uncooked, 1 half, .5 oz. ...............................................................31
uncooked, halves, 1 cup..............................................................382
stewed, 1 cup ..............................................................................199
**Peach, frozen, sliced,** sweetened, thawed, 1 cup ...................235
**Peach butter** (*Smucker's*), 1 tbsp. ...........................................45
**Peach nectar:**
(*Libby's*), 11.5-fl.-oz. can...........................................................200
(*Libby's*), 8 fl. oz. .....................................................................140
(*Libby's*), 5.5-fl.-oz. can..............................................................90
**Peanut,** shelled, except as noted:
(*Beer Nuts* Classic), 1 oz. .........................................................170
(*Frito-Lay* Salted), 3 tbsp., 1.1 oz.............................................200
(*Little Debbie* Salted), 1 oz. ......................................................160
(*Planters* Salted), 1 oz..............................................................170
all varieties, raw, ¼ cup..............................................................207
cocktail (*Planters/Planters* Salted/Unsalted), 1 oz....................170
dry roasted (*Planters*), 1 oz.......................................................160
dry roasted (*Planters* Lightly Salted), 1 oz.................................170
dry roasted, ¼ cup ......................................................................214

honey roasted (*Planters*), 1 oz. ..................................................160
honey roasted, and cashews (*Planters* Mix), 1 oz. ...................160
hot (*D. L. Jardine's* Texacali), ¼ cup, 1 oz. ...............................160
hot (*Frito-Lay*), 3 tbsp., 1.1 oz. .................................................190
hot spicy (*Planters Heat*), 1 oz. ................................................160
oil roasted, 1 oz. ........................................................................165
in shell, boiled, salted, 1 cup (edible yield 2.2 oz.) ...................200
in shell, roasted, salted (*Planters*), 1 oz. ..................................150
Spanish (*Planters*), 3 tbsp. ......................................................180
Spanish, oil roasted, 1 oz. .........................................................164
Valencia, oil roasted, 1 oz. .........................................................167
Virginia, oil roasted, 1 oz. ..........................................................164
**Peanut butter,** 2 tbsp.:
(*Laura Scudder's* Natural Style Reduced Fat) .............................220
(*Reese's* Pourable) ....................................................................220
(*Smucker's* Natural Style Reduced Fat) .....................................200
all varieties (*Arrowhead Mills*) ..................................................200
creamy or crunchy (*Adam's*) .....................................................200
creamy or crunchy (*Adam's* No Stir) ..........................................210
creamy or crunchy (*Reese's*) .....................................................200
creamy or chunky (*Smucker's* Natural) ......................................200
nutty or smooth (*Laura Scudder's* Old Fashioned) .....................200
**Peanut butter and jelly** (*Goober*), 2 tbsp. .............................230
**Peanut butter and jelly sandwich,** grape or strawberry
    (*Smucker's Uncrustables*), 2-oz. sandwich ..........................200
**Peanut butter baking chips,** ½ oz.:
(*Reese's*) ......................................................................................80
(*Reese's* Bits) ..............................................................................70
**Peanut butter sprinkles** (*Hershey's Reese's*), 2 tbsp. ............150
**Peanut butter topping** (*Smucker's Magic Shell*), 2 tbsp. ..........220
**Peanut sauce,** Oriental, 2 tbsp.:
(*Annie Chun's*) ...........................................................................120
(*San-J* Thai) ..................................................................................70
hot (*San-J*) ....................................................................................80
**Peanut sauce mix** (*A Taste of Thai*), ¼ pkt. ...........................45
**Peanut topping** (*Hershey's* Shell), 2 tbsp. ...............................220
**Pear** (see also specific listings), fresh:
(*Dole*), 1 medium .......................................................................100
1 large, approx. 2 per lb. ...........................................................123

**Pear** (*cont.*)
sliced, 1 cup..................................................................97
**Pear, Asian,** fresh, raw:
(*Frieda's*), 5 oz. ............................................................60
1 pear, 3⅜" by 3" diam., 9⅔ oz...................................116
1 pear, 2¼" by 2½" diam., 4.3 oz. ...............................51
**Pear, cactus,** see "Prickly pear"
**Pear, canned,** ½ cup, except as noted:
in juice, halves (*Del Monte Fruit Naturals*) .....................60
in juice, halves, 1 cup .................................................124
in lightly sweetened juice, Bartlett (*S&W* Natural Style) ............80
in extra light syrup, halves (*Del Monte*) ........................60
in extra light syrup, slices (*Del Monte* Lite) ..................60
in extra light syrup, diced (*Del Monte Fruit Cup* Lite), 4 oz. .......50
in light syrup, halves, 1 cup ........................................143
in light syrup, Bartlett (*Del Monte Orchard Select*)...............80
in heavy syrup, halves (*Del Monte*) .............................100
in heavy syrup, halves, Bartlett (*S&W*)............................90
in heavy syrup, diced (*Del Monte Fruit Cup*), 4 oz. ............80
cinnamon flavor, in light syrup (*Del Monte*)......................80
ginger flavor, halves (*Del Monte*) ..................................90
**Pear, dried,** halves, sulfured:
uncooked, 1 half ...........................................................47
uncooked, 1 cup ..........................................................472
stewed, 1 cup ..............................................................324
stewed, w/sugar, halves, 1 cup ...................................392
**Pear nectar:**
(*Libby's*), 11.5-fl.-oz. can...........................................210
(*Libby's*), 8 fl. oz.......................................................150
(*Libby's*), 5.5-fl.-oz. can............................................100
(*Natural Country*), 8 fl. oz. ........................................150
**Peas, black-eyed,** see "Black-eyed peas"
**Peas, butter,** frozen (*Birds Eye*), ½ cup .....................110
**Peas, creamed,** canned (*East Texas Fair*), ½ cup ..................100
**Peas, crowder,** ½ cup:
canned (*Allens/East Texas Fair*) ..................................110
frozen (*Birds Eye*) .....................................................120
**Peas, edible pod** (see also "Edamame"), fresh:
raw (*Frieda's* Snow Peas), 1 cup, 3 oz. ........................35

raw (*Frieda's* Sugar Snap), ⅔ cup, 3 oz. .......................................35
raw (*Mann's Stringless Sugar Snap*), 4 oz. ..............................50
raw, whole, 1 cup ...............................................................................27
raw, chopped, 1 cup ..........................................................................41
boiled, drained, 1 cup .......................................................................67
w/carrots (*Mann's*), 3 oz. ...............................................................40
**Peas, edible pod, frozen:**
(*Birds Eye* Deluxe Sugar Snap), ½ cup...................................40
(*Birds Eye/Freshlike* Sugar Snap Stir-Fry), ¾ cup....................35
(*Freshlike* Snow Peas), 1 cup...................................................50
(*Freshlike* Snow Pea Stir-Fry), 2 cups....................................100
(*Freshlike* Sugar Snap Select), ⅔ cup......................................45
boiled, drained, 1 cup ...................................................................83
**Peas, edible pod, combination, frozen:**
(*La Choy* Snow Pea Pods), 3 oz., approx. 42 pods ..................35
w/sweet peas and carrots (*Birds Eye* California Style)............100
w/water chestnuts (*Freshlike*), 1¼ cup ...................................50
**Peas, edible pod, pickled,** in jars (*Hogue Farms* Snappers),
   ¼ cup, 1 oz. ...............................................................................15
**Peas, field, canned,** ½ cup:
(*Sunshine*) ...................................................................................120
w/bacon (*Trappey's*) ......................................................................90
w/snaps (*Allens/East Texas Fair*) ...............................................120
w/snaps and bacon (*Trappey's*) ................................................110
**Peas, field, frozen,** w/snaps (*Birds Eye*), ⅔ cup....................130
**Peas, green,** fresh:
raw, 1 cup .....................................................................................118
raw, sugar (*Dole*), ½ cup, 2.5 oz. ...............................................30
boiled, drained, 1 cup ...................................................................134
**Peas, green, canned or in jars,** ½ cup:
early (*LeSueur*) ...............................................................................60
early June (*Crest Top*) ..................................................................100
garden (*Greene's Farm* Organic) ....................................................60
garden (*Twin Tree Gardens*) ...........................................................73
sweet (*Del Monte/Del Monte* No Salt) ............................................60
sweet (*Green Giant*) ........................................................................60
sweet (*Walnut Acres Organic Farms*) .............................................60
sweet, young, small (*Del Monte*).....................................................60
seasoned .........................................................................................57

**Peas, green, frozen,** ½ cup, except as noted:
(*Birds Eye* Deluxe) ...............................................................60
(*Freshlike/Freshlike* Select), ⅔ cup ..............................................70
(*Seabrook Farms*), ⅔ cup ..............................................70
boiled, drained, ½ cup..............................................62
baby (*Birds Eye*), ⅔ cup ..............................................70
baby, sweet (*Green Giant Le Sueur*), ⅔ cup ..............................70
baby, sweet, and butter sauce (*Green Giant Le Sueur*),
   ¾ cup ...............................................................90
petite (*Seabrook Farms* Extra Fancy), ⅔ cup............................70
**Peas, green, combination, canned or in jars:**
and carrots (*Del Monte*), ½ cup.....................................60
and carrots (*Twin Tree Gardens*), 4.5 oz. ............................78
and carrots, 1 cup.....................................................97
and onions, 1 cup.....................................................61
**Peas, green, combination, frozen:**
and carrots (*Birds Eye*), ⅔ cup.....................................50
and carrots, boiled, drained, ½ cup ...................................38
and carrots and corn (*Birds Eye* Baby Blend), ¾ cup................40
and onions, boiled, drained, 1 cup ...................................81
and onions, pearl (*Birds Eye*), ⅔ cup...............................90
w/potatoes, in cream sauce (*Birds Eye*), ½ cup ....................90
**Peas, pepper,** canned (*East Texas Fair*), ½ cup .....................120
**Peas, purple hull, canned** (*Allens/East Texas Fair*), ½ cup ....120
**Peas, purple hull, frozen** (*Birds Eye*)................................110
**Peas, snow or Chinese,** see "Peas, edible pod"
**Peas, split,** see "Split peas"
**Peas, sprouted,** mature seeds, 1 cup .....................................154
**Peas, sugar snap,** see "Peas, edible pod"
**Peas, sweet,** see "Peas, green"
**Peas, white acre,** canned (*East Texas Fair*), ½ cup ................100
**Peas and carrots or onions,** see "Peas, green, combination"
**Peas and pork,** canned (*East Texas Fair*), ½ cup ...................110
**Pecan,** shelled:
halves (*Planters*), 2-oz. pkg........................................390
halves, ¼ cup .............................................................187
chopped, ¼ cup...........................................................206
dry roasted, 1 oz..........................................................198

oil roasted, ¼ cup.................................................................197
oil roasted, 1 oz., 15 halves...............................................203
**Pecan topping** (*Smucker's* Spoonable Toppings), 2 tbsp. .......170
**Pectin,** see "Fruit pectin/protector"
**Penne,** dry, plain, see "Pasta"
**Penne dish, mix:**
black beans (*Marrakesh Express*), 1 cup*.............................170
rigate, Italian herb butter (*Land O Lakes International Pasta
    Collection*), 1 cup*.........................................................340
w/sausage flavored tomato sauce (*Classico It's Pasta
    Anytime!*), 15.25-oz. pkg............................................540
w/tomato and mushroom sauce (*Classico It's Pasta
    Anytime!*), 15.25-oz. pkg............................................510
tomato Parmesan (*Bowl Appetite!*), 1 bowl ............................350
sun-dried tomato Parmesan sauce (*Knorr*), ½ cup.................270
**Penne entree,** frozen, 1 pkg., except as noted:
and chicken bake (*Stouffer's*), 11.5 oz. ...............................350
marinara, w/Italian sausage (*Michelina's*), 8 oz. ....................250
w/meat sauce (*Freezer Queen*), 9 oz. .................................250
and meatballs (*Marie Callender's* Skillet Meals), ½ of
    24-oz. pkg. ...............................................................600
w/mushrooms (*Michelina's*), 8 oz........................................250
w/mushroom sauce (*Michelina's*), 8 oz. ...............................280
pollo (*Michelina's*), 8.5 oz. ...............................................290
primavera (*Michelina's*), 8.5 oz. ........................................280
w/tomato basil sauce (*Lean Cuisine Everyday Favorites*),
    10 oz. .......................................................................260
**Pepeao:**
raw, .2-oz. piece................................................................2
raw, sliced, 1 cup.............................................................25
dried, 1 cup.....................................................................72
**Pepper, seasoning,** 1 tsp., except as noted:
black, whole......................................................................8
black, ground....................................................................5
chili .................................................................................9
lemon, garlic, or seasoned (*Lawry's*), ¼ tsp. ..........................0
red or cayenne..................................................................6
white ...............................................................................7

**Pepper, ancho**, dried, .6-oz. pepper ........................................47
**Pepper, banana:**
fresh, raw, 1 small, 1.2 oz. .....................................................9
canned (*Trappey's*), 1 oz. ......................................................5
**Pepper, bell,** see "Pepper, sweet"
**Pepper, cherry,** mild, in jars (*Trappey's*), 1.1 oz. ..................10
**Pepper, chili,** fresh:
green or red, 1.6-oz. pepper ..................................................18
green or red, chopped or diced, 1 cup ..................................30
**Pepper, chili, canned or in jars:**
green, whole (*Ortega*), 1 pc. ................................................15
green, whole or diced (*Chi-Chi's*), 1 oz. .............................10
green, chopped (*Ortega*), 2 tbsp. ........................................10
green or red, 2.6-oz. pepper..................................................15
green or red, chopped or diced, ½ cup .................................14
red, minced (*A Taste of Thai*), 2 tbsp. .................................40
**Pepper, chili, dried,** 1 pepper ...........................................2
**Pepper, Hungarian,** fresh, raw, 1-oz. pepper .......................8
**Pepper, jalapeno,** fresh, raw:
.5-oz. pepper..........................................................................4
sliced, 1 cup..........................................................................27
**Pepper, jalapeno, canned:**
whole (*Ortega*), 2 pcs. .........................................................10
whole or wheels (*Chi-Chi's*), 1 oz. ......................................10
sliced (*Trappey's*), 1 oz. .......................................................5
sliced, 1 cup..........................................................................28
chopped (*Ortega*), 2 tbsp. ...................................................10
chopped, 1 cup......................................................................37
**Pepper, pasilla,** dried, ¼-oz. pepper..................................24
**Pepper, poblano,** canned (*Herdez*), 3.5 oz. .....................24
**Pepper, roasted,** see "Pepper, sweet, in jars"
**Pepper, serrano,** fresh, raw:
.2-oz. pepper..........................................................................2
chopped, 1 cup......................................................................34
**Pepper, stuffed, entree,** frozen:
(*Stouffer's*), 10-oz. pkg........................................................210
green (*Stouffer's*), ½ of 15.5-oz. pkg..................................180
green (*Stouffer's*), ¼ of 32-oz. pkg....................................200

**Pepper, sweet,** fresh:
(*Dole*), 1 medium, 5.3 oz. ..............................................30
green or red, raw, sliced, 1 cup ...................................25
green or red, raw, chopped, 1 cup ...............................40
green or red, boiled, drained, 1 tbsp. .............................3
green or red, boiled, drained, strips, 1 cup ..................38
yellow, raw, 1 large, 5" by 3" diam. .............................50
yellow, raw, 10 strips, 1.8 oz. ......................................14
**Pepper, sweet, canned or in jars:**
(*Trappey's* Tempero), 1 oz. ...........................................5
green or red, ½ cup ......................................................13
pickled (*Hogue Farms* Sweet Bells), ¼ cup ...............25
roasted (*Peloponnese* Florina), 1 oz. ..........................10
**Pepper, sweet, freeze-dried,** ¼ cup ...........................5
**Pepper, sweet, frozen:**
(*Birds Eye* Stir-Fry/*Freshlike* Stir-Fry), 1 cup ............25
green, diced (*Birds Eye*), ¾ cup .................................20
green, and onion (*Seabrook Farms* Stir-Fry), 1 cup .....25
**Pepper, tabasco,** in vinegar (*Trappey's*), 1 oz. ..........5
**Pepper, torrido** (*Trappey's*), 1.3 oz. ..........................10
**Pepper dip,** red (*Victoria*), ¼ cup ............................50
**Pepper relish:**
hot or sweet (*Cains*), 1 tbsp. .....................................20
chile (*Patak's*), 1 tbsp. ...............................................50
**Pepper sauce** (see also "Hot sauce"), 2 tbsp.:
cracked (*San-J*) ...........................................................35
lemon or tomato (*San-J*) .............................................45
**Pepper spread,** sweet, in jars (*Peloponnese*), 1 tbsp. ....15
**Pepper steak,** see "Beef entree"
**Peppercorn sauce mix,** dry (*Knorr* Classic), 2 tsp. ....25
**Peppermint,** fresh, 2 tbsp. ...........................................2
**Pepperoni** (see also "Turkey pepperoni"):
(*Hormel* Chunk/Twin), 1 oz. .....................................140
(*Sara Lee* Sandwich), 7 slices, 1.1 oz. ....................140
(*Sara Lee* Sandwich Size Deli), 7 slices, .9 oz. .......120
pork and beef, 1 oz. ..................................................141
pork and beef, .2-oz. slice ...........................................27
sliced (*Hormel*), 15 slices, 1 oz. ..............................140
sliced (*Hormel Pillow Pack*), 14 slices, 1 oz. ...........140

**Perch** (see also "Ocean perch"), meat only:
raw, 4 oz. ...............................................................................103
baked, broiled, or microwaved, 4 oz. ................................133
**Persimmon,** fresh:
(*Dole*), 1 medium ..................................................................32
(*Frieda's*), 5 oz. ....................................................................140
Japanese, 2½" diam., 5.9 oz. .............................................118
native, trimmed, 1 .9 oz. .......................................................32
**Persimmon, dried:**
fuyu (*Frieda's*), ⅓ cup .........................................................140
Japanese, trimmed, 1.2 oz. ...................................................93
**Pesto sauce, in jars:**
(*Christopher Ranch*), ¼ cup ...............................................190
(*Pasta Gusto*), ⅓ cup .........................................................320
basil and garlic (*Christopher Ranch*), ¼ cup .....................230
**Pesto sauce, refrigerated,** ¼ cup:
basil (*Di Giorno*) .................................................................320
w/basil (*Contadina Buitoni*) ...............................................290
w/basil (*Contadina Buitoni* Reduced Fat) ..........................230
garlic (*Di Giorno*) ...............................................................340
w/sun-dried tomatoes (*Contadina Buitoni*) ........................190
**Pesto sauce mix:**
(*Knorr*), 2 tsp. .......................................................................15
creamy (*Knorr*), 1 tbsp. ........................................................15
red bell pepper (*Knorr*), ⅔ tbsp. .........................................25
sun-dried tomato (*Knorr*), 1 tbsp. ........................................35
**Pheasant,** raw, 4 oz., except as noted:
meat w/skin ...........................................................................205
meat only ...............................................................................151
breast, meat only, ½ breast, 6.4 oz. ....................................242
breast, meat only .................................................................151
leg, meat only, 3.8 oz. .........................................................143
leg, meat only .......................................................................152
**Picante sauce** (see also "Salsa"), all varieties, 2 tbsp.:
(*Chi-Chi's*) .............................................................................10
(*Muir Glen* Organic) ..............................................................10
(*Ortega* Green Chile) .............................................................10
(*Pace*) ....................................................................................10

(*Taco Bell Home Originals* Smooth 'N Zesty) ..............................15
(*Shotgun Willie's* Hotter'n Hell) ........................................10
**Pickle, cucumber:**
bread and butter (*Claussen*), 4 slices, 1 oz. ........................20
bread and butter (*Mrs. Fanning's Bread'n Butter*), 1 oz. ..........25
cornichon (*Dessaux*), 5 pcs., .6 oz. ......................................0
dill, all varieties (*B&G*), 1 oz. .............................................0
dill, whole (*Claussen*), ½ pickle, 1 oz. ..................................5
dill, whole or tiny kosher (*Del Monte*), 1½ pcs., 1 oz. ............5
dill, halves (*Del Monte*), ¼ pickle, 1 oz. ................................5
dill, sliced (*Claussen* Super Slices for Burgers), 1 oz. ............5
dill, chips (*Del Monte* Hamburger), 5 pcs., 1 oz. ....................5
dill, chopped or diced, 1 cup ................................................26
kosher (*Hebrew National*), 1 pickle .....................................23
sour, 1 large, 4" long, 4¾ oz. ..............................................15
sweet, sliced, 1 cup .........................................................199
sweet, chips (*Del Monte*), 5 pcs., 1 oz. ...............................40
sweet, gherkin (*Del Monte* 12 oz.), 1 oz. .............................40
sweet, midget (*Del Monte*), 3 pickles, 1 oz. .........................40
**Pickle relish, cucumber** (see also "Chow chow relish"),
    1 tbsp.:
(*Crosse & Blackwell* Branston) ............................................25
hamburger ........................................................................19
hamburger or sweet (*Del Monte*) .........................................20
hot dog (*Del Monte*) ...........................................................15
hot dog .............................................................................14
India (*Heinz*) ....................................................................20
sweet .................................................................................20
**Pie:**
apple (*Entenmann's* Homestyle), ⅙ pie .............................370
coconut custard (*Entenmann's*), ⅕ pie ..............................340
lemon (*Entenmann's*), ⅙ pie ..............................................340
pumpkin (*Entenmann's*), ⅕ pie ...........................................270
sweet potato (*Entenmann's*), ⅙ pie ....................................290
**Pie, frozen:**
apple (*Amy's*), ½ pie ........................................................220
apple (*Mrs. Smith's*), ⅛ pie ...............................................340
apple (*Mrs. Smith's Special Recipe*), 1/12 pie ......................330
apple, Dutch (*Mrs. Smith's*), ⅛ pie .....................................360

**Pie, frozen (*cont.*)**

apple, Dutch (*Mrs. Smith's Special Recipe*), 1/10 pie .................320
apple (*Sara Lee* 45% Reduced Fat), 1/6 pie................................290
apple (*Sara Lee* Homestyle), 1/8 pie .......................................350
apple or cherry (*Mrs. Smith's* No Sugar Added), 1/8 pie ...........350
blueberry (*Mrs. Smith's*), 1/8 pie .............................................330
blueberry (*Sara Lee* Homestyle), 1/8 pie..................................360
cappuccino (*Mrs. Smith's Restaurant Classics*), 1/9 pie ............360
cherry (*Mrs. Smith's*), 1/8 pie ..................................................360
cherry or cherry-berry (*Mrs. Smith's Special Recipe*), 1/12 pie..330
cherry (*Sara Lee* Homestyle), 1/8 pie ......................................320
chocolate cream or lemon cream (*Mrs. Smith's*), 1/3 pie ..........440
chocolate mint (*Mrs. Smith's Cookies & Cream*), 1/6 pie ..........390
chocolate silk (*Sara Lee* Supreme), 1/5 pie ..............................500
coconut cream (*Sara Lee*), 1/5 pie............................................480
coconut custard (*Mrs. Smith's*), 1/8 pie ...................................250
French silk (*Mrs. Smith's Restaurant Classics*), 1/9 pie .............560
lemon meringue (*Sara Lee*), 1/6 pie .........................................350
lemony lemon (*Mrs. Smith's Cookies & Cream*), 1/6 pie ...........370
lime, Key (*Mrs. Smith's Restaurant Classics*), 1/9 pie................420
mince (*Mrs. Smith's*), 1/8 pie....................................................360
mince (*Sara Lee* Homestyle), 1/8 pie ........................................360
peach (*Mrs. Smith's*), 1/8 pie ...................................................320
peach (*Mrs. Smith's Special Recipe*), 1/12 pie ...........................300
peach (*Sara Lee* Homestyle), 1/8 pie ........................................320
peanut butter silk (*Mrs. Smith's Restaurant Classics*), 1/9 pie...600
pecan (*Mrs. Smith's*), 1/5 pie....................................................560
pecan (*Mrs. Smith's Special Recipe*), 1/8 pie .............................550
pecan (*Sara Lee* Homestyle), 1/8 pie ........................................520
pumpkin (*Sara Lee* Homestyle), 1/8 pie.....................................260
pumpkin (*Mrs. Smith's* Hearty), 1/8 pie.....................................260
pumpkin (*Mrs. Smith's Special Recipe* Homemade), 1/10 pie ....290
pumpkin custard (*Mrs. Smith's*), 1/8 pie ...................................240
raspberry (*Mrs. Smith's*), 1/8 pie ..............................................330
raspberry (*Sara Lee* Homestyle), 1/8 pie ..................................380
s'mores (*Mrs. Smith's Cookies & Cream*), 1/6 pie .....................410
strawberry banana (*Mrs. Smith's Cookies & Cream*), 1/6 pie ....380
sweet potato custard (*Mrs. Smith's*), 1/8 pie.............................330
**Pie, mix,** chocolate silk (*Jell-O* No Bake), 1/6 pie* ...................320

**Pie, snack:**
apple (*Drake's*), 2 pcs., 4 oz. .......................................................400
apple (*Hostess*), 4.5-oz. pc. .......................................................480
cherry (*Hostess*), 4.5-oz. pc. .......................................................470
**Pie crust:**
cookie, chocolate (*Oreo*), 1/6 crust......................................140
cookie, shortbread (*Ready Crust*), 1/8 crust .........................110
cookie, vanilla (*Nilla* Wafer), 1/6 crust ...................................140
graham cracker (*Honey Maid*), 1/6 crust ...............................140
graham cracker (*Ready Crust*), 1/8 crust................................110
graham cracker (*Ready Crust* Reduced Fat), 1/8 crust..................90
graham cracker (*Ready Crust* Single Serve), 1 crust................120
graham cracker, chocolate (*Ready Crust*), 1/8 crust...................110
**Pie crust, frozen or refrigerated:**
(*Pillsbury*), 1/8 crust......................................................................120
(*Mrs. Smith's*), 1/8 crust................................................................100
deep dish (*Mrs. Smith's*), 1/8 crust .............................................110
**Pie crust mix\*:**
(*Betty Crocker*), 1/8 crust ...........................................................110
(*"Jiffy"*), 1/7 pkg. .........................................................................180
(*Pillsbury*), 1/8 crust....................................................................100
**Pie filling,** canned:
apple (*Lucky Leaf* Lite), 3 oz., 1/7 can .....................................25
apple (*Lucky Leaf/Lucky Leaf* Premium), 3 oz., 1/7 can...............90
apple, blueberry, or peach (*Comstock* More Fruit), 1/3 cup .........80
apricot or blueberry (*Lucky Leaf*), 3 oz., 1/7 can.........................90
berry, triple (*Crosse & Blackwell*), 1/3 cup................................120
blueberry (*Lucky Leaf* Lite), 3 oz., 1/7 can ................................60
blueberry (*Lucky Leaf* Premium), 3 oz., 1/7 can .......................100
cherry (*Comstock* Original), 1/3 cup...........................................90
cherry (*Comstock* Original Lite), 1/3 cup....................................60
cherry (*Lucky Leaf/Lucky Leaf* Premium), 3 oz., 1/7 can...........100
cherry (*Lucky Leaf* Lite), 3 oz., 1/7 can .....................................35
lemon (*Comstock*), 1/3 cup........................................................130
lemon (*Lucky Leaf*), 3 oz., 1/7 can.............................................120
mincemeat, plain or rum/brandy (*Crosse & Blackwell*),
   1/4 cup .....................................................................................180
mincemeat (*Lucky Leaf*), 3 oz., 1/8 can....................................140
peach or strawberry (*Lucky Leaf*), 3 oz., 1/7 can ........................80

**Pie filling (*cont.*)**
pumpkin (*Comstock*), ⅓ cup......................................................90
raisin (*Lucky Leaf*), 3 oz., ⅟₇ can...........................................90
**Pie filling mix,** see "Pudding and pie filling mix"
**Pie glaze,** see "Glaze, fruit"
**Pierogi,** frozen:
"cheddar" and potato, nondairy (*Tofutti*), 4 pcs., 5.3 oz. .........185
cheese, American (*Mrs. T's*), 3 pcs., 4.25 oz............................220
jalapeno and cheddar (*Mrs. T's*), 3 pcs., 4.25 oz.....................190
jalapeno and cheddar, mini (*Mrs. T's 'Rogies*), 7 pcs., 3 oz. ....130
potato and cheddar, mini (*Mrs. T's 'Rogies*), 7 pcs., 3 oz. .......130
potato cheese (*Empire Kosher*), 5.3 oz. ..................................243
potato and cheese or potato and onion (*Mrs. T's*), 3 pcs.,
    4.25 oz. ...............................................................................180
potato onion (*Empire Kosher*), 5.3 oz. ....................................247
potato and roasted garlic (*Mrs. T's*), 3 pcs., 4.25 oz. ..............270
sauerkraut (*Mrs. T's*), 3 pcs., 4.25 oz. ...................................170
sweet potato (*Mrs. T's*), 3 pcs., 4.25 oz..................................270
**Pigeon peas,** immature, fresh:
raw, 10 pigeon peas ....................................................................5
raw, 1 cup................................................................................209
boiled, drained, 1 cup...............................................................170
**Pigeon peas, mature:**
dry, 1 cup.................................................................................703
boiled, 1 cup............................................................................203
**Pig's feet,** pickled (*Hormel*), 2 oz............................................80
**Pignolia nuts,** see "Pine nuts"
**Pike,** meat only:
northern, raw, 4 oz. ..................................................................100
northern, baked, broiled, or microwaved, 4 oz. .........................128
walleye, raw, 4 oz. ...................................................................106
walleye, baked, broiled, or microwaved, 4 oz. ...........................135
**Pili nuts,** dried, shelled, ¼ cup..............................................216
**Pimento,** canned:
1 cup..........................................................................................44
1 tbsp..........................................................................................3
**Piña colada mix,** bottled:
(*Daily's*), 3 fl. oz.....................................................................160
(*Mr & Mrs T*), 4.5 fl. oz. ..........................................................180

**Pine nuts,** dried:

(*Frieda's*), ¼ cup, 1.1 oz............................................150

pignolia, 1 oz. ...................................................161

pignolia, ¼ cup .................................................192

pignolia, 1 tbsp. ...............................................161

pinyon, 10 kernels ................................................6

pinyon, 1 oz. .....................................................178

**Pineapple,** fresh:

1 lb., whole ......................................................231

sliced (*Dole*), 2 slices ..........................................70

diced, 1 cup ......................................................76

sugar loaf, baby (*Frieda's*), 3 oz. ..............................70

**Pineapple, candied,** slices (*S&W*), 1 pc. .....................180

**Pineapple, canned,** ½ cup, except as noted:

in juice, chunks or tidbits .......................................60

in juice, crushed (*Dole*) ........................................70

in juice, crushed, sliced, or chunks ..............................75

in juice, slice or ring, 1 pc. w/liquid ...........................28

in juice, slices (*Del Monte*), 2 pcs. ............................60

in juice, slices (*Dole*), 2 pcs. .................................60

in juice, spears, wedges, chunks, tidbits, or crushed

   (*Del Monte*) .................................................70

in juice, tidbits (*Del Monte Fruit Cup*), 4 oz....................50

in juice, lightly sweetened, shapes (*Dole Fun Shapes*) ...........80

in light syrup, crushed, sliced or chunks .........................65

in light syrup, slice or ring, 1 pc. w/liquid .....................25

in heavy syrup, chunks or tidbits (*Dole*) ........................90

in heavy syrup, crushed (*Dole*) ..................................90

in heavy syrup, crushed or chunks (*Del Monte*) ...................90

in heavy syrup, crushed, sliced or chunks .........................99

in heavy syrup, slice or ring, 1 pc. w/liquid .....................38

in heavy syrup, slices (*Del Monte*), 2 pcs. ......................90

in heavy syrup, slices (*Dole*), 2 pcs. ...........................90

**Pineapple, frozen,** sweetened, chunks, 1 cup ...................208

**Pineapple apricot sauce** (*Sable & Rosenfeld*), 2 tbsp. .........80

**Pineapple drink blends,** guava mango or orange banana

   (*Chiquita*), 8 fl. oz.........................................120

**Pineapple drink mix,** 8 fl. oz.*:
(*Kool-Aid* Piña) ............................................................100
(*Kool-Aid* Piña Sugar Sweetened) ................................60
**Pineapple juice,** 8 fl. oz., except as noted:
(*Del Monte*)...............................................................130
(*Del Monte*), 6 oz. .......................................................80
(*Del Monte* Not from Concentrate)..............................110
(*Dole*)........................................................................120
frozen*, unsweetened..................................................130
**Pineapple juice blends,** 8 fl. oz.:
orange or orange banana (*Dole*) ................................120
orange strawberry (*Dole*) ..........................................130
**Pineapple topping,** 2 tbsp.:
(*Kraft*)........................................................................110
(*Smucker's* Spoonable Toppings)...............................110
**Pink bean,** mature:
dry, 1 cup...................................................................720
boiled, 1 cup...............................................................252
**Pinto bean,** mature:
dry (*Arrowhead Mills*), ¼ cup .....................................150
dry, 1 cup...................................................................656
boiled, 1 cup...............................................................234
**Pinto bean, canned** (*Allens/Brown Beauty*), ½ cup ............110
**Pinto bean, frozen,** boiled, drained, ⅓ of 10-oz. pkg. .........152
**Pistachio nut,** shelled, except as noted:
raw, 1 oz., 47 kernels .................................................156
raw, ¼ cup..................................................................176
dry roasted (*Planters*), ½ cup ....................................160
dry roasted, ¼ cup......................................................182
dry roasted, 1 oz.........................................................162
dry roasted, in shell (*Planters*), 2.25-oz. pkg............190
**Pita,** see "Bread"
**Pitanga,** fresh:
trimmed, ¼ oz. ................................................................3
1 cup............................................................................57
**Pizza,** frozen:
bacon cheeseburger (*Jack's Great Combinations* 12"),
    ¼ pie ....................................................................360
bacon cheeseburger (*Jack's Naturally Rising* 12"), ⅙ pie.........350

Canadian bacon (*Jack's Naturally Rising* 12"), ⅙ pie...............280
Canadian bacon (*Tombstone* Original 12"), ¼ pie.....................350
cheese (*Amy's*), ⅓ pie.............................................................300
cheese (*Celeste* Large), ¼ pie..............................................300
cheese (*Celeste* Pizza for One), 1 pie...................................420
cheese (*Empire Kosher*), 4-oz. pie.........................................220
cheese (*Empire Kosher* 10 oz.), ⅓ pie...................................340
cheese (*Jack's Naturally Rising* 12"), ⅙ pie............................290
cheese (*Jack's Naturally Rising* 9"), ⅓ pie..............................300
cheese (*Michelina's* Singles), 1 pie.......................................380
cheese (*Michelina's That'za Pizza!*), 1 pie.............................370
cheese, double (*Jack's Great Combinations* 12"), ¼ pie..........380
cheese, double (*Jack's Great Combinations* 9"), ½ pie.............430
cheese, extra (*Tombstone* Original 12"), ¼ pie.......................350
cheese, extra (*Tombstone* Original 9"), ½ pie.........................380
cheese, 4 (*Celeste* Pizza for One Original/Zesty), 1 pie............470
cheese, 4 (*Celeste* Rising Crust), ⅙ pie.................................320
cheese, 4 (*Di Giorno* 12"), ⅛ pie............................................320
cheese, 4 (*Di Giorno* 8"), ⅓ pie.............................................260
cheese, 3 (*Tombstone Oven Rising*), ⅙ pie.............................320
cheese, 3 (*Tombstone* Thin Crust), ¼ pie...............................360
cheese, 3 (*Tombstone* Double Top), ⅙ pie..............................380
"cheese," nondairy (*Amy's* Soy Cheeze), ⅓ pie.......................280
"cheese," nondairy (*Tofutti* Pizzaz), ⅓ pkg. ...........................175
chicken supreme (*Di Giorno* 8"), ⅓ pie...................................270
chicken supreme, zesty (*Celeste* Pizza for One), 1 pie.............380
combination (*Michelina's* Singles), 1 pie................................400
deluxe (*Celeste* Large), ¼ pie................................................340
deluxe (*Tombstone* Original 12"), ⅕ pie..................................310
deluxe (*Tombstone* Original 9"), ⅓ pie....................................280
hamburger (*Tombstone* Original 12"), ⅕ pie............................310
hamburger (*Tombstone* Original 9"), ⅓ pie..............................280
meat, 4 (*Tombstone* Thin Crust Combo), ¼ pie........................380
meat, 3 (*Celeste* Rising Crust), ⅙ pie....................................340
meat, 3 (*Di Giorno* 12"), ⅛ pie...............................................380
meat, 3 (*Di Giorno* 8"), ⅓ pie.................................................310
meat, 3 (*Tombstone Oven Rising*), ⅙ pie................................340
mushroom and olive (*Amy's*), ⅓ pie.......................................250
pepperoni (*Banquet*), 6.75 oz. ..............................................480

**Pizza (cont.)**

pepperoni (*Celeste* Large), ¼ pie ............................................350
pepperoni (*Celeste* Pizza for One), 1 pie ...............................470
pepperoni (*Celeste* Rising Crust), ⅙ pie ................................330
pepperoni (*Di Giorno* 12"), ⅛ pie ..........................................370
pepperoni (*Di Giorno* 8"), ⅓ pie ............................................300
pepperoni (*Jack's Great Combinations* 12"), ¼ pie .................410
pepperoni (*Jack's Naturally Rising* 9"), ⅓ pie ........................360
pepperoni (*Michelina's* Singles), 1 pie ..................................410
pepperoni (*Michelina's That'za Pizza!*), 1 pie........................400
pepperoni (*Tombstone* Double Top), ⅛ pie...............................340
pepperoni (*Tombstone* Thin Crust), ¼ pie ...............................400
pepperoni (*Tombstone* Original 12"), ¼ pie .............................400
pepperoni (*Tombstone* Original 9"), ⅓ pie ...............................300
pepperoni (*Tombstone* Oven Rising), ⅙ pie ............................340
pepperoni supreme (*Jack's Naturally Rising* 12"), ⅙ pie ..........340
pepperoni and mushroom (*Jack's Great Combinations* 12"),
   ¼ pie .................................................................................340
pepperoni and sausage:
   (*Jack's Great Combinations* 9"), ½ pie .............................380
   (*Tombstone* Original 9"), ⅓ pie.........................................300
pesto, w/tomato and broccoli (*Amy's*), ⅓ pie ........................300
sausage (*Celeste* Pizza for One), 1 pie ..................................480
sausage (*Jack's Great Combinations* 12"), ¼ pie ...................390
sausage (*Jack's Naturally Rising* 12"), ⅙ pie .........................340
sausage (*Jack's Naturally Rising* 9"), ⅓ pie ...........................360
sausage (*Tombstone* Double Top), ⅛ pie .................................320
sausage (*Tombstone* Original 12"), ⅕ pie ...............................300
sausage (*Tombstone* Original 9"), ⅓ pie ..................................310
sausage, Italian (*Di Giorno* 12"), ⅛ pie ..................................360
sausage, Italian (*Di Giorno* 8"), ⅓ pie ....................................300
sausage, Italian (*Tombstone* Oven Rising), ⅙ pie ...................320
sausage, Italian (*Tombstone* Thin Crust), ¼ pie .....................370
sausage, Italian, spicy (*Jack's Naturally Rising* 12"), ⅙ pie......330
sausage and mushroom (*Jack's Great Combinations* 12"),
   ¼ pie .................................................................................310
sausage and mushroom (*Tombstone* Original 12"), ⅕ pie .......300
sausage and pepperoni:
   (*Celeste* Pizza for One), 1 pie.........................................560

(*Jack's Great Combinations* 12"), ¼ pie................................350
(*Jack's Naturally Rising* Combination 12"), ⅙ pie .............360
(*Jack's Naturally Rising* Combination 9"), ¼ pie...............300
(*Tombstone* Double Top), ⅛ pie .....................................340
(*Tombstone* Original 12"), ⅕ pie.....................................320
spinach (*Amy's*), ⅓ pie.....................................................320
spinach (*Di Giorno* 8"), ⅓ pie.........................................250
supreme (*Celeste* Pizza for One Suprema), 1 pie...................530
supreme (*Celeste* Rising Crust), ⅙ pie .............................360
supreme (*Di Giorno* 12"), ⅛ pie.......................................380
supreme (*Di Giorno* 8"), ⅓ pie .......................................310
supreme (*Jack's Great Combinations* 12"), ¼ pie .............350
supreme (*Michelina's* Singles), 1 pie ................................400
supreme (*Tombstone* Double Top), ⅛ pie.........................330
supreme (*Tombstone* Original 12"), ⅕ pie .......................320
supreme (*Tombstone* Oven Rising), ⅙ pie .......................320
supreme (*Tombstone* Thin Crust), ¼ pie ..........................380
taco, supreme (*Tombstone* Thin Crust), ¼ pie .................370
vegetable (*Amy's* Veggie Combo), ⅓ pie ...........................250
vegetable (*Celeste* Pizza for One), 1 pie ............................430
vegetable (*Di Giorno* 12"), ⅛ pie.....................................310
vegetable (*Di Giorno* 8"), ⅓ pie .......................................250
vegetable, roasted (*Amy's*), ⅓ pie ....................................270
the works (*Jack's Naturally Rising* 12"), ⅙ pie .................330
the works (*Jack's Naturally Rising* 9"), ¼ pie....................280
**Pizza, bagel,** frozen:
(*Tofutti* Cheese Pizzaz), 1 pc..............................................175
cheese (*Empire* Kosher), 2.25-oz. pc.................................100
**Pizza, English muffin,** frozen, cheese (*Empire Kosher*),
  2-oz. pc. ........................................................................130
**Pizza, French bread,** frozen:
cheese (*Lean Cuisine Everyday Favorites*), 6-oz. pkg. ..............320
cheese (*Marie Callender's*), 7.2-oz. pkg. .....................................530
cheese (*Stouffer's*), ½ of 10⅜-oz. pkg. .....................................370
cheese, extra (*Stouffer's*), ½ of 11.75-oz. pkg.........................400
cheese, 5 (*Stouffer's*), ½ of 10.25-oz. pkg..............................410
cheese or pepperoni (*Healthy Choice Meals To Go*),
  6-oz. pkg. ......................................................................340
deluxe (*Lean Cuisine Everyday Favorites*), 6-oz. pkg. ...............290

**Pizza, French bread (*cont.*)**
deluxe (*Stouffer's*), ½ of 12⅜-oz. pkg. ...................................420
garlic, creamy (*Lean Cuisine*), 6-oz. pkg. ...........................310
meat, 3 (*Stouffer's*), ½ of 12.5-oz. pkg. ..............................460
pepperoni (*Lean Cuisine Everyday Favorites*), 5.25-oz. pkg. ....300
pepperoni (*Marie Callender's*), 7.5-oz. pkg. ..........................570
pepperoni (*Stouffer's*), ½ of 11.25-oz. pkg. ..........................390
pepperoni mushroom (*Stouffer's*), ½ of 12.25-oz. pkg. ...........440
sausage (*Healthy Choice Meals To Go*), 6-oz. pkg. ..................320
sausage (*Stouffer's*), ½ of 12-oz. pkg. .................................420
sausage and pepperoni (*Stouffer's*), ½ of 12.5-oz. pkg. ...........470
sun-dried tomato (*Lean Cuisine Everyday Favorites*),
   6-oz. pkg. ..................................................................340
supreme (*Healthy Choice Meals To Go*), 6-oz. pkg. .................330
supreme (*Marie Callender's*), 7.5-oz. pkg. .............................510
vegetable (*Healthy Choice Meals To Go*), 6-oz. pkg. ................280
vegetable, grilled (*Stouffer's*), ½ of 11⅝-oz. pkg. ..................350
white (*Stouffer's*), ½ of 10⅛-oz. pkg. ..................................470
**Pizza crust,** refrigerated (*Pillsbury*), ⅕ pkg. ...........................150
**Pizza crust mix:**
plain or Italian herb (*Betty Crocker Pouch*), ¼ crust* .............160
(*"Jiffy"*), ⅓ cup .................................................................160
***Pizza Hut,*** 1 slice of medium pie, except as noted:
Big New Yorker:
   cheese .............................................................................393
   pepperoni .........................................................................380
   supreme ...........................................................................459
*Edge:*
   chicken supreme ................................................................90
   *Meat Lover's* ....................................................................160
   *Veggie Lover's* ...................................................................70
   works ...............................................................................110
hand tossed:
   cheese .............................................................................309
   chicken supreme ...............................................................291
   beef .................................................................................347
   ham .................................................................................279
   *Meat Lover's* ....................................................................376
   pepperoni .........................................................................301

*Pepperoni Lover's* ........................................372
pork topping........................................342
sausage, Italian ...............................363
super supreme ...............................359
supreme ............................................333
taco......................................................280
taco, beef...........................................270
taco, chicken ....................................290
taco, meatless ..................................250
*Veggie Lover's*.................................281
Personal Pan Pizza, 1 pie:
   cheese ..................................................813
   pepperoni ............................................810
   supreme ...............................................808
   taco........................................................780
pan pizza:
   cheese ..................................................361
   chicken supreme ..............................343
   beef........................................................399
   ham ........................................................331
   *Meat Lover's*....................................428
   pepperoni ............................................353
   *Pepperoni Lover's* .........................370
   pork topping........................................394
   sausage, Italian ...............................415
   super supreme ...............................401
   supreme ...............................................385
   taco........................................................310
   taco, beef...........................................300
   taco, chicken ....................................320
   taco, meatless ..................................290
   *Veggie Lover's*.................................333
Sicilian:
   cheese ..................................................295
   chicken supreme ..............................269
   beef........................................................282
   ham ........................................................257
   *Meat Lover's*....................................344
   pepperoni ............................................227

**Pizza Hut**, Sicilian (*cont.*)

   *Pepperoni Lover's* ..............................................321
   pork topping..............................................314
   sausage, Italian ..............................................333
   super supreme ..............................................323
   supreme ..............................................307
   *Veggie Lover's*..............................................252
Stuffed Crust:
   cheese ..............................................295
   chicken supreme..............................................269
   beef..............................................282
   ham ..............................................257
   *Meat Lover's*..............................................344
   pepperoni ..............................................227
   *Pepperoni Lover's* ..............................................321
   pork topping..............................................314
   sausage, Italian ..............................................333
   super supreme ..............................................323
   supreme ..............................................307
   *Veggie Lover's*..............................................421
Thin 'N Crispy:
   cheese ..............................................243
   chicken supreme..............................................232
   beef..............................................305
   ham ..............................................212
   *Meat Lover's*..............................................339
   pepperoni ..............................................235
   *Pepperoni Lover's* ..............................................289
   pork topping..............................................298
   sausage, Italian ..............................................325
   super supreme ..............................................304
   supreme ..............................................284
   taco..............................................260
   taco, beef..............................................260
   taco, chicken ..............................................230
   taco, meatless..............................................260
   *Veggie Lover's*..............................................222
pasta, 1 serving:
   *Cavatini*..............................................480

*Cavatini Supreme*......................................................560
  spaghetti w/marinara ............................................490
  spaghetti w/meat sauce .......................................600
  spaghetti w/meatballs .........................................850
sandwiches, 1 serving:
  ham and cheese ..................................................550
  supreme ..............................................................640
starters/sides:
  Buffalo wings, hot, 4 pcs. ....................................210
  Buffalo wings, mild, 5 pcs. ..................................200
  breadstick, 1 serving...........................................130
  breadstick dipping sauce, 1 serving .....................30
  dessert pizza, apple or cherry, 1 slice................250
**Pizza pocket,** frozen, 1 pc.:
(*Croissant Pockets* Supreme), 4.5 oz......................350
cheese (*Amy's*), 4.5 oz. .........................................300
cheese, double (*Toaster Breaks*), 2.2 oz. ..............170
pepperoni (*Croissant Pockets*), 4.5 oz. .................360
pepperoni (*Deli Stuffs*), 4.5 oz. ..............................350
pepperoni (*Lean Pockets* Deluxe), 4.5 oz...............290
pepperoni (*Toaster Breaks*), 2.2 oz. ......................180
pepperoni or pepperoni and sausage (*Hot Pockets*), 4.5 oz.....340
sausage (*Hot Pockets*), 4.5 oz................................370
sausage and pepperoni (*Toaster Pockets*), 4.5 oz. ..................170
veggie, nondairy (*Amy's* Soy Cheeze), 4.5 oz. .........270
vegetarian (*Amy's*), 4.5 oz......................................250
**Pizza roll,** see "Pizza snack"
**Pizza sauce,** ¼ cup:
(*Contadina Pizza Squeeze*) .....................................30
(*Muir Glen* Organic)................................................40
(*Prince* Traditional) ................................................20
(*Ragú Pizza Quick* Traditional)................................40
mushroom, chunky or garlic and basil (*Ragú Pizza Quick*)........40
original or 4 cheese (*Contadina*) .............................30
pepperoni flavor (*Contadina*)...................................35
pepperoni flavor (*Ragú Pizza Quick*)........................60
tomato, chunky (*Ragú Pizza Quick*)..........................50
**Pizza snack,** frozen, 6 pcs., except as noted:
all varieties (*Hot Pockets Pizza Mini's*), 3.2 oz. .........280

**Pizza snack (*cont.*)**
all varieties, except pepperoni (*Jack's Pizza Bursts*) .................250
cheese (*Banquet* Munchers) ..................................................200
cheese, combination, or 4 meat (*Michelina's*) .....................230
hamburger or nacho cheese (*Michelina's*) ...........................220
pepperoni (*Banquet* Munchers) ............................................230
pepperoni (*Jack's Pizza Bursts*) ..........................................260
pepperoni (*Michelina's*) ......................................................240
pepperoni and sausage (*Banquet* Munchers) .......................210
**Plantain,** fresh:
raw (*Frieda's*), 3 oz. ............................................................100
raw, 1 medium, 6.3 oz. ..........................................................218
raw, sliced, 1 cup .................................................................181
cooked, sliced, 1 cup ...........................................................179
cooked, mashed, 1 cup .........................................................232
**Plum,** fresh:
(*Dole*), 2 medium ...................................................................70
2⅛" diam., 2⅓ oz. ...................................................................36
sliced, 1 cup ..........................................................................91
**Plum, canned,** purple:
in juice, 1 plum w/liquid .........................................................27
in juice, pitted, 1 cup ...........................................................146
in light syrup, 1 plum w/liquid ................................................29
in light syrup, pitted, 1 cup ..................................................159
in heavy syrup, 1 plum w/liquid ..............................................41
in heavy syrup (*Oregon*), ½ cup ..........................................100
in heavy syrup, pitted, 1 cup ................................................230
**Plum pudding** (*Crosse & Blackwell*), ⅓ pkg., 4.66 oz. ...........460
**Plum sauce,** 1 tbsp. ..................................................................35
**Poi,** fresh, 1 cup ......................................................................269
**Pocket sandwich,** see specific listings
**Poke greens,** canned (*Allens*), ½ cup .......................................35
**Pokeberry shoots:**
raw, 1 cup ..............................................................................37
boiled, drained, 1 cup ............................................................33
**Polenta, canned** (*Greene's Farm* Organic), ½ cup ...................80
**Polenta, refrigerated,** plain (*San Gennaro's*), 2 slices ½" .........70
**Polish sausage** (see also "Kielbasa"), pork, 1 oz. ...................92

**Pollock,** meat only:
Atlantic, raw, 4 oz. .................................................................104
Atlantic, baked, broiled, or microwaved, 4 oz. .........................134
walleye, raw, 4 oz. ...................................................................92
walleye, baked, broiled, or microwaved, 4 oz. ........................128
**Pomegranate,** fresh:
(*Dole*), 1 medium ....................................................................104
(*Frieda's*), 5 oz. .....................................................................100
3⅜" diam. ...............................................................................105
**Pompano,** Florida, meat only:
raw, 4 oz. ...............................................................................184
baked, broiled, or microwaved, 4 oz. ......................................239
**Popcorn,** unpopped, except as noted:
(*Arrowhead Mills*), ¼ cup ......................................................180
(*Pop•Secret* Homestyle/Natural), 1 cup* ..................................35
butter/butter flavor:
   (*Chester's* Microwave), 5 cups* ...........................................160
   (*Jolly Time America's Best/Healthy Pop* Microwave),
      2 tbsp., 5 cups* .............................................................90
   (*Jolly Time Blast O Butter* Light Microwave), 2 tbsp.,
      4 cups* .........................................................................130
   (*Jolly Time Blast O Butter* Microwave), 2 tbsp.,
      3½ cups* .......................................................................150
   (*Jolly Time Butter 'Licious* Light Microwave), 2 tbsp.,
      5 cups* .........................................................................120
   (*Jolly Time Butter 'Licious* Microwave), 2 tbsp., 4 cups* ...140
   (*Pop•Secret*), 1 cup* .............................................................35
   (*Pop•Secret* Light/Natural 94% Fat Free/94% Fat Free),
      1 cup* ............................................................................20
   (*Pop•Secret* Movie Theater/Homestyle Extra Butter/*Jumbo
      Pop/Jumbo Pop* Movie Theater), 1 cup* .........................40
   white (*Jolly Time White & Buttery* Microwave), 2 tbsp.,
      4 cups* .........................................................................150
cheddar cheese (*Jolly Time* Microwave), 2 tbsp., 3 cups* .......160
white (*Jolly Time Crispy 'n White* Microwave), 2 tbsp.,
   4 cups* ..............................................................................150
white (*Jolly Time Crispy 'n White* Light Microwave), 2 tbsp.,
   5 cups* ..............................................................................120
white or yellow (*Jolly Time*), 2 tbsp., 5 cups air popped..........100

**Popcorn, popped:**
(*Herr's* Regular), 1 oz., approx. 2 cups .....................................140
butter (*Chester's*), 3 cups .............................................................160
butter (*Smartfood* Reduced Fat), 3⅓ cups ...............................130
caramel, w/peanuts (*Cracker Jack*), ½ cup ...............................120
caramel, w/peanuts (*Cracker Jack* Fat Free), ¾ cup .................120
cheddar (*Chester's*), 3 cups..........................................................190
cheddar, white (*Smartfood* Reduced Fat), 3 cups.....................140
cheddar, white (*Smartfood*), 2 cups ...........................................190
toffee, butter (*Cracker Jack* Fat Free), ¾ cup............................110
**Poppy seed,** 1 tsp. ........................................................................15
**Porgy,** see "Scup"
**Pork** (see also "Ham"), 4 oz., except as noted:
loin, whole, braised, lean w/fat.....................................................271
loin, whole, braised, lean only .....................................................231
loin, whole, broiled, lean w/fat......................................................274
loin, whole, broiled, lean only........................................................238
loin, whole, roasted, lean w/fat.....................................................281
loin, whole, roasted, lean only ......................................................237
loin, blade, chop, bone-in, braised or roasted, lean w/fat.........366
loin, blade, chop, bone-in, braised, lean only............................255
loin, blade, roast, bone-in, broiled, lean w/fat...........................363
loin, blade, chop, bone-in, broiled, lean only ............................265
loin, blade, chop, bone-in, pan-fried, lean only .........................273
loin, blade, roast, bone-in, roasted, lean only ...........................280
loin, center, chop, bone-in, braised, lean w/fat .........................280
loin, center, chop, bone-in, braised or broiled, lean only ..........229
loin, center, chop, bone-in, broiled, lean w/fat...........................272
loin, center, roast, bone-in, roasted, lean w/fat.........................265
loin, center, roast, bone-in, roasted, lean only ..........................226
loin, center rib, chop, bone-in, braised, lean w/fat....................284
loin, center rib, chop, bone-in, braised, lean only .....................234
loin, center rib, chop, bone-in, broiled, lean w/fat .....................298
loin, center rib, chop, bone-in, broiled, lean only.......................248
loin, center rib, roast, bone-in, roasted, lean w/fat ...................289
loin, center rib, roast, bone-in, roasted, lean only ....................253
loin, sirloin, chop, bone-in, braised, lean w/fat .........................278
loin, sirloin, chop, bone-in, braised, lean only ..........................223
loin, sirloin, chop, bone-in, broiled, lean w/fat..........................294

loin, sirloin, chop, bone-in, broiled, lean only ...........................242
loin, sirloin, roast, bone-in, roasted, lean w/fat......................296
loin, sirloin, roast, bone-in, roasted, lean only .........................245
loin, tenderloin, roasted, lean only .............................................186
loin, top loin, chop, boneless, braised, lean w/fat....................264
loin, top loin, chop, boneless, braised, lean only .....................229
loin, top loin, chop, boneless, broiled, lean w/fat.....................260
loin, top loin, chop, boneless, broiled, lean only......................230
loin, top loin, roast, boneless, roasted, lean w/fat ...................256
loin, top loin, roast, boneless, roasted, lean only.....................220
shoulder, whole, roasted, lean w/fat..........................................331
shoulder, whole, roasted, lean w/fat, diced, 1 cup...................394
shoulder, whole, roasted, lean only.............................................261
shoulder, whole, roasted, lean only, diced, 1 cup .....................311
shoulder, arm, picnic, braised, lean w/fat..................................373
shoulder, arm, picnic, braised, lean w/fat, diced, 1 cup...........444
shoulder, arm, picnic, braised, lean only...................................281
shoulder, arm, picnic, roasted, lean w/fat .................................359
shoulder, arm, picnic, roasted, lean w/fat, diced, 1 cup...........428
shoulder, arm, picnic, roasted, lean only...................................259
shoulder, Boston blade, steak, braised, lean w/fat....................362
shoulder, Boston blade, steak, braised, lean only .....................310
shoulder, Boston blade, steak, broiled, lean w/fat.....................294
shoulder, Boston blade, steak, broiled, lean only......................257
shoulder, Boston blade, roast, roasted, lean w/fat....................305
shoulder, Boston blade, roast, roasted, lean only .....................263
spareribs, braised, lean w/fat .....................................................450
**Pork, pickled** (see also "Pig's feet"):
hocks (*Hormel*), 2 oz. ................................................................110
tidbits (*Hormel*), 2 oz..................................................................100
**Pork, refrigerated,** 4 oz., except as noted:
blade steak (*Hormel Always Tender*) .........................................260
chop, center cut (*Hormel Always Tender*) .................................140
chops, center cut (*Hormel Always Tender*)................................190
loin, center cut, boneless (*Hormel Always Tender*) ..................160
loin, center cut, chops (*Hormel Always Tender*)........................190
loin filet and roast:
      (*Hormel Always Tender* Original) .........................................130

**Pork, refrigerated (*cont.*)**

   honey mustard or salsa (*Hormel Always Tender*)...............140

   lemon garlic or mesquite barbecue (*Hormel Always*
      *Tender*)...........................................................................130

rib (*Hormel Always Tender*) ............................................240

rib (*Hormel Always Tender* Countrystyle) ........................260

rib (*Hormel Always Tender* Special Trim)..........................280

roast, w/au jus (*Hormel Always Tender*), 5 oz.........................180

roast, boneless (*Hormel Always Tender* Chef's Prime) .............160

shoulder roast, boneless (*Hormel Always Tender* Country
   Roast)..............................................................................130

shoulder roast, boneless, onion garlic (*Hormel Always*
   *Tender*)...........................................................................200

spareribs (*Hormel Always Tender*) ...................................280

tenderloin, peppercorn (*Hormel Always Tender*) .....................130

tenderloin, teriyaki (*Hormel Always Tender*)............................140

**Pork backfat,** raw, 1 oz. ...................................................230

**Pork and beans,** see "Baked beans" and specific bean listings

**Pork belly,** raw, 1 oz. ......................................................147

**Pork dinner,** frozen, 1 pkg.:

rib, boneless (*Swanson Hungry-Man*), 14.1 oz. .......................750

riblet, boneless (*Banquet Extra Helping*), 15.25 oz. .................720

**Pork ear,** simmered, 1 ear, 3.9 oz.....................................182

**Pork entree,** frozen, 1 pkg.:

chop suey, w/rice (*Yu Sing*), 8.5 oz....................................320

cutlet (*Banquet*), 10.25 oz.................................................420

cutlet, breaded (*Stouffer's* Homestyle), 10 oz. .....................370

patty, breaded, herb (*Healthy Choice* Entree), 8 oz. .................280

rib, boneless (*Banquet*), 10 oz.........................................400

roasted, honey (*Lean Cuisine Cafe Classics*), 9.5 oz. .............250

and roasted potatoes (*Stouffer's Hearty Portions*), 15⅜ oz. ....510

**Pork gravy,** in jars, ¼ cup:

(*Franco-American*).............................................................45

(*Heinz* Home Style)..........................................................25

**Pork gravy mix,** roasted (*Knorr*), 1 tbsp. or ¼ cup*...........25

**Pork lunch meat** (see also "Ham lunch meat"):

roast (*Healthy Deli* 98% Fat Free), 2 oz.................................70

roast, oven roasted (*Sara Lee*), 2 oz. .................................70

**Pork rind snack,** ½ oz.:
(*Baken-ets*) ..................................................................80
(*Baken-ets* Cracklins)....................................................40
barbecue or hot and spicy (*Baken-ets*) ........................70
hot and spicy (*Baken-ets* Cracklins)..............................80
**Pork sandwich,** frozen, 1 pc.:
barbecue (*Hormel Quick Meal*), 4.3 oz. .......................360
barbecue, rib shaped (*Hormel Quick Meal*), 4.8 oz. .................430
**Pork seasoning and coating mix,** ⅛ pkt.:
(*Shake 'n Bake* Original Recipe) ...................................45
extra crispy (*Oven Fry*) .................................................60
**Pot pie,** see specific entree listings
**Pot roast,** see "Beef dinner" and "Beef entree"
**Potato,** fresh:
raw (*Dole*), 1 medium, 5.3 oz. ....................................100
raw (*Frieda's* Baby/Fingerling/Purple/Red/Yellow Finnish/
    Yukon Gold), ½ cup, 3 oz. ........................................70
raw, unpeeled, 1 large, 3–4¼" diam., 6.5 oz. ..............145
raw, unpeeled, 1 long type, 2⅓" diam. by 4¾", 7.1 oz. .............160
baked, unpeeled, 2⅓" by 4¾", 7.1 oz. ..........................220
baked, unpeeled, ½ cup ................................................67
baked, w/out skin, 1 potato, 2⅓" by 4¾", 5.5 oz. .........145
baked, w/out skin, ½ cup ..............................................57
baked, skin only, from 1 potato, 2 oz. ...........................115
boiled in skin, peeled, 2½" diam., 4.8 oz........................118
boiled in skin, peeled, ½ cup...........................................68
boiled, skin only, from 1 potato, 1.2 oz...........................27
boiled w/out skin, 2½" diam.............................................116
boiled w/out skin, ½ cup .................................................67
microwaved in skin, unpeeled, 2½" diam., 7.1 oz..........212
microwaved in skin, peeled, 1 potato, 2⅓" by 4¾", 5.5 oz. ......156
microwaved in skin, peeled, ½ cup..................................78
microwaved in skin, skin only, 2 oz.................................77
**Potato, canned:**
16-oz. can..................................................................200
whole (*Butterfield/Sunshine*), 2½ pcs.............................90
whole, 1 cup ...............................................................132
drained, 1.2-oz. potato .................................................21
sliced (*Butterfield*), ½ cup ...........................................100

**Potato, canned (*cont.*)**
sticks (*Butterfield*), ⅔ cup ........................................................150
diced (*Butterfield*), ⅔ cup........................................................100
new, whole (*Del Monte*), 2 med., w/liquid................................60
new, sliced (*Del Monte*), ⅔ cup ................................................60
**Potato, frozen** (see also "Potato dish, frozen"):
french fried:
    (*Empire Kosher* Crinkle Cut), 3 oz., approx. 17 pcs. ...........120
    (*Ore-Ida Crispy Crunchies!*), 3 oz., approx. 13 pcs. ...........160
    (*Ore-Ida* Deep Fries), 3 oz., approx. 15 pcs........................140
    (*Ore-Ida* Fast Food Fries), 3 oz., approx. 35 pcs. ................160
    (*Ore-Ida* Crispy Crinkles/Golden Fries), 3 oz., 13 pcs. ........120
    (*Ore-Ida* Golden Twirls), 3 oz., approx. 17 pcs...................160
    (*Ore-Ida* Waffle Fries), 3 oz., approx. 9 pcs.......................150
    (*Ore-Ida* Wedges), 3 oz., approx. 8 pcs..............................100
    oven heated, 1¾ oz., 10 pcs................................................100
hash brown (*Ore-Ida Toaster*), 2 patties, 3.6 oz. ......................220
hash brown, Southern style (*Ore-Ida*), ⅔ cup ...........................70
O'Brien (*Ore-Ida*), ¾ cup ...........................................................60
patty (*Ore-Ida Golden Patties*), 2.2-oz. patty............................130
puffs (*Ore-Ida Tater Tots*), 3 oz., 9 pcs. ...................................170
puffs, onion (*Ore-Ida Tater Tots*), 3 oz., 9 pcs. .........................150
**Potato, stuffed,** see "Potato dish, frozen"
**Potato, sweet,** see "Sweet potato"
**Potato chips and crisps,** 1 oz., except as noted:
(*Herr's*)......................................................................................140
(*Lay's* Baked) ...........................................................................110
(*Lay's* Classic/Deli Style) .........................................................150
(*Lay's* Wavy/Unsalted) .............................................................160
(*Lay's Wow!/Ruffles Wow!*).......................................................75
(*Ruffles*)....................................................................................150
(*Ruffles* Baked) ........................................................................130
(*Ruffles* Buffalo Style/The Works) ............................................160
(*Ruffles* Reduced Fat)...............................................................140
all flavors (*Barbara's*)................................................................150
all flavors (*Chester's Fries*) ......................................................140
all flavors (*Sun Chips*) ..............................................................140
barbecue (*Lay's KC Masterpiece/Lay's* Spicy)...........................150
barbecue (*Lay's KC Masterpiece* Baked) ..................................120

barbecue (*Lay's Wow!* Mesquite)................................................75
barbecue (*Lay's KC Masterpiece* Mesquite) ............................150
barbecue and cheddar (*Ruffles* Flavor Rush)............................160
cheese (*Lay's* Cracker Barrel)...............................................150
cheddar and sour cream (*Ruffles*) ........................................160
cheddar and sour cream (*Ruffles* Baked)...............................130
cheddar and sour cream (*Ruffles Wow!*) ..................................75
hot (*Lay's* Flamin')..............................................................150
hot (*Ruffles* Flamin')...........................................................150
onion, French (*Ruffles*)........................................................150
onion, toasted, and cheese (*Lay's*).......................................160
salt and vinegar (*Lay's*)......................................................150
sour cream and chive (*Lay's Wow!*) ........................................80
sour cream and onion (*Air Crisps*)........................................120
sour cream and onion (*Lay's*)...............................................160
sour cream and onion (*Lay's* Baked)......................................120
sour cream and onion (*Ruffles* Flavor Rush) ..........................150
**Potato dish, canned or packaged:**
au gratin, w/*Cure 81* ham (*Dinty Moore American Classics*),
  1 bowl ................................................................................290
scalloped, w/ham (*Hormel* Microcup Meals), 1 cup .................240
**Potato dish, frozen** (see also "Potato pancake"):
au gratin (*Marie Callender's* Skillet Meals), ⅔ cup ..................190
au gratin (*Stouffer's* 11.5 oz.), ½ cup ..................................130
au gratin, ham and broccoli (*Banquet* Family Size), ⅔ cup......210
cheddar (*Lean Cuisine Everyday Favorites* Deluxe),
  10⅜-oz. pkg.......................................................................250
cheddar broccoli (*Healthy Choice* Entree), 10.5-oz. pkg...........330
cheddar broccoli (*Michelina's*), 8-oz. pkg. ..............................380
mashed (*Boston Market*), ½ cup.............................................180
mashed, w/beef gravy (*Larry's* Classic), 4.46-oz. tray .............160
mashed, w/chicken gravy (*Larry's* Classic), 4.46-oz. tray.........170
pot pie, and broccoli w/ham, cheesy (*Banquet*), 7-oz. pie .......410
roasted, w/broccoli and cheddar cheese (*Lean Cuisine*
  *Everyday Favorites*), 10.25-oz. pkg....................................260
roasted, w/ham (*Healthy Choice* Bowl), 8.5-oz. pkg. ...............210
scalloped (*Stouffer's* 40 oz.), ½ cup .....................................140
scalloped (*Stouffer's* 11.5 oz.), ½ cup ..................................170

**Potato dish, frozen (*cont.*)**

scalloped, w/hickory smoked turkey ham (*Lean Cuisine Café
   Classics*), 10-oz. pkg............................................................250
stuffed, cheddar (*OhBoy!*), 1 potato ........................................130
stuffed, onion, sour cream, and chives (*OhBoy!*), 1 potato .....110
whipped, w/bacon and cheese (*Ore-Ida*), 5-oz. tray ................190
whipped, w/cheese (*Ore-Ida*), 5-oz. tray ..................................190
**Potato dish, mix,** ½ cup*, except as noted
Alfredo (*Knorr* Skillet Potatoes), ½ cup ...................................110
au gratin (*Betty Crocker*)............................................................150
au gratin, broccoli (*Betty Crocker* Homestyle) ..........................140
cheddar, cheesy (*Knorr* Skillet Potatoes), ½ cup......................130
cheddar cheese (*Betty Crocker* Homestyle) ..............................120
cheddar and bacon (*Betty Crocker*)............................................150
cheddar and bacon, twice baked (*Betty Crocker*), ⅔ cup* ......210
cheddar and sour cream (*Betty Crocker*) ..................................130
cheese, 3 (*Betty Crocker*)............................................................150
chicken and vegetable, creamy (*Betty Crocker*), ⅔ cup*.........160
garlic, roasted (*Knorr* Skillet Potatoes), ⅔ cup .......................120
hash browns (*Betty Crocker*).......................................................190
hash brown, cheesy (*Knorr* Skillet Potatoes), ⅓ cup................120
hash brown, onion (*Knorr* Skillet Potatoes), ⅓ cup..................100
julienne (*Betty Crocker*) ..............................................................150
mashed:
   (*Barbara's*), ⅓ cup ...............................................................70
   (*Hungry Jack*) ........................................................................80
   (*Pillsbury Idaho*) ...................................................................90
   (*Potato Buds*).......................................................................160
   butter, creamy or butter and herb (*Betty Crocker*)..............160
   cheddar and bacon or 4 cheese (*Betty Crocker*).................150
   chicken and herb (*Betty Crocker*).........................................150
   garlic, roasted (*Betty Crocker*) .............................................160
   sour cream and chives (*Betty Crocker*).................................150
mashed, w/gravy:
   beef, hearty or roasted chicken (*Betty Crocker*), ¾ cup* ...170
   brown or chicken (*Hungry Jack*), ⅓ cup flakes plus 1 tbsp.
      gravy mix.........................................................................100
ranch (*Betty Crocker*)..................................................................160

scalloped:
   (*Betty Crocker* 8.25 oz.) .....................................................150
   (*Betty Crocker* 5 oz./20 oz.) ..........................................160
   cheese and bacon (*Knorr* Skillet Potatoes), ½ cup .............110
   cheesy (*Betty Crocker* Homestyle)...................................140
sour cream and chive (*Betty Crocker*) ....................................160
Southwestern style (*Knorr* Skillet Potatoes), ½ cup .................140
**Potato flour,** 1 cup ..............................................................571
**Potato knish,** refrigerated (*Joshua's Coney Island*), 1 pc. .......380
**Potato pancake,** frozen:
(*Dr. Praeger's* Homestyle), 1.5-oz. pc. ..................................80
(*Empire Kosher* Latkes), 2-oz. pc.........................................80
(*Ratner's*), 1.5-oz. pc. ..........................................................110
(*Tofutti*), 1.33-oz. pc.............................................................71
mini (*Empire Kosher* Latkes), 12 pcs., 3 oz. ...........................150
**Potato salad,** refrigerated:
(*Blue Ridge Farms*), ½ cup ...................................................180
(*Chef's Express*), 4 oz.............................................................260
**Potato seasoning mix,** ⅙ pkg.:
cheddar, creamy (*Shake 'n Bake Perfect Potatoes*) ...................30
herb and garlic, home fries or savory onion (*Shake 'n Bake*
   *Perfect Potatoes*)................................................................20
Parmesan peppercorn (*Shake 'n Bake Perfect Potatoes*)............25
**Poultry,** see specific listings
**Poultry seasoning,** 1 tsp. ...................................................5
**Pout,** ocean, meat only:
raw, 4 oz. ...............................................................................90
baked, broiled, or microwaved, 4 oz. .....................................116
**Preserves,** see "Jam and preserves"
**Pretzels,** 1 oz., except as noted:
(*Air Crisps* Original)..............................................................110
(*Little Debbie* Mini Twists), 1.5 oz. ......................................180
(*Rold Gold* Classic Sticks).....................................................100
(*Rold Gold* Classic Thin Sticks/Classic Tiny Twists/Rods)........110
(*Rold Gold* Fat Free Thins/Fat Free Tiny Twists)......................100
cheddar cheese (*Combos*), 1.8-oz. bag ...................................240
cheddar cheese or honey mustard (*Rold Gold* Classic Tiny
   Twists)..................................................................................110
nacho cheese (*Combos*), 1.8-oz. bag......................................230

**Pretzels (*cont.*)**

pizzeria (*Combos*), 1.8-oz. bag..................................................230
soft, w/ or w/out salt (*Act II* Big Softy), 2.3-oz. pretzel.............200
sourdough (*Herr's* Hard) ..........................................................100
sourdough (*Rold Gold* Hard/Nuggets) .....................................100

**Prickly pear,** fresh

(*Frieda's* Cactus Pear), 5 oz.......................................................60
trimmed, 1 prickly pear, 3.6 oz.....................................................42
1 cup..............................................................................................61

**Prosciutto** (*Boar's Head*), 1 oz..................................................60

**Prune, canned:**

in heavy syrup, 5 prunes w/2 tbsp. liquid ...................................90
in heavy syrup, 1 cup .................................................................246

**Prune, dehydrated:**

uncooked, 1 oz. ............................................................................96
uncooked, 1 cup ..........................................................................448
stewed, 1 cup .............................................................................316

**Prune, dried:**

pitted (*Dole*), ¼ cup, 1.4 oz. .....................................................110
uncooked, .3-oz. prune..................................................................20
uncooked, pitted, 1 cup..............................................................406
stewed, pitted, 1 cup .................................................................265
stewed, w/sugar, pitted, 1 cup....................................................308

**Prune juice** (*Sunsweet*), 8 fl. oz...............................................170

**Pudding,** ready-to-eat, 1 cont.:

all flavors:

    (*Jell-O Free*), 4 oz. ...............................................................100
    (*Kraft Handi-Snacks* Fat Free), 3.5 oz. ...................................90
    except chocolate fudge (*Kraft Handi-Snacks*), 3.5 oz..........120
    except tapioca (*Jell-O*), 4 oz. ...............................................160
banana or vanilla (*Kozy Shack*), 4 oz.......................................130
chocolate (*Kozy Shack*), 4 oz....................................................140
chocolate or vanilla (*Kozy Shack* No Sugar Added), 4 oz. .......130
chocolate fudge (*Kraft Handi-Snacks*), 3.5 oz...........................130
flan (*Kozy Shack*), 4 oz. ...........................................................150
tapioca (*Jell-O*), 4 oz. ..............................................................140
tapioca (*Kozy Shack*), 4 oz.......................................................140

**Pudding and pie filling mix,** ½ cup*:

all flavors (*Jell-O* Fat Free Instant) .........................................140

all flavors (*Jell-O* Sugar Free)......................................................130
all flavors, except chocolate and chocolate fudge
   (*Jell-O* Fat/Sugar Free Instant) ...........................................70
banana cream (*Jell-O*)...............................................................140
banana cream (*Jell-O* Instant) ...............................................150
butterscotch (*Jell-O*) ................................................................160
butterscotch (*Jell-O* Instant)...................................................150
chocolate or chocolate fudge (*Jell-O* Instant) .....................160
chocolate or chocolate fudge (*Jell-O* Fat/Sugar Free Instant) .....80
chocolate, chocolate fudge or milk, chocolate (*Jell-O*)............150
coconut cream (*Jell-O*) .............................................................150
coconut cream (*Jell-O* Instant)................................................160
custard (*Jell-O Americana*) .......................................................140
flan (*Jell-O*)...............................................................................140
lemon (*Jell-O*) ..........................................................................140
lemon (*Jell-O* Instant)...............................................................150
pistachio (*Jell-O* Instant) .........................................................160
rice, see "Rice pudding mix"
tapioca (*Jell-O Americana*) .......................................................130
vanilla (*Jell-O*) ..........................................................................140
vanilla (*Jell-O* Instant)...............................................................150
vanilla, French (*Jell-O* Instant)................................................160
**Puff pastry,** frozen:
sheet (*Pepperidge Farm*), 1/6 sheet......................................190
shell (*Pepperidge Farm*), 1.7-oz. shell..................................170
**Pummelo,** fresh:
(*Frieda's*), 5 oz. .........................................................................50
trimmed, 1 1/3-lb. ......................................................................231
sections, 1 cup .........................................................................72
**Pumpkin,** fresh:
raw, cubed, 1 cup .....................................................................30
boiled, drained, mashed, 1 cup ...............................................49
mini (*Frieda's*), 3/4 cup, 3 oz....................................................20
**Pumpkin, canned** (see also "Pie filling"), 1 cup.........................83
**Pumpkin flower,** fresh, raw, 1 cup.............................................5
**Pumpkin leaf,** fresh:
raw, 1 cup ...................................................................................7
boiled, drained, 1 cup ...............................................................15
**Pumpkin pie spice,** 1 tsp..........................................................6

**Pumpkin/squash seeds:**
dried, shelled, 1 oz., 142 kernels................................................154
roasted, in shell, 1 cup ...............................................................285
roasted, in shell, 1 oz., 85 seeds..............................................126
roasted, shelled, ¼ cup ...............................................................296
**Purslane:**
raw, 1 cup .........................................................................................7
boiled, drained, 1 cup ....................................................................21
**Quail,** raw:
whole, meat w/skin, 3.8 oz. (4.3 oz. w/bone) .........................209
whole, meat only, 3.3 oz............................................................123
meat w/skin, 4 oz.........................................................................218
meat only, 4 oz. ...........................................................................152
breast, meat only, 2 oz. ................................................................69
**Quesadillas,** frozen (*Cedarlane*), 3 pcs. ...................................250
**Quince,** fresh, raw:
(*Frieda's*), 5 oz. .............................................................................80
trimmed, 1 quince, 3.2 oz............................................................52
**Quinoa,** dry (*Frieda's*), ⅓ cup.....................................................170

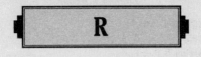

**FOOD AND MEASURE**    **CALORIES**

**Rabbit,** meat only, 4 oz.:
domestic, roasted ................................................................223
domestic, stewed.................................................................234
wild, stewed.........................................................................196
**Radiatore dish, mix,** 1 cup\*:
Alfredo primavera (*Land O Lakes International Pasta
    Collection*) ...................................................................350
and mixed beans (*Marrakesh Express*) .....................................200
**Radicchio,** fresh:
(*Frieda's*), ⅔ cup, 3 oz. ...............................................................20
shredded, 1 cup......................................................................9
**Radish,** fresh, raw:
1 large, 1–1¼" diam................................................................2
sliced, 1 cup.........................................................................23
**Radish, black** (*Frieda's*), ¾ cup, 3 oz. ......................................15
**Radish, Chinese** (*Frieda's* Lo Bok), ⅔ cup, 3 oz. ......................25
**Radish, Korean** (*Frieda's*), ⅔ cup, 3 oz. .....................................15
**Radish, Oriental,** fresh:
(*Frieda's* Daikon), ½ cup, 1.1 oz. ...............................................15
raw, 7" long, 11.9 oz. .............................................................62
boiled, drained, sliced, 1 cup....................................................25
**Radish, Oriental, dried,** ½ cup.................................................157
**Radish, white icicle,** fresh, raw:
1 medium, .6 oz.......................................................................2
sliced, ½ cup .........................................................................7
**Radish seeds, sprouted,** fresh, raw, 1 cup ..............................16
**Raisin:**
golden seedless, 1 oz. .............................................................86
golden seedless, not packed, 1 cup .........................................438
seeded, 1 oz.........................................................................84
seedless (*Dole* California), ¼ cup.............................................130
seedless (*Sun•Maid*), ¼ cup....................................................130

**Raisin (*cont.*)**
seedless, 1 oz. ....................................................................85
seedless, not packed, 1 cup ...........................................435
**Raisin sauce** (*Reese*), ¼ cup ......................................150
**Rambutan,** canned, in syrup, drained, 1 cup ...............123
**Ranch dip,** 2 tbsp.:
(*Breakstone's Free/Knudsen Free/Kraft Free*) ................25
(*Kraft*) ................................................................................60
(*Kraft* Premium)................................................................50
**Ranch dip mix,** cracked pepper, dry (*Knorr*), ½ tsp........5
**Rapini,** see "Broccoli rabe"
**Raspberry,** fresh:
(*Dole*), 3 oz...................................................................... 40
(*Dole*), 1 cup ..................................................................45
1 cup ...................................................................................60
**Raspberry, canned,** in heavy syrup, ½ cup ................117
**Raspberry, frozen** (*Birds Eye*), ½ cup .......................90
**Raspberry drink,** 8 fl. oz.:
(*Welch's* Wild) ................................................................140
blue (*Kool-Aid Splash*).................................................120
**Raspberry drink mix,** 8 fl. oz.*:
(*Kool-Aid*).......................................................................100
(*Kool-Aid* Sugar Sweetened) .........................................60
cranberry (*Kool-Aid Roarin'*)........................................100
cranberry (*Kool-Aid Roarin'* Sugar Sweetened) .............70
**Raspberry juice blend** (*Mott's*), 11.5-fl.-oz. can ......160
**Raspberry syrup,** red, ¼ cup:
(*Knott's Berry Farm*) .....................................................210
(*Smucker's*) ...................................................................210
**Ratatouille,** in jars (*Life in Provence*), ½ cup ...........100
**Ravioli** (see also "Ravioli entree"), frozen or refrigerated:
artichoke, in lemon parsley pasta (*Cafferata*), 10 pcs..............210
beef (*Contadina Buitoni*), 1¼ cups .............................330
black bean, in fiesta pasta (*Cafferata*), 7 pcs. .............220
cheese (*Contadina Buitoni*), 1 cup.............................290
cheese (*Di Giorno* Light), 1 cup .................................280
cheese, 4 (*Contadina Buitoni* Light), 1 cup ...............230
cheese, 4 (*Di Giorno*), 1 cup ......................................350
chicken, roasted, and garlic (*Contadina Buitoni*), 1¼ cups......330

chicken herb parmigiana (*Contadina Buitoni*), 1¼ cups ..........310
sausage, Italian (*Di Giorno*), 1¼ cups......................................350
sun-dried tomato (*Di Giorno*), 1⅓ cups...................................380
vegetable, garden (*Contadina Buitoni*), 1 cup..........................250
**Ravioli entree, canned or packaged,** 1 cup, except as noted:
beef (*Chef Boyardee*) ................................................................230
beef (*Chef Boyardee* Overstuffed) .............................................280
beef (*Chef Boyardee Mini Ravioli*) ............................................240
beef (*Dinty Moore American Classics*), 1 bowl .....................300
beef (*Kid's Kitchen* Mini) ...........................................................240
beef, in meat sauce (*Franco-American Superiore*)....................280
beef, in tomato and cheese sauce (*Franco-American*)..............230
beef or cheese (*Chef Boyardee* 99% Fat Free) .........................210
Italian sausage (*Chef Boyardee* Overstuffed) ...........................290
in tomato sauce (*Hormel* Microcup Meals)...............................220
**Ravioli entree, frozen,** 1 pkg., except as noted:
(*Freezer Queen*), 7.75 oz. .........................................................350
cheese (*Lean Cuisine Everyday Favorites*), 8.5 oz. ..................270
cheese (*Michelina's* Jumbo), 11 oz. ..........................................400
cheese (*Stouffer's*), 10⅝ oz. .....................................................450
cheese, Alfredo, w/broccoli (*Michelina's*), 8 oz. .......................390
cheese, in marinara sauce (*Marie Callender's*), 16 oz..............750
cheese, parmigiana (*Healthy Choice* Entree), 9 oz. ..................260
cheese, w/tomato sauce (*Freezer Queen*), 1 cup .....................280
meat, w/pomodoro sauce (*Michelina's*), 8 oz. ..........................300
(*Michelina's* Ravin'), 8.5 oz. ......................................................320
with sauce (*Amy's*), 8 oz. ..........................................................340
**Red bean** (see also "Kidney bean"), canned (*Allens*), ½ cup...100
**Red kuri squash** (*Frieda's*), ¾ cup, 3 oz. ...............................30
**Red snapper,** see "Snapper"
**Redfish,** see "Ocean perch"
**Refried beans,** canned, ½ cup:
(*Allens*) ......................................................................................150
(*Chi-Chi's* Fat Free) ...................................................................120
(*Chi-Chi's* Fiesta).......................................................................130
(*Greene's Farm* Organic)............................................................100
(*Ortega* Traditional)....................................................................130
(*Taco Bell Home Originals*).........................................................140
all varieties (*Shari Ann's* Organic) .............................................110

**Refried beans (*cont.*)**
black bean (*Greene's Farm* Organic) ........................................110
black bean, w/green chilies and spices (*Greene's Farm* Spicy)...80
w/green chilies and spices (*Greene's Farm* Spicy)....................100
plain or w/chilies (*Taco Bell Home Originals* Fat Free)..............110
vegetable (*Chi-Chi's*)..............................................................100
**Relish,** see "Pickle relish, cucumber" and other specific listings
**Relish, mixed,** Indian (*Patak's*), 1 tbsp. .....................................40
**Remoulade sauce** (*Zatarain's*), ¼ cup.......................................80
**Rennet** (*Junket*), 1 tablet ...............................................................1
**Rhubarb,** fresh, raw:
1.8-oz. stalk ................................................................................11
diced, 1 cup ................................................................................26
**Rhubarb, canned,** in heavy syrup (*Oregon*), ½ cup ................180
**Rhubarb, frozen,** unsweetened, diced, 1 cup.............................29
**Rice** (see also "Wild rice"), dry, ¼ cup, except as noted:
(*Lundberg Christmas*) ...............................................................170
arborio, white (*Lundberg Nutra-Farmed* California) ..................160
basmati, brown (*Arrowhead Mills*).............................................150
basmati, brown (*Lundberg* California Organic).........................160
basmati, brown (*Lundberg Nutra-Farmed* California) ...............170
basmati, white (*Lundberg Nutra-Farmed* California)................180
basmati, white (*Lundberg* California Organic)...........................180
blend:
    (*Lundberg* Black Japonica/Organic Black Japonica/
       Jubilee) ............................................................................170
    (*Lundberg* Countrywild).........................................................170
    (*Lundberg* Wild Blend/Organic Wild Blend)..........................150
    brown basmati and wild (*Lundberg* Organic California)......150
brown:
    (*Lundberg* Royal) ...................................................................170
    (*Minute*), approx. ⅔ cup* ......................................................170
    (*River*)......................................................................................150
    instant (*Success* Boil-in-Bag), ½ cup ...................................150
    long grain (*Arrowhead Mills*).................................................150
    long grain (*Carolina/Mahatma*) ............................................150
    long or short grain (*Lundberg Nutra-Farmed/*Organic) .......170
    medium grain (*Lundberg* Organic Golden Rose) .................160
    short grain (*Arrowhead Mills*)................................................170

glutinous or sweet.............................................................171
jasmine (*A Taste of Thai*) ...........................................160
jasmine (*Mahatma* Thai Fragrant) .............................160
jasmine, white (*Lundberg* California Organic/*Lundberg*
    *Nutra-Farmed* California).........................................160
sushi (*Lundberg* Organic)...........................................160
wehani (*Lundberg/Lundberg* Organic) .......................170
white:
    (*River*).................................................................160
    instant (*Minute* Boil-in-Bag), approx. 1 cup*.....190
    instant (*Success* Boil-in-Bag), ½ cup.................190
    long grain (*Arrowhead Mills*)...............................150
    long grain (*Carolina/Mahatma*)...........................150
    long grain, instant (*Carolina/Mahatma*)..............160
    long grain, instant (*Minute*), approx. ¾ cup*......160
    long grain, instant (*Minute* Premium), approx. 1 cup*.......160
    long grain, instant................................................90
    parboiled (*Carolina* Gold/*Mahatma* Gold) ..........160
    short grain (*Mahatma* Valencia)...........................160
**Rice bran,** crude, 1 cup .............................................373
**Rice cake,** 1 cake:
all varieties except multigrain and koku seaweed
(*Lundberg* Organic) .....................................................70
multigrain or koku seaweed (*Lundberg* Organic).........80
apple cinnamon, caramel, or honey nut (*Lundberg*
    *Nutra-Farmed*) ....................................................80
brown, mochi, sesame tamari, or wild (*Lundberg*
    *Nutra-Farmed*) ....................................................70
**Rice dish, canned or packaged,** w/chicken and vegetables
(*Chef Boyardee* Microwave Bowl), 1 bowl...........220
**Rice dish, frozen,** 1 pkg., except as noted:
and beans (*Lean Cuisine Everyday Favorites* Santa Fe),
    10⅜ oz...............................................................300
broccoli, onion, and pasta in cheese sauce (*Freezer Queen*),
    1 cup .................................................................190
and broccoli, in cheese sauce (*Birds Eye*), 10 oz......290
cheesy, w/broccoli (*Green Giant*), approx. ½ cup.....100
fried, chicken (*Yu Sing*), 8 oz....................................360
fried, w/chicken and egg rolls (*Banquet*), 8.5 oz......330

**Rice dish, frozen (*cont.*)**
fried, pork (*Yu Sing*), 8 oz......................................................450
fried, pork and shrimp (*Yu Sing*), 8 oz. ...............................410
fried, shrimp (*Yu Sing*), 8 oz.................................................350
risotto, parmigiano (*Michelina's*), 8 oz.................................450
stir-fry, teriyaki (*Amy's*), 1 cup ............................................320
stir-fry, Thai (*Amy's* Skillet Meals), 9.5 oz...........................270
white and wild (*Birds Eye*), 1 cup.........................................180
white and wild, w/broccoli, in cheese sauce
    (*Marie Callender's* Skillet Meals), 1 cup............................300
**Rice dish, mix,** 1 cup*, except as noted:
(*A Taste of Thai* Golden), ¾ cup...........................................180
and beans, black (*Carolina*) .................................................200
and beans, black (*Mahatma*) ................................................200
and beans, pinto or red (*Mahatma*).......................................190
and beans, red (*Carolina*) ....................................................190
and beans, red (*Rice-A-Roni*), approx. 1 cup* ......................290
and beans, red (*Success*).....................................................240
beef flavor (*Lipton* Rice & Sauce) .........................................280
beef flavor (*Rice-A-Roni*), approx. 1 cup* .............................310
beef flavor (*Success*)............................................................190
beef and mushroom (*Rice-A-Roni*), approx. 1 cup* ...............290
broccoli (*Rice-A-Roni*), approx. 1 cup*..................................280
broccoli au gratin (*Rice-A-Roni*), approx. 1 cup* ..................370
broccoli and cheese (*Mahatma*) ...........................................200
broccoli and cheese (*Success*)..............................................210
brown, all varieties, except hearty harvest
    (*Lundberg* Organic Quick).................................................260
brown, hearty harvest (*Lundberg* Organic Quick)...................140
brown and wild (*Success*).....................................................190
Cajun style (*Lipton* Rice & Sauce).........................................270
cheddar, white, and herbs (*Rice-A-Roni*), approx. 1 cup* .......340
cheddar broccoli (*Bowl Appetite*), 1 bowl .............................300
cheddar broccoli (*Lipton* Rice & Sauce) ................................280
chicken/chicken flavor:
    (*Carolina/Mahatma*) ........................................................190
    (*Lipton* Rice & Sauce)......................................................290
    (*Rice-A-Roni*), approx. 1 cup* .........................................310
    (*Rice-A-Roni* Low Fat), approx. 1 cup* .............................210

(*Success* Classic)..............................................150
broccoli (*Lipton* Rice & Sauce)..........................280
and broccoli (*Rice-A-Roni*), approx. 1 cup*......230
and garlic (*Rice-A-Roni*), approx. 1 cup*.........260
grilled (*Success*)............................................190
herb roasted (*Rice-A-Roni*), approx. 1 cup*......260
w/mushrooms (*Rice-A-Roni*), approx. 1 cup*......360
vegetable, herb (*Bowl Appetite*), 1 bowl.............260
vegetable, savory (*Rice-A-Roni* Low Fat), approx.
   1 cup*......................................................210
and vegetables (*Rice-A-Roni*), approx. 1 cup*......290
coconut ginger (*A Taste of Thai*), ¾ cup............190
fried (*Rice-A-Roni*), approx. 1 cup*...................329
fried, chicken (*Lipton* Rice & Sauce).................290
garlic basil (*A Taste of Thai*), ¾ cup.................160
gumbo (*Mahatma*)............................................160
herb and butter (*Lipton* Rice & Sauce)...............280
herb and butter (*Rice-A-Roni*), approx. 1 cup*......320
jambalaya (*Mahatma*).......................................190
and lentils, chili (*Lundberg* One Step)................180
and lentils, garlic basil or curry (*Lundberg* One Step)..............160
long grain and wild:
   (*Mahatma*)..............................................190
   (*Rice-A-Roni* Original/Pilaf), approx. 1 cup*......240
   (*Success*)...............................................190
   chicken w/almonds (*Rice-A-Roni*), approx. 1 cup*......300
   w/herbs (*Minute*)......................................230
medley (*Lipton* Rice & Sauce)............................270
Mexican style (*Rice-A-Roni*), approx. 1 cup*......260
nacho cheese (*Mahatma*)..................................250
Oriental stir-fry (*Rice-A-Roni*), approx. 1 cup*......290
pilaf (*Carolina* Classic/*Mahatma* Classic)............190
pilaf (*Lipton* Rice & Sauce)...............................260
pilaf (*Rice-A-Roni*), approx. 1 cup*....................310
pilaf (*Success*)................................................200
pilaf, lemon herb, w/jasmine rice (*Knorr*), ⅓ cup......260
risotto:
   (*Knorr* Original Recipe), ⅓ cup....................210
   all varieties (*Lundberg*), ¼ box....................140

**Rice dish, mix, risotto** (*cont.*)

    all varieties, except eggplant (*Real Torino* Dinner), ¼ cup ..240

    broccoli au gratin or Milanese (*Knorr* Italian), ⅓ cup .........260

    chicken flavor (*Knorr*), ⅓ cup ...............................................210

    eggplant (*Real Torino* Dinner), ¼ cup.................................220

    garlic, roasted, primavera (*Marrakesh Express*)..................210

    Milanese, w/saffron (*Marrakesh Express*) ...........................200

    mushroom, wild (*Marrakesh Express*) ..................................210

    mushroom or vegetable primavera (*Knorr* Italian), ⅓ cup..280

    onion herb (*Knorr* Italian), ⅓ cup.......................................300

    tomato, sun-dried (*Marrakesh Express*) ..............................200

Southwestern (*Bowl Appetite*), 1 bowl......................................260

Spanish (*Carolina/Mahatma*) ....................................................180

Spanish (*Lipton* Rice & Sauce) ..................................................270

Spanish (*Rice-A-Roni*), approx. 1 cup*.....................................270

Spanish (*Success*)......................................................................190

Stroganoff (*Rice-A-Roni*), approx. 1 cup*.................................360

yellow, saffron (*Carolina/Mahatma*) ..........................................190

yellow, spicy (*Mahatma*).............................................................180

**Rice flour,** ¼ cup:

brown (*Arrowhead Mills*)............................................................120

brown (*Lundberg Nutra-Farmed*)................................................120

brown (*Lundberg* Organic)..........................................................110

white (*Arrowhead Mills*)..............................................................130

**Rice pudding,** ready-to-eat (*Kozy Shack*), 4-oz. cont..............130

**Rice pudding mix:**

(*Jell-O Americana*), ½ cup*.......................................................140

all varieties (*Lundberg* Elegant), ½ cup ....................................70

**Rice seasoning mix,** Mexican (*Lawry's* Spices & Seasonings),

    1½ tbsp..................................................................................40

**Rice syrup** (*Lundberg* Sweet Dreams *Nutra-Farmed/*Organic),

    ¼ cup .................................................................................170

**Rigatoni dish, mix,** white cheddar and broccoli sauce

    (*Pasta Roni*), approx. 1 cup*..............................................400

**Rigatoni entree, frozen,** 1 pkg., except as noted:

jumbo, w/meatballs (*Lean Cuisine Hearty Portions*),

    15⅜ oz...................................................................................440

w/meat sauce (*Freezer Queen*), 1 cup .....................................250

pomodoro (*Michelina's*), 8 oz....................................................220

pomodoro, w/broccoli and olives (*Michelina's*), 9 oz. ..............240
stuffed cheese (*Michelina's*), 8.5 oz. ..............................300
w/vegetables in cheese sauce (*Marie Callender's* Skillet Meals),
   1 cup ...............................................................290
**Risotto,** see "Rice dish, mix"
**Rockfish,** meat only:
raw, 4 oz. ............................................................107
baked, broiled, or microwaved, 4 oz. ...............................137
**Roe** (see also "Caviar"):
raw, 1 oz. .............................................................40
raw, 1 tbsp. ..........................................................20
baked, broiled, or microwaved, 1 oz. .................................58
**Roll** (see also "Biscuit"), 1 pc.:
dinner, all varieties (*Awrey's*), .9 oz. ...........................120
hamburger (*Arnold*), 1.8 oz. .......................................140
hamburger (*Pepperidge Farm*), 1.5 oz. ..............................120
hamburger (*Sunbeam*), 1.4 oz. ......................................100
hoagie (*Awrey's*), 3.25 oz. ........................................230
hot dog/frankfurter (*Arnold*), 1.5 oz. .............................120
hot dog/frankfurter (*Sunbeam*), 1.4 oz. ............................100
hot dog/frankfurter, presliced (*Pepperidge Farm*), 1.8 oz. ........140
kaiser (*Awrey's*), 2.5 oz. .........................................190
kaiser (*Francisco International*), 2.2 oz. .........................180
sandwich, potato sesame (*Arnold*), 2 oz. ...........................170
sandwich, sesame (*Arnold*), 1.8 oz. ................................140
sandwich, sesame (*Pepperidge Farm*), 1.6 oz. .......................130
**Roll, refrigerated,** 1 pc.:
crescent (*Grands!*) ................................................270
crescent (*Pillsbury*) ..............................................110
crescent (*Pillsbury* Reduced Fat) ..................................100
dinner (*Pillsbury*) ................................................110
**Roll, sweet,** see "Bun, sweet"
**Roll mix** (*Pillsbury* Hot Roll Mix), 1 roll* ....................150
**Roselle,** fresh, trimmed, 1 cup....................................28
**Rosemary,** fresh, 1 tbsp. ..........................................2
**Rosemary, dried,** 1 tsp.............................................4
**Rotini dish, mix:**
and cheese, w/broccoli (*Kraft Velveeta*), approx. 1 cup* ..........400
cheese, 3 (*Bowl Appetite*), 1 bowl..................................370

**Rotini dish, mix (*cont.*)**
w/4 cheese sauce (*Knorr*), ⅓ cup ...........................................130
w/mushroom sauce (*Knorr*), ⅔ cup........................................260
**Roughy,** orange, meat only:
raw, 4 oz. ...........................................................................78
baked, broiled, or microwaved, 4 oz. ....................................101
**Rum sauce,** in jars (*Sable & Rosenfeld*), 2 tbsp. ...................130
**Rutabaga,** fresh:
raw, 1 large, 1.7 lb. ...............................................................278
raw, cubed, 1 cup ...................................................................50
boiled, drained, cubed, 1 cup.................................................66
boiled, drained, mashed, 1 cup .............................................94
**Rutabaga, canned,** diced (*Sunshine*), ½ cup ...........................30
**Rye,** whole grain (*Arrowhead Mills*), ¼ cup ...........................160
**Rye flakes,** rolled (*Arrowhead Mills*), ⅓ cup..........................110
**Rye flour:**
(*Arrowhead Mills*), ¼ cup......................................................100
(*Hodgson Mill* Organic), ¼ cup...............................................90
(*Robin Hood*), ¼ cup .............................................................122
whole grain (*Hodgson Mill*), scant ¼ cup ...............................90

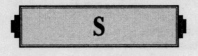

**FOOD AND MEASURE**                                    **CALORIES**

**Sablefish,** meat only:
raw, 4 oz. ...............................................................221
baked, broiled, or microwaved, 4 oz. ...................284
smoked, 4 oz. .......................................................291
**Saffron,** 1 tsp. .......................................................2
**Sage, ground,** 1 tsp. ............................................2
**Salad dressing,** 2 tbsp.:
(*Wish-Bone* Sweet 'n Spicy) ................................140
all varieties (*Nasoya Veggie-Dressing*) ...............60
bacon and tomato (*Kraft*) ....................................140
balsamic vinaigrette (*Wish-Bone*) .......................60
berry vinaigrette (*Wish-Bone*) .............................50
blue cheese (*Just 2 Good!*) .................................45
blue cheese (*Kraft Roka*) ....................................130
blue cheese, chunky (*Seven Seas*) .....................130
blue cheese, chunky (*Wish-Bone*) .......................170
blue cheese, chunky (*Wish-Bone* Fat Free) ..........35
blue cheese flavored (*Kraft Free*) ........................45
Caesar (*Just 2 Good!* Classic) .............................40
Caesar (*Kraft* Classic) .........................................110
Caesar (*Kraft Free* Classic) .................................45
Caesar (*Seven Seas* Classic) ..............................100
Caesar (*Wish-Bone* Classic) ...............................110
Caesar, cilantro pepita (*El Torito*) .......................120
Caesar, creamy (*Just 2 Good!*) ............................40
Caesar, creamy (*Wish-Bone*) ...............................180
coleslaw (*Kraft*) ...................................................130
French (*Catalina*) .................................................120
French (*Catalina Free*) ..........................................35
French (*Catalina* ⅓ Less Fat) ...............................80
French (*Just 2 Good!* Sweet 'n Spicy) ..................50
French (*Wish-Bone* Deluxe) .................................120
French, creamy (*Kraft*) .........................................160

**Salad dressing (*cont.*)**

French, w/honey (*Catalina*) ...................................................130
French style (*Just 2 Good!* Deluxe) ........................................45
French style (*Kraft Free*) .......................................................45
garlic, creamy (*Kraft*) ..........................................................110
garlic, roasted, vinaigrette (*Wish-Bone*) ...............................50
green goddess (*Seven Seas*) ................................................130
herb vinaigrette (*Seven Seas*) .............................................140
herbs and spices (*Seven Seas*) ...........................................90
honey Dijon (*Just 2 Good!*) ...................................................50
honey Dijon (*Kraft*) .............................................................110
honey Dijon (*Kraft Free*) ......................................................45
honey mustard (*Seven Seas*) ..............................................110
Italian (*Just 2 Good!*) ..........................................................35
Italian (*Just 2 Good!* Country) ..............................................30
Italian (*Kraft Free*) ..............................................................20
Italian (*Kraft* ⅓ Less Fat) ....................................................70
Italian (*Kraft* Presto/Viva) ...................................................90
Italian (*Kraft* Zesty) ...........................................................110
Italian (*Viva Free*) ...............................................................10
Italian (*Viva* ⅓ Less Fat) .....................................................45
Italian (*Wish-Bone*) .............................................................80
Italian (*Wish-Bone* Classic House) .....................................140
Italian (*Wish-Bone* Fat Free) ...............................................10
Italian (*Wish-Bone* Robusto) ...............................................90
Italian, Caesar (*Kraft*) .........................................................100
Italian, Caesar (*Kraft Free*) ..................................................25
Italian, 2 cheese (*Seven Seas*) .............................................70
Italian, creamy (*Kraft*) .........................................................110
Italian, creamy (*Kraft Free/Seven Seas Free*) ......................50
Italian, creamy (*Seven Seas*) ..............................................120
Italian, creamy (*Seven Seas* ⅓ Less Fat) .............................60
Italian, creamy (*Wish-Bone*) ...............................................110
Italian, w/olive oil blend (*Kraft* House) ...............................120
Italian, w/olive oil blend (*Seven Seas* ⅓ Less Fat) ..............45
Italian, Parmesan basil (*Just 2 Good!*) .................................40
Italian, tomato and herb (*Kraft*) ..........................................100
mango lime vinaigrette (*Chi-Chi's*) ....................................120
olive oil vinaigrette (*Wish-Bone*) .........................................60

Oriental (*Wish-Bone*) ................................................35
Parmesan and onion (*Wish-Bone*) ...........................110
ranch (*Kraft*) .........................................................170
ranch (*Kraft Free*) ...................................................50
ranch (*Kraft* ⅓ Less Fat) ........................................110
ranch (*Seven Seas*) ...............................................160
ranch (*Seven Seas Free*) ..........................................45
ranch (*Seven Seas* ⅓ Less Fat) .............................100
ranch (*Wish-Bone*) .................................................160
ranch (*Wish-Bone* Fat Free) ......................................40
ranch, buttermilk (*Kraft*) .........................................150
ranch, Caesar (*Kraft*) ..............................................110
ranch, cucumber (*Kraft*) ..........................................140
ranch, cucumber (*Kraft* ⅓ Less Fat) ..........................60
ranch, garlic (*Kraft*) ................................................180
ranch, garlic (*Kraft Free*) ..........................................45
ranch, peppercorn (*Kraft*) ........................................170
ranch, peppercorn (*Kraft Free*) ..................................45
ranch, serrano (*Chi-Chi's/El Torito*) ..........................140
ranch, sour cream and onion (*Kraft*) .........................170
ranch, sour cream and onion (*Kraft Free*) ...................50
raspberry vinaigrette (*Seven Seas Free*) ......................30
red wine vinaigrette (*Wish-Bone*) ..............................90
red wine vinaigrette (*Wish-Bone* Fat Free) ..................35
red wine vinegar (*Kraft Free/Seven Seas Free*) ............15
red wine vinegar and oil (*Seven Seas*) ........................90
red wine vinegar and oil (*Seven Seas* ⅓ Less Fat) .......45
Russian (*Kraft*) .......................................................130
Russian (*Viva*) ........................................................150
Russian (*Wish-Bone*) ..............................................110
salsa vinaigrette (*Chi-Chi's*) ...................................110
serrano grape vinaigrette (*El Torito*) ...........................25
sesame cilantro (*Annie Chun's*), 1 tbsp ......................15
sun-dried tomato vinaigrette (*Wish-Bone*) ....................60
tamari mustard (*San-J*) .............................................45
tamari peanut or vinaigrette (*San-J*) ............................60
tamari sesame (*San-J*) ..............................................40
Thousand Island (*Just 2 Good!*) .................................60
Thousand Island (*Kraft*) ..........................................110

**Salad dressing (*cont.*)**

Thousand Island (*Kraft Free*).......................................................40
Thousand Island (*Kraft* ⅓ Less Fat).......................................70
Thousand Island, w/bacon (*Kraft*) ........................................130
white wine vinaigrette (*Wish-Bone*).......................................60

**Salad dressing mix,** 2 tbsp.*:

cheese garlic or garlic and herbs (*Good Seasons*) ..................140
Caesar (*Good Seasons* Gourmet)............................................150
French, honey (*Good Seasons*) .............................................160
garlic, roasted, or honey mustard (*Good Seasons*) ................150
honey mustard or honey French (*Good Seasons* Fat Free)........20
Italian, mild (*Good Seasons*) ...............................................150
Italian, Parmesan (*Good Seasons* Gourmet)...........................150
Italian or zesty herb (*Good Seasons* Fat Free) .......................10
Italian or zesty Italian (*Good Seasons*)..................................140
Italian or zesty Italian (*Good Seasons* Reduced Calorie) ...........50
Mexican spice (*Good Seasons*) ............................................140
Oriental sesame (*Good Seasons*) ..........................................150

**Salad seasoning mix,** taco (*Lawry's* Spices & Seasonings),
  1 tsp. ...........................................................................15

**Salami** (see also "Turkey salami"):

beef (*Boar's Head*), 2 oz....................................................120
beef (*Hebrew National*), 3 slices, 2 oz. ...............................150
beef (*Hebrew National* Lean), 4 slices, 2 oz. .........................90
beef (*Sara Lee* Deli), 3 slices, 2.2 oz. ..................................70
cooked (*Boar's Head*), 2 oz................................................130
cooked (*Russer*), 2 oz......................................................120
cooked (*Russer* Light), 2 oz. ...............................................90
dry or hard (*Oscar Mayer*), 3 slices, 1 oz. ...........................100
Genoa (*Boar's Head*), 2 oz.................................................180
Genoa (*Di Lusso*), 2 oz.....................................................210
Genoa (*Hormel Pillow Pack*), 5 slices, 1 oz. ........................120
Genoa or hard (*Russer*), 1 oz. ............................................100
Genoa or hard (*Sara Lee*), 4 slices, 1.1 oz.............................160
Genoa or hard (*Sara Lee* Deli), 4 slices, .9 oz.........................130
hard (*Boar's Head*), 2 oz...................................................110
hard (*Homeland*), 2 oz......................................................110

**Salisbury steak,** see "Beef dinner" and "Beef entree"

**Salmon,** fresh, meat only:
Atlantic, farmed, raw, 4 oz. ................................................207
Atlantic, farmed, baked, broiled, or microwaved, 4 oz. ............234
Atlantic, wild, raw, 4 oz. ...................................................161
Atlantic, wild, baked, broiled, or microwaved, 4 oz. ..................206
Chinook, raw, 4 oz. .........................................................204
Chinook, baked, broiled, or microwaved, 4 oz. .......................262
chum, raw, 4 oz. .............................................................136
chum, baked, broiled, or microwaved, 4 oz. ...........................175
coho, farmed, raw, 4 oz. ...................................................182
coho, farmed, baked, broiled, or microwaved, 4 oz. .................202
coho, wild, raw, 4 oz. .......................................................166
coho, wild, baked, broiled, or microwaved, 4 oz. .....................158
coho, wild, boiled, poached, or steamed, 4 oz. ........................209
pink, raw, 4 oz. ...............................................................132
pink, baked, broiled, or microwaved, 4 oz. .............................169
sockeye, raw, 4 oz. ..........................................................191
sockeye, baked, broiled, or microwaved, 4 oz. ........................245
**Salmon, canned:**
chum w/bone, drained, 13-oz. can .......................................520
pink (*Bumble Bee* Alaska/*Libby's*), 2.2 oz., about ¼ cup ...........90
red, sockeye, w/bone, drained, 13-oz. can .............................565
red, sockeye (*Bumble Bee* Alaska/*Libby's*), 2.2 oz., about
   ¼ cup .......................................................................110
**Salmon, smoked,** 2 oz., except as noted:
(*Ocean Beauty*) ...............................................................86
Atlantic (*Ducktrap River* Kendall Brook/Winter Harbor) ............130
Atlantic (*Ducktrap River* Spruce Point) .................................110
Chinook, regular or lox, 4 oz. .............................................133
roasted (*Ducktrap River*) ..................................................100
**Salmon, smoked, pâté** (*Ducktrap River*), ¼ cup ...................150
**Salmon burger,** frozen (*Ocean Beauty*), 3.2-oz. burger ............80
**"Salmon" burger, vegetarian** (*Dr. Praeger's* Veggie),
   2.8-oz. burger .............................................................100
**Salmon entree,** frozen:
croquettes (*Dr. Praeger's*), 2.2 oz. ......................................120
grilled, creamy dill or honey mustard (*Mrs. Paul's*),
   3.2-oz. pc. ...................................................................90
**Salmon nuggets,** frozen, heated, 4 oz. ................................240

**Salsa** (see also "Picante sauce"), 2 tbsp., except as noted:

(*D. L. Jardine's* Bobos) ................................................................15
(*D. L. Jardine's* Greenhorn Salsa & Dip) .............................10
(*Tostitos* Mild/Medium/Hot), 2.3 oz. .....................................30
(*Tostitos* Restaurant Style), 2.2 oz. ......................................30
all varieties:
    (*El Torito* Fire Roasted/Original Restaurant) ...................10
    (*Ortega*) .........................................................................10
    (*Pace* Thick & Chunky) ..................................................10
    (*Shotgun Willie's* Hotter'n Hell) .....................................10
    (*Taco Bell Home Originals* Thick 'N Chunky) .................15
    except black bean and corn (*Muir Glen* Organic) ...........10
    except garden and con queso (*Chi-Chi's*) .....................10
black bean (*D. L. Jardine's* Buckaroo Whistle-Berries) ........35
black bean, medium (*D. L. Jardine's* Buckaroo Buckshot) ....15
black bean and corn (*D. L. Jardine's* Buckaroo) ..................20
black bean and corn (*Muir Glen* Organic) ...........................15
cherry (*D. L. Jardine's* Wild & Woolly) ..................................20
garden (*Chi-Chi's*) ...............................................................15
garlic, roasted (*D. L. Jardine's* Buckaroo) ..........................10
garlic, roasted (*Tostitos*), 2.4 oz. ........................................30
habanero, hot (*D. L. Jardine's* XXX) ...................................10
medium (*D. L. Jardine's* Texacante) ....................................10
peach (*D. L. Jardine's*) .........................................................20
peach (*D. L. Jardine's* Twenty-Four Kick) ...........................10
pinto bean, spicy (*D. L. Jardine's* Buckaroo Cowboy
    Thunder) ..........................................................................15
raspberry (*D. L. Jardine's*) ...................................................15
verde (*D. L. Jardine's* Green Tomatillo Dip) ........................10
**Salsa dip** (see also "Cheese dip" and "Salsa"), 2 tbsp.:
(*Kraft Free*) ..........................................................................20
creamy (*Breakstone's Free/Knudsen Free*) .........................20
**Salsify,** fresh:
raw (*Frieda's*), ¾ cup, 3 oz. ................................................70
raw, sliced, 1 cup .................................................................109
boiled, drained, sliced, 1 cup ..................................................92
**Salt** (see also specific listings), table, 1 tbsp. .......................0
**Salt, seasoned,** all varieties (*Lawry's*) .................................0
**Salt substitute** (*Lawry's* Salt Free 17), ¼ tsp. .....................0

**Sandwich,** see specific listings
**Sandwich sauce,** see "Sloppy joe sauce"
**Sandwich spread** (see also "Meat spread"), 1 tbsp.:
(*Hellmann's/Best Foods*).................................................................50
(*Kraft*) ...............................................................................................50
(*Kraft* Reduced Fat).........................................................................35
**Sapodilla,** fresh (*Frieda's*), 3 oz...................................................70
**Sapote,** fresh, raw, trimmed, 7.9 oz. .....................................302
**Sardine,** fresh, see "Herring"
**Sardine, canned:**
Atlantic, in oil, w/bone, drained, 4 oz. .....................................236
Atlantic, in oil, w/bone, drained, 1 cup.....................................310
in olive oil, boneless, skinless (*Granadaisa*), ¼ cup .................120
lightly smoked, in hot sauce (*Bella*), ¼ cup .............................110
lightly smoked, in lemon sauce (*Bella*), ¼ cup ........................130
lightly smoked, in tomato sauce (*Bella*), ¼ cup.......................120
in mustard sauce (*Underwood* Fancy), 3.7-oz. can ..................180
Pacific, in tomato sauce, w/bone, drained, 13-oz. can..............659
**Sauce,** see specific listings
**Sauerkraut,** 2 tbsp., except as noted:
refrigerated (*Boar's Head*) ...............................................................5
refrigerated (*Claussen*), ¼ cup .......................................................5
refrigerated (*Hebrew National*).......................................................5
canned (*Del Monte*) ..........................................................................0
canned, w/liquid, 1 cup .................................................................45
canned, Bavarian style (*Del Monte*)...............................................15
**Sausage** (see also specific sausage listings):
(*Jones Dairy Farm* Light), 2 links...............................................130
(*Jones Dairy Farm* Patties), 1.13-oz. patty................................130
breakfast:
    raw, all flavors (*Johnsonville* Lower Fat), 3 links, 2.4 oz.....180
    pan-fried, all flavors (*Johnsonville/Perri*), 3 links, 1.9 oz. ..190
    pan-fried (*Johnsonville* Original/Maple), 2 patties, 2 oz. ......130
    pork and turkey (*Healthy Choice*), 2 links..............................50
brown and serve, precooked:
    (*Jones Dairy Farm* Golden Brown), 2 links.........................170
    (*Jones Dairy Farm* Golden Brown), 2 patties......................150
    (*Jones Dairy Farm* Golden Brown Light), 2 links .................100
    (*Jones Dairy Farm* Golden Brown Sandwich), 2 patties......170

**Sausage, brown and serve (*cont.*)**
    (*Little Sizzler*), 3 links........................................................230
    (*Little Sizzler*), 2 patties.....................................................190
    (*Swift Premium Brown 'N Serve* Original), 2 links..............210
    (*Swift Premium Brown 'N Serve* Original), 2 patties...........170
    apple cinnamon or pork and bacon (*Jones Dairy Farm*
       Golden Brown), 2 links.....................................................170
    maple (*Jones Dairy Farm* Golden Brown), 2 links...............190
chicken, raw:
    and apple, fresh (*Aidells*), 1.9-oz. link...............................100
    Romano, garlic, and parsley (*Perdue*), 2 oz. ......................110
    Romano, garlic, and parsley (*Perdue*), 1 link.....................150
    teriyaki, fresh (*Aidells*), 3.5-oz. link ................................210
chicken and turkey, see "turkey and chicken" and "smoked
    turkey and chicken," p. 227
dinner (*Jones Dairy Farm*), 1.44-oz. link.................................150
Italian:
    chicken, sweet, raw (*Perdue*), 2 oz. ..................................100
    chicken, sweet, raw (*Perdue*), 1 link .................................140
    pork, raw, 4-oz. link .............................................................391
    pork, cooked, 4-oz. link........................................................216
    pork, hot or sweet, raw (*Perri*), 4-oz. patty.......................340
    pork, mild, precooked (*Johnsonville*), 2.72-oz. link ...........250
    pork, mild or hot, raw (*Aidells*), 3.5-oz. link......................230
    pork, mild or hot, raw (*Perri*), 2.72-oz. link ......................230
    pork, mild or hot, grilled (*Johnsonville*), 3-oz. link .............290
    pork, pan-fried (*Johnsonville*), 2.5-oz. patty .....................240
    turkey, mild, raw (*Aidells*), 3.5-oz. link .............................190
    turkey, sweet or hot (*Perdue*), 1 link ................................150
lamb and beef, rosemary, fresh, raw (*Aidells*), 3.5-oz. link ......220
pork:
    link, raw, 1 oz. .....................................................................117
    link (*Jones Dairy Farm* Little Links), 3 links ......................190
    link, cooked (*Perri*), 3 links ...............................................190
    patty, cooked, 1 oz. .............................................................100
    roll (*Jones Dairy Farm* All Natural Original/Hot), 2 oz. .........230
smoked, beef (*Healthy Choice*), 2 oz. ....................................70
smoked, beef, 1.5-oz. sausage................................................134

smoked, chicken, precooked:
    and apple (*Aidells*), 3.5-oz. link ..............................210
    and apple (*Aidells* Mini), 6 links, 2 oz...................100
    lemon (*Aidells*), 3.5-oz. link................................210
smoked, duck and turkey (*Aidells*), 3.5-oz. link ......................220
smoked, hot (*Boar's Head*), 3.2-oz. link.....................................280
smoked, pork, whiskey fennel (*Aidells*), 3.5-oz. link................220
smoked, pork and beef:
    (*Johnsonville* Beddar with Cheddar Light), 2.32-oz. link.....240
    (*Johnsonville* Hot Links), 2.72-oz. link ...............................240
    (*Johnsonville* Light), 2.3-oz. link .........................................140
    (*Johnsonville* Little Smokies), 6 links, 2 oz. .......................180
    (*Johnsonville/Johnsonville* Beddar with Cheddar),
      2.72-oz. link.................................................................240
smoked, pork and veal, precooked (*Aidells* Bier), 3.5-oz. link .240
smoked, turkey, cranberry (*Aidells*), 3.5-oz. link......................210
smoked, turkey and chicken, 1 link:
    artichoke, precooked (*Aidells*), 3.5 oz. ...............................220
    Burmese curry or Thai, precooked (*Aidells*), 3.5 oz............220
    habanero and green chili (*Aidells*), 3.2 oz. .........................160
    New Mexico, precooked (*Aidells*), 3.5 oz. ...........................210
    sun-dried tomato basil, precooked (*Aidells*), 3.5 oz............200
smoked, turkey, pork, and beef (*Healthy Choice*), 2 oz.............70
turkey, scallion and herbs, fresh, raw (*Aidells*), 3.5-oz. link .....200
turkey and chicken, sun-dried tomatoes and basil, raw
    (*Aidells*), 3.5-oz. link.............................................................100
turkey and chicken, Thai, fresh, raw (*Aidells*), 3.5-oz. link .......200
**Sausage, canned:**
pickled, smoked, regular or hot (*Hormel*), 6 links, 2 oz...........140
Vienna (*Armour*), 3 links.............................................................150
Vienna (*Libby's*), 3 links .............................................................150
Vienna (*Hormel*), 2 oz..................................................................150
Vienna, chicken (*Hormel*), 2 oz...................................................110
**Sausage hash,** canned (*Mary Kitchen*), 1 cup .........................410
**Sausage sandwich,** frozen, 4.5-oz. piece:
biscuit, and egg (*Hormel Quick Meal*) .......................................390
muffin, egg and cheese (*Hormel Quick Meal*) ...........................260
**Sausage stick,** 1 pc., except as noted:
beef jerky (*Rustler's Roundup*), .3 oz..........................................40

**Sausage stick (*cont.*)**
hot (*Rustler's Roundup Flamin' Hot*), .3 oz. ...............................40
smoked/smoky (*Rustler's* Smoky Steak Strip), .8 oz. ................60
spicy (*Rustler's Roundup* Stick), .6 oz. ...................................100
**Savory, ground,** 1 tsp. ...................................................................4
**Scallion,** see "Onion, green"
**Scallop,** meat only:
raw, 2 large or 5 small, 1.1 oz. ...................................................26
raw, 4 oz. .....................................................................................100
breaded, fried, 2 large, 1.1 oz. .....................................................67
**Scallop, smoked** (*Ducktrap River*), ¼ cup ...............................60
**"Scallop," imitation,** from surimi, 4 oz. ...................................113
**Scallop entree,** frozen, fried (*Mrs. Paul's*), 13 pcs., 3.7 oz. ....220
**Scallop squash,** fresh:
raw, baby (*Frieda's* Sunburst), ⅔ cup, 3 oz. ..............................15
raw, sliced, 1 cup ........................................................................23
boiled, drained, sliced, 1 cup .......................................................29
**Scrapple** (*Jones Dairy Farm* Country Style), 2 oz. ..................120
**Scrod,** see "Cod, Atlantic"
**Scup,** meat only:
raw, 4 oz. .....................................................................................119
baked, broiled, or microwaved, 4 oz. ..........................................153
**Sea bass,** meat only:
raw, 4 oz. .....................................................................................110
baked, broiled, or microwaved, 4 oz. ..........................................141
**Sea breeze mix,** bottled (*Mr & Mrs T*), 4 fl. oz. .......................80
**Sea trout,** meat only:
raw, 4 oz. .....................................................................................118
baked, broiled, or microwaved, 4 oz. ..........................................151
**Seafood,** see specific listings
**Seafood sauce** (see also specific listings), cocktail, ¼ cup:
(*Crosse & Blackwell*) ..................................................................100
(*Del Monte*) ................................................................................100
(*Kraft*) ...........................................................................................60
shrimp (*Crosse & Blackwell*) ......................................................110
**Seafood seasoning,** see "Fish seasoning and coating mix"
**Seasoning and coating mix** (see also specific listings):
country (*Shake 'n Bake*), ⅛ pkt. .................................................35
peanut (*A Taste of Thai* Bake), ¼ pkt. .......................................25

**Seaweed:**

| | |
|---|---|
| agar, raw, 2 tbsp. | 3 |
| kelp, raw, 2 tbsp. | 4 |
| laver, raw, 10 sheets | 2 |
| laver, raw, 2 tbsp. | 4 |
| nori (*Eden*), 1 sheet | 10 |
| spirulina, dried, 1 cup | 44 |
| wakame, raw, 2 tbsp. | 5 |

**Semolina,** whole grain, 1 cup ... 601

**Semolina flour:**

| | |
|---|---|
| (*Arrowhead Mills*), ½ cup | 240 |
| pasta (*Hodgson Mill*), scant ¼ cup | 110 |

**Serrano chili,** see "Pepper, chili"

**Sesame butter,** see "Tahini"

**Sesame flour,** low fat, 1 oz. ... 95

**Sesame meal,** partially defatted, 1 oz. ... 161

**Sesame paste,** see "Tahini"

**Sesame seeds:**

| | |
|---|---|
| whole, dried, 1 tbsp. | 52 |
| whole, roasted/toasted, 1 oz. | 160 |
| kernels, decorticated, whole, 1 tbsp. | 47 |
| mechanically hulled (*Arrowhead Mills*), ¼ cup | 210 |
| whole brown (*Arrowhead Mills*), ¼ cup | 200 |

**Sesbania flower,** steamed, 1 cup ... 23

**Shad,** American, meat only:

| | |
|---|---|
| raw, 4 oz. | 223 |
| baked, broiled, or microwaved, 4 oz. | 286 |

**Shallot,** fresh:

| | |
|---|---|
| raw (*Frieda's*), 1 tbsp. | 20 |
| raw, chopped, 1 tbsp. | 7 |

**Shallot, freeze-dried,** 1 tbsp. ... 3

**Shark,** meat only, raw, 4 oz. ... 147

**Sheepshead,** meat only:

| | |
|---|---|
| raw, 4 oz. | 123 |
| baked, broiled, or microwaved, 4 oz. | 143 |

**Shell, pasta,** dry, see "Pasta"

**Shell, pasta, dinner,** frozen, stuffed (*Healthy Choice* Meal),
10.35-oz. pkg. ... 370

**Shell, pasta, entree,** frozen:
and cheese (*Freezer Queen*), 8.5-oz. pkg. ................................270
and cheese, American (*Stouffer's*), 1 cup ..............................280
and cheese, w/jalapenos (*Michelina's*), 8-oz. pkg. ................360
**Shell, pasta, mix:**
w/cheddar, white (*Pasta Roni*), approx. 1 cup* ......................310
w/cheese (*Kraft Velveeta* Original/Bacon), about 1 cup* ..........360
w/cheese (*Kraft Velveeta* Salsa), about 1 cup* ......................380
and cheese, creamy (*Land O Lakes*), 1 cup* ..........................350
**Shellie beans,** canned, 1 cup ..................................................74
**Sherbet,** ½ cup:
lemon bar or Swiss orange (*Edy's/Dreyer's*) ..........................150
orange, rainbow, or raspberry (*Breyers* All Natural) ................130
orange vanilla swirl (*Edy's/Dreyer's*) ......................................150
rainbow, berry, or tropical (*Edy's/Dreyer's*) ............................130
raspberry chocolate swirl (*Edy's/Dreyer's*) ............................130
**Sherbet bar,** 1 bar:
chocolate:
    (*Fudgsicle* 8 Pack), 2.5 fl. oz. ..............................................90
    (*Fudgsicle* 10/12 Pack) 1.75 fl. oz. .....................................60
    (*Fudgsicle* No Sugar Added 12 Pack), 1.75 fl. oz. ................45
    (*Fudgsicle Banana Bananza!* 8 Pack), 1.8 fl. oz. ..................60
    (*Popsicle Sherbet Cyclone* 8 Pack), 1.8 fl. oz. ....................50
and vanilla ice cream, all flavors:
    (*Creamsicle* 8 Pack), 2.5 fl. oz. ..........................................110
    (*Creamsicle* 12 Pack), 1.75 fl. oz. .......................................80
    (*Creamsicle* No Sugar Added), 1.75 fl. oz. ...........................25
**Shortening** (*Wesson*), 1 tbsp. ................................................110
**Shrimp,** mixed species, meat only:
raw, 4 oz. ..............................................................................120
raw, 4 large, 1 oz. ...................................................................30
boiled, poached, or steamed, 4 oz. ........................................112
boiled, poached, or steamed, 4 large, .8 oz. ............................22
breaded, fried, 4 large, 1.1 oz. .................................................73
**Shrimp,** canned:
medium, drained (*Bumble Bee*), ½ of 6-oz. can ......................45
tiny cocktail, drained (*Orleans*), ½ of 6-oz. can ......................44
1 cup ....................................................................................154
**Shrimp, smoked** (*Ducktrap River*), ¼ cup ..............................60

**Shrimp dinner,** frozen, and vegetables (*Healthy Choice* Meal),
    11.8-oz. pkg. .........................................................................270
**Shrimp entree,** frozen:
Alfredo, w/fettuccine (*Michelina's*), 8-oz. pkg. ........................310
w/angel hair pasta (*Lean Cuisine Cafe Classics*), 10-oz. pkg....240
buffalo (*Mrs. Paul's/Van de Kamp's*), 20 pcs., 4 oz. ...............320
butterfly (*Mrs. Paul's*), 7 pcs., 4 oz. ......................................270
butterfly (*Van de Kamp's*), 7 pcs., 4 oz. ................................300
linguine (*Mrs. Paul's/Van de Kamp's*), 1½ cups ......................180
lo mein (*Yu Sing*), 8-oz. pkg. .................................................210
popcorn (*Mrs. Paul's*), 20 pcs., 4 oz. .....................................290
popcorn (*Van de Kamp's*), 20 pcs., 4 oz. ...............................270
stir-fry (*Mrs. Paul's/Van de Kamp's*), 1⅔ cups ......................260
stuffed (*Van de Kamp's*), 3 pcs., 4.5 oz. ...............................290
**Shrimp sauce,** see "Seafood sauce"
**Sisymbrium seeds,** whole, dried, 1 tbsp. ................................15
**Sloppy joe sauce,** canned:
(*Heinz*), ½ cup ..........................................................................70
(*Manwich* Original), ¼ cup .......................................................30
**Smelt, rainbow,** meat only:
raw, 4 oz. ..................................................................................110
baked, broiled, or microwaved, 4 oz. .......................................141
**Snack mix** (see also "Trail mix"):
(*Cheez-It* Baked Big Crunch), ¾ cup .......................................110
(*Chex* Bold Party Blend/Peanut Lovers), ½ cup......................140
(*Chex* Traditional), ½ cup .......................................................130
(*D. L. Jardine's* Buckaroo Saddlebag Hunter's Mix), 1 oz.........170
(*Doo Dads*), ½ cup ..................................................................150
(*Planters* Caribbean Crunch), ¼ cup .......................................170
(*Ritz* Cheddar Flavor/Traditional), ½ cup ................................150
all varieties (*Act II*), ¾ cup ......................................................130
cheddar cheese (*Chex*), ½ cup ................................................140
cheese (*Cheez-It* Baked), ½ cup..............................................130
cheese, double (*Cheez-It* Baked), ¾ cup .................................110
honey, toasted (*Wheatables*), ½ cup .......................................130
honey nut (*Chex*), ½ cup .........................................................130
hot 'n spicy (*Chex*), ⅔ cup ......................................................130
nacho fiesta (*Chex*), ⅔ cup .....................................................120
w/nuts (*Cheez-It* Baked Get Nutty), ½ cup..............................150

**Snack mix (*cont.*)**
peanut butter (*Wheatables*), ½ cup................................160
**Snail, sea,** see "Whelk"
**Snapper,** meat only:
raw, 4 oz. ..............................................................113
baked, broiled, or microwaved, 4 oz. ......................145
**Snow pea,** see "Peas, edible pod"
**Soft drinks,** carbonated, 8 fl. oz., except as noted:
all flavors, except orange mango (*Koala*).................90
apple raspberry (*Fruit Works*), 12 fl. oz. ...............160
birch beer, brown (*Canada Dry*)..............................110
birch beer, clear (*Canada Dry*) ...............................100
blueberry (*Minute Maid*)........................................110
(*Canada Dry* Cactus Cooler/Half & Half/Hi-Spot).....100
(*Canada Dry* Tahitian Treat)...................................110
cherries n' cream (*Stewart's* Old Fashioned), 12 fl. oz..............190
cherry (*Crush*) ......................................................120
cherry (*Sunkist*) ...................................................130
cherry, black (*Canada Dry* Wish)............................120
cherry, black (*Minute Maid*)...................................110
cherry, wild (*Canada Dry*) ......................................100
cherry lime (*Slice*), 12 fl. oz. ...............................160
cherry spice (*Slice*), 12 fl. oz. ..............................150
(*Citra*)...................................................................90
citrus (*Orangina*)...................................................90
citrus (*Sunkist*) .....................................................90
club soda (*Canada Dry*)............................................0
cola (*Canada Dry* Jamaica).....................................120
cola (*Cherry Coke*).................................................105
cola (*Coca-Cola* Classic/Caffeine Free)..................100
cola (*Pepsi* Regular/Caffeine Free), 12 fl. oz. ........150
cola (*Slice*), 12 fl. oz. ...........................................160
cola, wild cherry (*Pepsi*), 12 fl. oz. .......................160
collins mixer (*Canada Dry/Schweppes*) ...................90
cream/creme soda:
    (*A&W*) .............................................................110
    (*Hires*) ............................................................120
    (*Mug*), 12 fl. oz. ...........................................170
    (*Stewart's*), 12 fl. oz. .....................................180

red (*Barq's*) ...........................................................115
vanilla (*Canada Dry*) ..............................................110
vanilla, French (*Barq's*) ..........................................110
(*Dr Pepper*) ..........................................................100
fruit punch (see also "Fruit drink blend"):
    (*Crush* Fruity Red)..........................................120
    (*Minute Maid* Carbonated) .............................115
    (*Slice*), 12 fl. oz...............................................190
    (*Sunkist*) .......................................................120
    tropical (*Crush*) .............................................110
    tropical (*Welch's*) ..........................................130
ginger ale (*Canada Dry/Schweppes*) .......................80
ginger ale (*Canada Dry* Golden) ...............................90
ginger ale (*Vernors*).................................................100
ginger ale, cherry (*Canada Dry*) .............................100
ginger ale, cranberry or lemon (*Canada Dry*) .............90
ginger ale, grape or raspberry (*Schweppes*)...............90
ginger beer (*Schweppes*) ..........................................90
grape (*Canada Dry* Concord)..................................110
grape (*Crush*) .........................................................130
grape (*Minute Maid*) ...............................................125
grape (*Schweppes*)...................................................120
grape (*Slice*), 12 fl. oz. ..........................................190
grape (*Stewart's* Classic), 12 fl. oz. .......................190
grape (*Sunkist/Welch's*)...........................................130
grapefruit (*Schweppes*) ...........................................100
grapefruit (*Squirt*) ...................................................100
grapefruit, ruby red (*Squirt*) ....................................120
guava berry (*Fruit Works*), 12 fl. oz. .......................170
lemon, bitter (*Schweppes*) .......................................110
lemon lime (*Schweppes*) ............................................90
lemon lime (*Slice*), 12 fl. oz. ..................................150
lemon meringue (*Stewart's*), 12 fl. oz. .....................200
lemon sour (*Canada Dry*)............................................90
lemon sour (*Schweppes*) ..........................................100
lemonade, pink (*Fruit Works*), 12 fl. oz.....................170
lime (*Canada Dry* Island) .........................................120
lime, key (*Stewart's*), 12 fl. oz. ...............................190
(*Mello Yello*)...........................................................120

**Soft drinks (*cont.*)**

(*Mountain Dew* Regular/Caffeine Free), 12 fl. oz. .....................170
(*Mr. Pibb*)............................................................................100
orange (*Crush/Welch's*)......................................................120
orange (*Fanta/Minute Maid*)...............................................120
orange (*Slice* Citrus Taste), 12 fl. oz. .................................170
orange (*Slice* New Bold Taste), 12 fl. oz. .............................190
orange (*Sunkist*) ................................................................130
orange n' cream (*Stewart's* Country), 12 fl. oz. ....................190
orange mango (*Koala*)...........................................................80
orange passion (*Fruit Works*), 12 fl. oz. ...............................160
peach (*Canada Dry*).............................................................110
peach (*Crush*) .....................................................................120
peach (*Stewart's*), 12 fl. oz. ................................................190
peach (*Sunkist*) ..................................................................110
peach (*Welch's*) ..................................................................130
peach papaya (*Fruit Works*), 12 fl. oz. .................................170
pineapple (*Canada Dry*).......................................................100
pineapple (*Crush/Sunkist*) ..................................................120
pineapple (*Minute Maid*)......................................................110
pineapple (*Slice*), 12 fl. oz...................................................190
pineapple (*Welch's*).............................................................130
(*Red Flash*) ........................................................................105
root beer (*A&W*) .................................................................120
root beer (*Barq's*) ...............................................................110
root beer (*Barrelhead*).........................................................100
root beer (*Hires*).................................................................120
root beer (*Mug*), 12 fl. oz....................................................160
root beer (*Stewart's*), 12 fl. oz. ...........................................160
seltzer, plain or flavored (*Canada Dry/Schweppes*).................0
(*7UP/Cherry 7UP*)..............................................................100
sour mixer (*Canada Dry*)........................................................80
(*Sprite*)...............................................................................100
strawberry (*Canada Dry* California) .....................................100
strawberry (*Crush*)..............................................................110
strawberry (*Minute Maid*) ...................................................120
strawberry (*Slice*), 12 fl. oz.................................................170
strawberry (*Sunkist*) ...........................................................120
strawberry (*Welch's*) ...........................................................120

strawberry melon (*Fruit Works*), 12 fl. oz. ...............160
(*Surge*)...............................................................115
tangerine citrus (*Fruit Works*), 12 fl. oz. ...............150
tonic water (*Canada Dry*) .......................................90
tonic water (*Schweppes*) ........................................80
(*Wink II*).............................................................110
**Sole,** see "Flatfish"
**Sole entree,** frozen, 5-oz. pc.:
au gratin (*Oven Poppers*) .....................................220
stuffed, w/broccoli and cheese (*Oven Poppers*) ......150
stuffed, w/crab (*Oven Poppers*) ............................250
stuffed, w/garlic shrimp and almonds (*Oven Poppers*) ..........250
stuffed, w/shrimp and lobster (*Oven Poppers*)........150
**Sopressata sausage:**
hot (*Beretta*), 2 oz...............................................230
w/wine (*Fiorucci*), 1 oz..........................................80
**Sorbet** (see also "Ice" and "Sherbet"), ½ cup:
(*Ben & Jerry's Doonesberry*) ...............................140
boysenberry (*Edy's/Dreyer's*)................................150
chocolate (*Ben & Jerry's Devil's Food*) .................170
chocolate (*Edy's/Dreyer's*) ...................................160
chocolate (*Häagen-Dazs*).....................................120
chocolate, Dutch (*Sharon's Sorbet*) ......................130
coconut (*Sharon's Sorbet*)....................................160
lemon (*Edy's/Dreyer's*)..........................................140
lemon (*Häagen-Dazs Zesty Lemon*) ......................120
lemon (*Sharon's Sorbet*)........................................75
lemon swirl (*Ben & Jerry's*)...................................120
mango, peach, or raspberry (*Edy's/Dreyer's*)...........130
mango or raspberry (*Sharon's Sorbet*).....................80
orange (*Häagen-Dazs*)..........................................120
peach (*Häagen-Dazs* Orchard)...............................140
*Purple Passion Fruit* (*Ben & Jerry's*) ...................140
raspberry (*Häagen-Dazs*)......................................120
strawberry (*Edy's/Dreyer's*) ..................................120
strawberry (*Häagen-Dazs*).....................................130
vanilla (*Häagen-Dazs*)..........................................120
vanilla, dark (*Sharon's Sorbet*) .............................110
**Sorbet bar** (*Frozfruit Cool Cotton Candy*), 1 bar ......100

**Sorghum,** whole grain, 1 cup....................................................651
**Sorghum syrup** (*Arrowhead Mills*), 1 tbsp.............................60
**Sorrel,** see "Dock"
**Soup, canned, ready-to-serve,** 1 cup, except as noted:
asparagus, cream of (*Baxters*) ...............................................130
bean (*Dominique's* U.S. Senate)..............................................170
bean, black (*Greene's Farm*)....................................................160
bean, black (*Progresso* Hearty)...............................................170
bean, black, Indian, w/rice (*Shari Ann's* Organic) ..................150
bean, 5, w/barley (*Coco Pazzo* Tuscan)..................................220
bean, 3, w/sage (*Coco Pazzo* Tuscan).....................................240
bean, white, w/escarole (*Coco Pazzo* Tuscan).........................210
bean, white, Italian (*Shari Ann's* Organic) ..............................170
bean, Mexican, spicy (*Shari Ann's* Organic).............................210
bean and ham (*Campbell's Chunky*) .........................................190
bean and ham (*Campbell's Home Cookin'*) ...............................180
bean and ham (*Healthy Choice*) ...............................................150
bean and pasta (*Baxters* Healthy Reward Italian)......................110
bean and pasta (*Healthy Choice* Mediterranean).......................130
beef barley (*Progresso/Progresso* 99% Fat Free) .....................130
beef broth (*College Inn* No Fat)..................................................20
beef broth (*Swanson*)..................................................................20
beef and mushroom (*Progresso*) ..............................................100
beef pasta (*Campbell's Chunky*)................................................140
beef and potato (*Healthy Choice*) .............................................110
beef and potato, baked (*Progresso*)..........................................130
beef and vegetable (*Progresso*).................................................100
beef vegetable, country (*Campbell's Chunky*) ...........................150
broccoli cheddar (*Healthy Choice*) .............................................90
chicken (*Healthy Choice* Hearty) ..............................................130
chicken Alfredo (*Healthy Choice*) ..............................................110
chicken barley (*Progresso*)........................................................110
chicken, broccoli, cheese, and potato (*Campbell's Chunky*).....200
chicken broth (*Campbell's Healthy Request*)..............................20
chicken broth (*College Inn*)........................................................20
chicken broth (*College Inn* Low Salt)..........................................25
chicken broth (*College Inn* No Fat).............................................10
chicken broth (*Swanson*) ...........................................................20
chicken broth (*Swanson* Clear) .................................................10

chicken broth (*Swanson* Fat Free).................................................15
chicken broth, w/Italian herbs or roasted garlic (*Swanson*) .......20
chicken broth, w/onion (*Swanson*) .................................................25
chicken corn chowder (*Campbell's Chunky*) .............................250
chicken corn chowder (*Campbell's Healthy Request* Hearty) ...150
chicken corn chowder (*Healthy Choice*)......................................150
chicken garden herb, roasted (*Progresso*)....................................70
chicken w/meatballs (*Progresso* Chickarina) .............................130
chicken mushroom chowder (*Campbell's Chunky*)..................210
chicken noodle (*Campbell's Chunky* Classic)............................130
chicken noodle (*Campbell's Healthy Request* Hearty)..............100
chicken noodle (*Campbell's Simply Home*)..................................80
chicken noodle (*Healthy Choice*).................................................120
chicken noodle (*Progresso/Progresso* 99% Fat Free) ...............90
chicken noodle, egg (*Campbell's Home Cookin'*) .......................90
chicken noodle, egg (*Wolfgang Puck's*).....................................150
chicken pasta (*Campbell's Simply Home*).....................................90
chicken pasta (*Healthy Choice*)...................................................110
chicken pasta and mushroom (*Campbell's Chunky*) ...............120
chicken pasta w/roasted garlic (*Campbell's Home Cookin'*).....120
chicken rice (*Campbell's Healthy Request*)................................110
chicken rice (*Campbell's Home Cookin'*) ...................................100
chicken rice (*Healthy Choice*) .....................................................100
chicken rice (*Rienzi*).....................................................................110
chicken rice, white/wild (*Campbell's Chunky*) ..........................140
chicken rice, white/wild (*Campbell's Simply Home*) .................100
chicken rice, wild (*Progresso*).....................................................100
chicken rice, wild (*Progresso* 99% Fat Free) ..............................90
chicken and rotini (*Progresso* Hearty) ..........................................80
chicken vegetable (*Campbell's Chunky* Hearty)...........................90
chicken vegetable (*Campbell's Healthy Request*) .....................110
chicken vegetable (*Campbell's Home Cookin'*)..........................120
chicken vegetable (*Progresso*) ......................................................90
chicken vegetable, Italian (*Campbell's Home Cookin'*) .............130
chicken vegetable, roast (*Wolfgang Puck's*)..............................140
chicken vegetable, spicy (*Campbell's Chunky*) ...........................90
chicken vegetable, w/pasta (*Progresso* Homestyle)....................90
chili beef (*Healthy Choice*)...........................................................190
chili beef w/beans (*Campbell's Chunky*), 1 can .......................300

**Soup, canned, ready-to-serve (*cont.*)**
clam chowder:
    Manhattan (*Campbell's Chunky*) ............................................130
    Manhattan (*Progresso*) .............................................................110
    New England (*Campbell's Chunky*) .....................................240
    New England (*Campbell's Healthy Request* Hearty) ............120
    New England (*Campbell's Home Cookin'*) .........................190
    New England (*Campbell's Home Cookin'* 98% Fat Free) .....110
    New England (*Dominique's*) ................................................200
    New England (*Healthy Choice*) ............................................120
    New England (*Progresso*) .....................................................190
    New England (*Snow's*) ..........................................................170
consommé, clear (*Dominique's* Madrilène) ...............................30
consommé, red (*Dominique's* Madrilène) .................................35
corn chowder (*Greene's Farm*) ................................................120
corn tortilla (*D. L. Jardine's* Buckaroo) ..................................130
crab, cream of (*Chincoteague*) ................................................200
crab, red, vegetable (*Chincoteague*) .........................................90
escarole (*Progresso*) ..................................................................25
gazpacho (*Dominique's*) .............................................................60
gumbo, zesty (*Healthy Choice*) ...............................................100
leek, Scotch (*Baxters*) ................................................................80
lentil (*Amy's* Organic) ..............................................................130
lentil (*Progresso* Classics) ......................................................140
lentil (*Progresso* 99% Fat Free) ..............................................130
lentil (*Rienzi*) ...........................................................................130
lentil, green, French, spicy (*Shari Ann's* Organic) ...................130
lentil, sausage (*Dominique's*) .................................................200
lentil, savory (*Campbell's Home Cookin'*) ...............................130
lobster bisque (*Baxters*) ..........................................................120
macaroni and bean (*Progresso* Classics) ................................160
macaroni and bean (*Rienzi*) ....................................................150
minestrone (*Amy's* Organic) .....................................................90
minestrone (*Baxters* Healthy Reward Homestyle) .....................110
minestrone (*Campbell's* Plus! Hearty) .....................................130
minestrone (*Campbell's Healthy Request* Hearty) ....................120
minestrone (*Campbell's Home Cookin'* Old World) ..................120
minestrone (*Campbell's Simply Home*) ....................................110
minestrone (*Healthy Choice*) ...................................................120

minestrone (*Progresso* 99% Fat Free) ......................................110
minestrone (*Rienzi*) ............................................................130
minestrone (*Shari Ann's* Organic) ........................................120
minestrone, Tuscany (*Campbell's Home Cookin'*) ...................190
mushroom, cream of (*Amy's* Organic), ¾ cup ........................120
mushroom, cream of (*Campbell's Home Cookin'* 98%
    Fat Free) ......................................................................80
mushroom rice (*Campbell's Home Cookin'* Country) .................90
noodle (*Amy's* Organic No Chicken) .......................................90
noodle, Oriental, vegetable (*Campbell's Home Cookin'*) ..........100
onion, French (*Progresso* Distinctive Recipe) ..........................50
onion, French, vegetarian (*Shari Ann's* Organic) .....................60
onion, French (*Wolfgang Puck's* Country) ..............................140
pasta and vegetables (*Campbell's* Plus! Hearty) .....................110
pea, split (*Amy's* Organic) ...................................................100
pea, split, green (*Progresso* Classics) ...................................170
pea, split (*Shari Ann's* Organic Great Plains) .........................150
pea, split, and ham (*Campbell's Chunky*) ...............................190
pea, split, and ham (*Campbell's Healthy Request*) ..................170
pea, split, w/ham (*Campbell's Home Cookin'*) .........................170
pea, split, w/ham (*Healthy Choice*) .......................................170
pea, split, w/ham (*Progresso* Distinctive Recipe) ...................150
penne (*Progresso* Hearty) ......................................................80
pepper steak (*Campbell's Chunky*) ........................................130
potato, baked:
    w/bacon bits and chives (*Campbell's Chunky*) ...................170
    w/cheddar and bacon bits (*Campbell's Chunky*) .................180
    w/steak and cheese (*Campbell's Chunky*) ..........................200
    style (*Healthy Choice*) ....................................................120
potato, creamy, w/roasted garlic (*Campbell's Home Cookin'*)..180
potato w/broccoli and cheese chowder (*Progresso*) ................160
potato and cheddar (*Shari Ann's* Organic) .............................100
potato and ham, creamy (*Healthy Choice*) .............................140
potato ham chowder (*Campbell's Chunky* Old Fashioned) .......220
potato and leek (*Baxters* Healthy Reward) ..............................80
potato w/roasted garlic (*Campbell's Healthy Request*) .............110
rotini tomato, basil (*Progresso*) ............................................120
sirloin burger w/country vegetables (*Campbell's Chunky*) ........210
steak and potato (*Campbell's Chunky*) ..................................150

**Soup, canned, ready-to-serve (*cont.*)**

| | |
|---|---|
| tomato (*Campbell's*) | 100 |
| tomato (*Muir Glen* Organic Fresh Pack) | 60 |
| tomato, cream of (*Amy's* Organic) | 100 |
| tomato, creamy (*Campbell's*) | 130 |
| tomato, garden (*Campbell's Home Cookin'*) | 100 |
| tomato, garden (*Healthy Choice*) | 110 |
| tomato, ravioli, cheese, w/vegetables (*Campbell's Chunky*) | 150 |
| tomato, ravioli, w/vegetables (*Campbell's Healthy Request* Hearty) | 140 |
| tomato, w/red bell pepper (*Shari Ann's* Organic) | 100 |
| tomato, w/roasted garlic (*Shari Ann's* Organic) | 50 |
| tomato, w/vegetables (*Wolfgang Puck's* Country) | 150 |
| tortellini, cheese and herb (*Progresso*) | 140 |
| tortellini, cheese, w/chicken, vegetables (*Campbell's Chunky*) | 110 |
| turkey, w/wild rice (*Healthy Choice*) | 100 |
| turkey noodle (*Progresso*) | 90 |
| turkey rice w/vegetables (*Progresso*) | 110 |
| turkey and wild rice (*Greene's Farm*) | 110 |
| vegetable (*Campbell's Chunky*) | 130 |
| vegetable (*Progresso* Classics) | 90 |
| vegetable (*Campbell's Healthy Request* Hearty) | 100 |
| vegetable (*Campbell's Home Cookin'* Country) | 110 |
| vegetable (*Campbell's Home Cookin'* Fiesta) | 140 |
| vegetable, country or garden (*Healthy Choice*) | 100 |
| vegetable, garden (*Campbell's Simply Home*) | 110 |
| vegetable, Indian, hot (*Patak's* Sabzi Mulligatawny) | 100 |
| vegetable, Indian, mild, tomato and lentil (*Patak's*) | 120 |
| vegetable, w/pasta (*Campbell's Chunky* Hearty) | 140 |
| vegetable, w/pasta (*Rienzi*) | 100 |
| vegetable, roasted, w/barley and wild rice (*Campbell's* Plus!) | 130 |
| vegetable, southwestern (*Campbell's Healthy Request*) | 140 |
| vegetable, thick (*Wolfgang Puck's* Country) | 180 |
| vegetable barley (*Shari Ann's* Organic) | 100 |
| vegetable beef (*Campbell's Chunky* Old Fashioned) | 150 |
| vegetable beef (*Campbell's Healthy Request* Hearty) | 140 |
| vegetable beef (*Campbell's Home Cookin'*) | 110 |
| vegetable beef (*Healthy Choice*) | 120 |

vegetable beef, pasta (*Campbell's Simply Home*) ....................120
vegetable broth (*Swanson* Clear) .................................................20
vegetable broth, garden (*College Inn*) ..........................................20
vichyssoise (*Dominique's*)............................................................130
**Soup, canned, condensed,** undiluted, ½ cup:
asparagus, cream of (*Campbell's*)..................................................90
bean, black (*Campbell's*).............................................................110
bean w/bacon (*Campbell's*) .........................................................180
bean w/ham and bacon (*Campbell's Healthy Request*) .............150
beef broth, double rich (*Campbell's*) ............................................15
beef consommé (*Campbell's*) ........................................................25
beef noodle (*Campbell's*) ..............................................................70
beef w/vegetables and barley (*Campbell's*) ..................................80
beefy mushroom (*Campbell's*) .......................................................70
broccoli, cream of (*Campbell's*) ...................................................100
broccoli, cream of (*Campbell's* 98% Fat Free) .............................80
broccoli, cream of (*Campbell's Healthy Request*)........................70
broccoli cheese (*Campbell's*)........................................................110
broccoli cheese, cream of (*Campbell's* 98% Fat Free) ................80
(*Campbell's Souper Stars*)..............................................................50
celery, cream of (*Campbell's*) ......................................................110
celery, cream of (*Campbell's* 98% Fat Free)................................80
celery, cream of (*Campbell's Healthy Request*) ..........................70
cheese, cheddar (*Campbell's*)........................................................90
cheese, nacho (*Campbell's* Fiesta) ..............................................140
chicken:
    alphabet w/vegetables (*Campbell's*)......................................80
    broth (*Campbell's*).....................................................................30
    cream of (*Campbell's*).............................................................130
    cream of (*Campbell's* 98% Fat Free).......................................80
    cream of (*Campbell's Healthy Request*) .................................70
    cream of, and broccoli (*Campbell's*)......................................120
    cream of, and broccoli (*Campbell's Healthy Request*) ..........80
    cream of, w/herbs (*Campbell's*)...............................................80
    dumplings (*Campbell's*) .............................................................80
    gumbo (*Campbell's*)...................................................................60
    noodle (*Campbell's*)...................................................................70
    noodle (*Campbell's* Homestyle) ................................................70
    noodle (*Campbell's Healthy Request*) .....................................70

**Soup, canned, condensed, chicken (*cont.*)**

noodle (*Campbell's NoodleO's*) ...............................................80
noodle, creamy (*Campbell's*) ...............................................130
noodle, curly (*Campbell's*) ...............................................80
noodle, double, in broth (*Campbell's*) ...............................................100
mushroom, cream of (*Campbell's*) ...............................................130
rice (*Campbell's*) ...............................................70
rice (*Campbell's Healthy Request*) ...............................................60
rice, white/wild (*Campbell's*) ...............................................70
and stars (*Campbell's*) ...............................................70
vegetable (*Campbell's*) ...............................................80
vegetable (*Campbell's Healthy Request*) ...............................................80
vegetable, southwestern style (*Campbell's*) ...............................................110
chili beef w/beans (*Campbell's Fiesta*) ...............................................170
clam bisque (*Chincoteague*) ...............................................100
clam chowder, Manhattan style (*Campbell's*) ...............................................60
clam chowder, Manhattan style (*Chincoteague*) ...............................................100
clam chowder, New England (*Campbell's*) ...............................................90
clam chowder, New England (*Campbell's 98% Fat Free*) ...............................................90
clam chowder, New England (*Chincoteague*) ...............................................80
clam chowder, New England (*Olde Cape Cod* All Natural) ...............................................80
corn chowder (*Chincoteague*) ...............................................100
corn chowder (*Olde Cape Cod* All Natural Old Fashioned) .......110
crab and cheddar (*Chincoteague* Chesapeake Bay) ...............................................90
lobster bisque (*Chincoteague*) ...............................................90
lobster bisque (*Olde Cape Cod* All Natural Gourmet) ...............................................60
minestrone (*Campbell's*) ...............................................90
minestrone (*Campbell's Healthy Request*) ...............................................90
mushroom, cream of (*Campbell's*) ...............................................110
mushroom, cream of (*Campbell's 98% Fat Free*) ...............................................70
mushroom, cream of (*Campbell's Healthy Request*) ...............................................70
mushroom, cream of, w/roasted garlic (*Campbell's*) ...............................................70
mushroom, golden (*Campbell's*) ...............................................80
noodle and ground beef (*Campbell's*) ...............................................100
onion, cream of (*Campbell's*) ...............................................110
onion, French (*Campbell's*) ...............................................70
oyster chowder (*Olde Cape Cod*) ...............................................70
oyster stew (*Campbell's*) ...............................................90
pea, green (*Campbell's*) ...............................................180

pea, split, w/ham (*Campbell's*) .................................................180
pepperpot (*Campbell's*) ...........................................................100
potato, cream of (*Campbell's*) ..................................................90
Scotch broth (*Campbell's*) ........................................................80
shrimp, cream of (*Campbell's*) ................................................100
shrimp bisque (*Chincoteague*) ..................................................80
shrimp and tomato bisque, garlic (*Olde Cape Cod*) ..................60
tomato (*Campbell's*) .................................................................80
tomato (*Campbell's Healthy Request*) ......................................90
tomato, Italian, w/basil and oregano (*Campbell's*) ..................100
tomato bisque (*Campbell's*) ...................................................130
tomato rice (*Campbell's* Old Fashioned) ................................120
turkey noodle (*Campbell's*) .......................................................80
turkey vegetable (*Campbell's*) ..................................................80
vegetable (*Campbell's*) .............................................................80
vegetable (*Campbell's* Old Fashioned) .....................................70
vegetable (*Campbell's Healthy Request*) ..................................90
vegetable, California style (*Campbell's*) ...................................60
vegetable, and pasta (*Campbell's Healthy Request* Hearty) ........90
vegetable, w/pasta (*Campbell's* Hearty) ...................................90
vegetable, vegetarian (*Campbell's*) ..........................................90
vegetable beef (*Campbell's*) .....................................................80
vegetable beef (*Campbell's Healthy Request*) ...........................80
won ton (*Campbell's*) ...............................................................45
**Soup, canned, semicondensed,** undiluted, ⅔ cup:
bean, black (*Pepperidge Farm*) ...............................................120
chicken, w/wild rice (*Pepperidge Farm*) ...................................80
chicken curry (*Pepperidge Farm*) ...........................................170
clam chowder or corn chowder (*Pepperidge Farm*) ..................70
consommé (*Pepperidge Farm* Madrilène) .................................50
gazpacho or vichyssoise (*Pepperidge Farm*) ............................70
lobster bisque (*Pepperidge Farm*) ..........................................160
mushroom, shiitake (*Pepperidge Farm*) ....................................80
onion, French (*Pepperidge Farm*) ............................................50
watercress (*Pepperidge Farm*) .................................................80
**Soup mix** (see also "Soup base mix"):
bean (*Hodgson Mill* Choice), ¼ cup...................................150
bean, navy (*Knorr* TasteBreaks), 1 cont. ..............................130
bean and ham (*Hormel* Microcup Soups), 1 cup.....................190

**Soup mix (*cont.*)**
bean, 7, and barley (*Arrowhead Mills*), ¼ cup ..........................170
bean, white, and spinach spirals (*Marrakesh Express* Zuppa),
    1 cup ...................................................................................130
beef noodle (*House of Tsang*), 1 cont. ...................................120
beef noodle vegetable (*Herb-Ox*), 1 cont. ............................130
beef vegetable (*Hormel* Microcup Soups), 1 cup.......................90
black bean (*Knorr* TasteBreaks), 1 cont. ................................190
black bean, spicy, w/orzo (*Marrakesh Express* Zuppa),
    1 cup ...................................................................................160
broccoli, cream of (*Knorr Recipe Classics*), 3 tbsp. ...................70
broccoli cheese, w/ham (*Hormel* Microcup Soups), 1 cup.......170
chicken/chicken flavor:
    creamy (*Knorr*), 3 tbsp.....................................................90
    noodle (*Herb-Ox*), 1 cont. ..............................................110
    noodle (*Hormel* Microcup Soups), 1 cup ..........................110
    noodle (*House of Tsang*), 1 cont. ....................................120
    noodle (*Mrs. Grass* Homestyle), ¼ pkg............................70
    rice (*Hormel* Microcup Soups), 1 cup ..............................110
    rice (*Mrs. Grass*), ¼ pkg.................................................80
chili (*Herb-Ox*), 1 cont. .........................................................200
chili, w/out beans (*Herb-Ox*), 1 cont.....................................210
clam chowder, New England (*Hormel* Microcup Soups),
    1 cup ...................................................................................130
corn chowder (*Knorr* TasteBreaks), 1 cont. ...........................140
corn, velvet (*House of Tsang*), 1 cont. ...................................170
couscous, toasted onion (*Marrakesh Express* Zuppa), 1 cup...160
eggplant, tomato, and mushroom (*Marrakesh Express*
    Zuppa), 1 cup.......................................................................160
garlic, roasted, herb (*Knorr Recipe Classics*), 3 tbsp. .............80
herb, fiesta, w/red pepper (*Lipton Recipe Secrets*), 1⅓ tbsp. ....30
herb, savory, w/garlic (*Lipton Recipe Secrets*), 1 tbsp. .............30
hot and sour (*Knorr Recipe Classics*), 2 tbsp. .........................45
leek (*Knorr Recipe Classics*), 2 tbsp. .....................................70
lentil (*Herb-Ox*), 1 cont. ........................................................140
lentil, hearty (*Knorr* TasteBreaks), 1 cont. .............................200
minestrone, savory (*Knorr* Mediterranean Style), 3 tbsp..........100
miso, dark (*San-J*), 1 cont......................................................40
miso, mild (*San-J*), 1 cont.......................................................50

mushroom, beefy (*Lipton Recipe Secrets*), 1½ tbsp. ..................35
mushroom, garlic (*Lipton Recipe Secrets*), 1⅓ tbsp. .................20
mushroom and noodle (*House of Tsang*), 1 cont. .....................120
noodle:
    all flavors except creamy chicken, tomato, and noodles
       only (*Maruchan* Ramen), ½ pkg. .....................................190
    beef (*Maruchan* Instant Lunch), 1 cont. ..............................290
    chicken or pork (*Maruchan* Instant Lunch), 1 cont. .............280
    chicken, creamy (*Maruchan* Instant Lunch), 1 cont. ...........290
    chicken, creamy (*Maruchan* Ramen), ½ pkg. ......................200
    chicken, savory (*Knorr*), 3 tbsp. ..........................................70
    chicken broth (*Mrs. Grass*), ¼ pkg. .....................................60
    chicken curry (*Maruchan* Instant Lunch), 1 cont. ...............290
    chicken flavor, hearty (*Knorr* TasteBreaks), 1 cont. ............120
    chicken mushroom (*Maruchan* Instant Lunch), 1 cont. .......270
    chili w/beans (*Maruchan* Instant Lunch), 1 cont. ................290
    Italian (*Maruchan* Instant Lunch), 1 cont. ...........................270
    noodles only (*Maruchan* Ramen), ½ pkg. ...........................189
    picante, all flavors, except vegetable (*Maruchan* Instant
       Lunch), 1 cont. .............................................................280
    picante, beef or chicken (*Maruchan*), 1 cont. .....................290
    picante, shrimp (*Maruchan*), 1 cont. ...................................280
    picante, vegetable (*Maruchan*), 1 cont. ..............................270
    picante, vegetable (*Maruchan* Instant Lunch), 1 cont. ........270
    shrimp (*Maruchan* Instant Lunch), 1 cont. ..........................290
    tomato (*Maruchan* Ramen), ½ pkg. .....................................200
    tomato vegetable (*Maruchan* Instant Lunch), 1 cont. .........290
    vegetable, California (*Maruchan* Instant Lunch), 1 cont. .....260
onion (*Lipton Recipe Secrets*), 1 tbsp. ...................................20
onion (*Mrs. Grass* Recipe Soup/Dip Mix), ¼ pkg. ...................30
onion (*Mrs. Grass* Reduced Sodium Recipe Soup/Dip Mix),
    ¼ pkg. ..............................................................................30
onion, beefy (*Lipton Recipe Secrets*), 1 tbsp. ..........................25
onion, French (*Knorr Recipe Classics*), 2 tbsp. ........................35
onion, golden (*Lipton Recipe Secrets*), 1⅔ tbsp. ......................50
onion-mushroom (*Lipton Recipe Secrets*), 2 tbsp. ...................30
onion-mushroom (*Mrs. Grass* Recipe Soup/Dip Mix), ¼ pkg. ....50
pasta fagioli/red beans (*Marrakesh Express* Zuppa), 1 cup ......140
pea, split (*Knorr* TasteBreaks), 1 cont. ...................................150

**Soup mix (*cont.*)**

potato cheese, w/ham (*Hormel* Microcup Soups), 1 cup .........190
potato leek (*Herb-Ox*), 1 cont. ...................................................140
potato leek (*Knorr* TasteBreaks), 1 cont. ...................................130
roasted red pepper and rice (*Marrakesh Express* Zuppa),
   1 cup .........................................................................................140
rice, Spanish (*Herb-Ox*), 1 cont. ...............................................250
rice, wild (*Herb-Ox*), 1 cont. .....................................................230
rice, wild, and herb (*Arrowhead Mills*), ⅓ cup...........................140
spinach, cream of (*Knorr Recipe Classics*), 2 tbsp....................70
tomato, w/basil (*Knorr Recipe Classics*), 3 tbsp. .......................80
tomato beef/oxtail (*Knorr Recipe Classics*), 2 tbsp....................60
vegetable:
   (*Knorr Recipe Classics*), 2 tbsp. .............................................60
   (*Lipton Recipe Secrets*), 1⅔ tbsp. .........................................30
   (*Mrs. Grass* Homestyle Recipe Soup/Dip Mix), ¼ pkg..........35
   chicken flavor (*Knorr* TasteBreaks), 1 cont....................120
   cream of, savory (*Knorr*), 3 tbsp...............................100
   herb (*Arrowhead Mills*), ⅓ cup.................................150
   spring (*Knorr Recipe Classics*), 2 tbsp. ...............................25
   vegetarian (*Knorr* TasteBreaks), 1 cont. ...........................160
vegetable and noodle (*House of Tsang*), 1 cont.......................120
wonton, 1 cont.:
   chicken, shrimp, or pork (*Maruchan* Instant).....................200
   hot and sour (*Maruchan* Instant)...........................................200
   Oriental (*Maruchan* Instant)................................................190
   skins only (*Maruchan* Instant)..............................................110
**Soup base mix,** dry, ⅛ pkg., except as noted:
beef stew (*Wyler's Soup Starter*).................................................70
beef vegetable flavor (*Wyler's Soup Starter*) ............................100
chicken noodle flavor (*Wyler's Soup Starter*) ............................80
chicken vegetable, hearty (*Wyler's Soup Starter*)......................70
chicken w/white and wild rice (*Wyler's Soup Starter*), ...............70
chili, 3 bean, hearty (*Wyler's Soup Starter*), ⅙ pkg. ...............150
potato garlic and chives (*Wyler's Soup Starter*), ⅙ pkg. .........130
**Sour cream,** see "Cream, sour"
**Soy beverage,** 1 cup:
(*NutraBlend* Original)...................................................................120
(*Soy Dream* Original)...................................................................140

apple (*NutraBlend*) ................................................110
orange (*NutraBlend*) ..............................................100
vanilla (*NutraBlend*) ..............................................140
**Soy flour:**
(*Arrowhead Mills*), ½ cup .......................................200
(*Hodgson Mill*), scant ¼ cup ...................................80
(*Hodgson Mill* Organic), scant ¼ cup .....................110
**Soy meal,** defatted, raw, 1 cup ..............................414
**Soy nut,** roasted:
all varieties (*Tofutti* Totally Nuts), 1 oz. ...............130
salted or unsalted (*Frieda's*), ⅓ cup, 1.1 oz. ...........140
**Soy sauce,** 1 tbsp.:
(*House of Tsang* Light/Low Sodium) ............................5
(*Kikkoman* Lite) ......................................................10
dark (*House of Tsang*) ..............................................10
ginger flavored (*House of Tsang*) ............................20
ginger flavored (*House of Tsang* Low Sodium) .........10
tamari (*San-J*) ........................................................15
tamari (*San-J* Reduced Sodium) ...............................20
tamari, wheat free (*San-J* Organic) ..........................15
shoyu (*San-J* Organic) .............................................15
**Soybean** (see also "Edamame"), green:
raw, 1 cup ...............................................................376
boiled, drained, 1 cup .............................................254
**Soybean, dried** (*Arrowhead Mills*), ¼ cup ...............170
**Soybean, fermented,** see "Miso" and "Natto"
**Soybean, mature:**
dry, 1 cup ...............................................................322
boiled, 1 cup ...........................................................298
dry roasted, 1 cup ...................................................774
roasted, salted or unsalted, 1 cup ...........................810
**Soybean, mature, sprouted,** raw, ½ cup ..................43
**Soybean cake or curd,** see "Tofu"
**Soybean kernels,** roasted, toasted, whole, 1 cup ....490
**Spaghetti,** see "Pasta"
**Spaghetti dish, mix,** dry, except as noted:
cheese, zesty (*Kraft Spaghetti Classics*), about 1 cup* ...........240
meat sauce (*Kraft Spaghetti Classics*), about 1 cup* ..............330
mild or tangy (*Kraft Spaghetti Classics* Italian), about 1 cup* 240

**Spaghetti dish, mix (*cont.*)**
tomato sauce (*Classico It's Pasta Anytime!*), 15.25-oz. pkg....490
tomato sauce, beef flavor (*Classico It's Pasta Anytime!*),
 15.25-oz. pkg. ...................................................................490
**Spaghetti entree, canned or packaged,** 1 cup, except as noted:
and meatballs (*Chef Boyardee*) ......................................270
and meatballs (*Chef Boyardee* Microwave Bowl), 1 bowl........210
and meatballs (*Dinty Moore American Classics*), 1 bowl ........290
and meatballs (*Franco-American Superiore*)...........................260
and meatballs (*Kid's Kitchen*) ........................................220
rings, and franks (*Franco-American SpaghettiOs*) ..................260
rings, and franks (*Kid's Kitchen*) ...................................240
rings, and meatballs (*Franco-American SpaghettiOs*)..............260
rings, and meatballs (*Kid's Kitchen*)................................230
rings, in tomato cheese sauce (*Franco-American
 SpaghettiOs*)...................................................................260
**Spaghetti entree, frozen,** 1 pkg.:
bake, cheesy (*Stouffer's*), 12 oz. ..................................460
Bolognese (*Michelina's*), 8.5 oz....................................280
marinara (*Michelina's*), 8 oz. .......................................240
w/meat sauce (*Lean Cuisine Everyday Favorites*), 11.5 oz. ......290
w/meat sauce (*Morton*), 8.5 oz. ....................................200
w/meat sauce, garlic bread (*Marie Callender's*), 17 oz. ...........670
w/meatballs (*Lean Cuisine Everyday Favorites*), 9.5 oz. ...........270
w/meatballs and sauce (*Michelina's*), 9 oz..............................300
w/meatballs in sauce (*Stouffer's*), 12⅝ oz................................390
w/onions (*Michelina's*), 9 oz...........................................270
and sauce, w/beef (*Healthy Choice* Entree), 10 oz. .................280
w/tomato basil sauce (*Michelina's*), 8 oz. .............................250
**Spaghetti sauce,** see "Pasta sauce"
**Spaghetti squash,** fresh:
raw (*Frieda's*), ¾ cup, 3 oz...........................................30
raw, cubed, 1 cup ............................................................31
baked or boiled, drained, 1 cup....................................42
**Spareribs,** see "Pork" and "Pork, refrigerated"
**Spearmint,** 2 tbsp. fresh or 1 tbsp. dried ....................5
**Spelt flour,** ¼ cup:
(*Arrowhead Mills*) ........................................................100
(*Hodgson Mill* Organic) ...............................................115

**Spinach,** fresh:
raw (*Mann's* Salad Spinach), 3 oz..................................................40
raw, 12-oz. bunch.....................................................................75
raw, chopped (*Dole*), 1 cup, 2 oz...........................................15
boiled, drained, 1 cup..............................................................41
**Spinach, canned,** ½ cup:
all styles (*Del Monte/Del Monte* No Salt) .............................30
all styles (*Popeye/Sunshine*) ................................................30
**Spinach, frozen:**
(*Green Giant*), ½ cup..............................................................25
leaf, whole (*Birds Eye*), 1 cup................................................20
leaf, chopped (*Seabrook Farms*), ⅓ cup...............................20
leaf, cut (*Freshlike*), 1 cup.....................................................20
leaf, cut, and butter (*Green Giant*), ½ cup.............................35
chopped (*Birds Eye/Freshlike*), ⅓ cup...................................20
chopped (*Seabrook Farms*), 1 cup.........................................20
boiled, drained, ½ cup.............................................................27
**Spinach, malabar,** fresh, cooked, 1 cup ...............................10
**Spinach, mustard:**
raw, chopped, 1 cup.................................................................33
boiled, drained, chopped, 1 cup...............................................29
**Spinach, New Zealand:**
raw, chopped, 1 cup...................................................................8
boiled, drained, chopped, 1 cup...............................................22
**Spinach dish,** frozen, ½ cup:
creamed (*Birds Eye*) ............................................................100
creamed (*Boston Market*) .....................................................190
creamed (*Green Giant*)...........................................................80
creamed (*Seabrook Farms*) ..................................................120
soufflé (*Stouffer's*)................................................................140
**Spinach-feta pocket,** frozen (*Amy's*), 4.5-oz. pc................250
**Spinach pancake,** frozen (*Dr. Praeger's*), 1.3-oz. pc.................70
**Spiny lobster,** meat only:
raw, 4 oz...............................................................................127
boiled, poached, or steamed, 1 lobster, 5.7 oz. ......................233
boiled, poached, or steamed, 4 oz..........................................162
**Spiral pasta entree,** frozen, spicy tomato sauce w/
(*Michelina's*), 8-oz. pkg........................................................210
**Spleen,** beef, braised, 4 oz.................................................164

**Split peas,** mature:

dry, 1 cup.....................................................................672

boiled, 1 cup .................................................................231

green, dry (*Arrowhead Mills*), ¼ cup .............................170

**Sports drink,** 8 fl. oz.:

all varieties (*All Sport*)....................................................70

all varieties (*Gatorade*)...................................................50

**Spot,** meat only:

raw, 4 oz. .....................................................................140

baked, broiled, or microwaved, 4 oz. .............................179

**Spring onion,** see "Onion, green"

**Squab,** raw:

whole, meat w/skin, 7 oz........................................................585

whole, meat only, 5.9 oz........................................................239

meat w/skin, 4 oz..................................................................333

meat only, 4 oz. ...................................................................161

breast, meat only, 3.6 oz. .....................................................135

**Squash,** see specific listings

**Squid,** meat only:

raw, 4 oz. .....................................................................104

fried, 4 oz......................................................................199

**Starfruit,** see "Carambola"

**Steak,** see "Beef"

**Steak sauce,** 1 tbsp.:

(*A.1.*)............................................................................15

(*A.1.* Bold & Spicy).........................................................20

(*A.1.* Sweet & Tangy)......................................................30

(*A.1.* Thick & Hearty)......................................................25

(*Crosse & Blackwell*).....................................................130

peppercorn (*Lawry's* Weekday Gourmet)..........................40

**Stir-fry sauce,** 1 tbsp.:

(*House of Tsang* Classic)................................................25

(*House of Tsang* Saigon Sizzle/Bangkok Padang) .............45

(*Kikkoman*)....................................................................20

herb and roasted garlic (*Lawry's*).....................................5

lemon basil (*Lawry's*)......................................................10

sesame ginger (*Lawry's*)..................................................15

sweet and sour (*House of Tsang*) ....................................35

sweet and spicy (*Lawry's*)...............................................20

spicy (*House of Tsang* Szechuan) ...............................................20
**Straightneck squash,** fresh:
raw, sliced, 1 cup ................................................................25
boiled, drained, sliced, 1 cup ...............................................36
**Straightneck squash, canned,** drained, diced, 1 cup ...............27
**Straightneck squash, frozen,** boiled, drained, sliced, 1 cup ......48
**Strawberry,** fresh:
(*Dole*), 8 medium, 5.3 oz. .....................................................45
halves, 1 cup .......................................................................46
**Strawberry, canned,** in light syrup (*Oregon*), ½ cup ...............100
**Strawberry, dried** (*Frieda's*), ½ cup .....................................150
**Strawberry,** frozen:
whole (*Birds Eye*), ½ cup ...................................................100
halves (*Birds Eye*), ½ cup ..................................................120
halves, in light syrup (*Birds Eye*), ½ cup .............................70
**Strawberry banana nectar** (*Libby's*), 11.5-fl.-oz. can .............220
**Strawberry drink:**
(*Capri Sun All Natural Strawberry Cooler*), 6.76 fl. oz. ..............90
(*Hershey's*), 1 box .............................................................170
(*Welch's* Breeze), 8 fl. oz. ..................................................130
kiwi (*Capri Sun All Natural*), 6.76 fl. oz. ...............................100
kiwi (*Kool-Aid Bursts Slammin'*), 6.76 fl. oz. .........................100
punch (*Hawaiian Punch Strawberry Surfin'*), 8 fl. oz. ............120
**Strawberry drink mix,** 8 fl. oz.*:
(*Kool-Aid*) .........................................................................100
(*Kool-Aid* Sugar Sweetened) ................................................60
kiwi (*Kool-Aid Slammin'*) ....................................................100
kiwi (*Kool-Aid Slammin'* Sugar Sweetened) .............................70
raspberry (*Kool-Aid*) ..........................................................100
raspberry (*Kool-Aid* Sugar Sweetened) ...................................60
**Strawberry juice blend** (*Juicy Juice*), 8 fl. oz. ......................120
**Strawberry kiwi nectar** (*Libby's*), 11.5-fl.-oz. can ...................200
**Strawberry milk,** 1 cup:
(*Hershey's* Reduced Fat) ....................................................200
(*Nesquik*) .........................................................................230
**Strawberry milk drink mix,** powder (*Nesquik*), 2 tbsp. ............90
**Strawberry syrup:**
(*Knott's Berry Farm*), ¼ cup ...............................................210
(*Nesquik*), 2 tbsp. .............................................................110

**Strawberry topping,** 2 tbsp.:
(*Kraft*).................................................................110
(*Smucker's* Spoonable Toppings)..............................100
(*Smucker's* Sundae Syrup)........................................110
**String bean,** see "Green bean"
**Stuffing** (see also "Stuffing mix"), dry:
corn bread (*Arnold*), ¾ cup.......................................140
herb seasoned (*Pepperidge Farm*), ¾ cup.................170
**Stuffing mix,** ½ cup*:
beef (*Stove Top*).......................................................180
chicken (*Stove Top/Stove Top* Flexible Serve).............170
chicken (*Stove Top* Microwave).................................160
chicken or turkey (*Pepperidge Farm* One Step)...........190
cornbread (*Stove Top*)...............................................170
cornbread (*Stove Top* Flexible Serve/Microwave).......160
herb, homestyle (*Stove Top* Flexible Serve)...............170
herbs, savory (*Stove Top*)..........................................170
long grain and wild rice (*Stove Top*)...........................180
mushroom and onion or traditional sage (*Stove Top*)....180
pork or turkey (*Stove Top*).........................................170
San Francisco style (*Stove Top*).................................170
**Sturgeon,** fresh, meat only:
raw, 4 oz. ................................................................119
baked, broiled, or microwaved, 4 oz. ........................153
smoked, 4 oz. ..........................................................196
***Subway,*** 1 serving:
*7 Under 6 subs,* w/out cheese or mayo:
   chicken breast, roasted...........................................311
   ham.........................................................................261
   roast beef................................................................264
   *Subway Club*...........................................................273
   turkey breast ..........................................................254
   turkey breast and ham.............................................267
   *Veggie Delite* .........................................................200
*7 Under 6 deli sandwiches,* w/out cheese or mayo:
   ham.........................................................................194
   roast beef................................................................206
   turkey breast ..........................................................200

*7 Under 6* salads:
  ham ................................................................112
  roast beef ......................................................114
  roasted chicken ............................................137
  *Subway Club* ...............................................123
  turkey breast .................................................105
  turkey breast and ham ..................................117
  *Veggie Delite* ................................................50
classic subs, 6":
  *Cold Cut Trio* ...............................................415
  *Italian BMT* ..................................................453
  meatball ........................................................501
  *Subway Seafood & Crab* w/light mayo .......378
  steak and cheese .........................................362
  *Subway Melt* ................................................380
  tuna, w/light mayo ........................................419
classic deli style sandwich, tuna .......................289
classic salads, w/out dressing:
  *Cold Cut Trio* ...............................................234
  *Italian BMT* ..................................................273
  meatball ........................................................320
  *Subway Seafood & Crab*, w/light mayo .......198
  steak and cheese .........................................182
  *Subway Melt* ................................................200
  tuna w/light mayo .........................................238
select subs, 6":
  asiago Caesar chicken ..................................407
  honey mustard melt ......................................373
  horseradish roast beef ..................................401
  southwest steak and cheese ........................412
wraps:
  select, asiago chicken ...................................411
  steak and cheese .........................................356
  turkey breast and bacon ...............................321
breads:
  deli style roll .................................................150
  6" Italian .......................................................178
  6" whole wheat ..............................................186
  6" Parmesan oregano ...................................195

*Subway,* **breads** (*cont.*)
　　6" hearty Italian ........................................................191
　　6" harvest wheat..........................................................203
　　6" sesame Italian .........................................................210
　　wrap ............................................................................200
condiments:
　　bacon, 2 strips ...............................................................42
　　cheese, 2 triangles .........................................................41
　　mayonnaise, 1 tbsp. ......................................................111
　　mayonnaise, light, 1 tbsp.................................................46
　　mustard, 2 tsp. .................................................................8
　　olive oil blend, 1 tsp........................................................45
　　vinegar, 1 tsp. ...................................................................1
select sauces, 1 tbsp.:
　　asiago Caesar .................................................................77
　　honey mustard .................................................................20
　　horseradish ...................................................................100
　　Southwest ancho.............................................................61
salad dressing, 2-oz. pkt.:
　　French, fat free ...............................................................70
　　Italian, fat free ................................................................20
　　ranch, fat free .................................................................60
cookies, 1 pc.:
　　chocolate chip ...............................................................209
　　chocolate chunk ............................................................210
　　oatmeal raisin.................................................................197
　　peanut butter .................................................................220
　　*M&M's*........................................................................210
　　sugar ............................................................................222
　　white macadamia nut......................................................221
**Succotash, canned,** ½ cup:
cream style corn ...................................................................103
kernel corn (*Seneca*) .............................................................90
kernel corn.............................................................................82
**Succotash, frozen,** kernel corn, boiled, drained, 1 cup............158
**Sucker,** white, meat only:
raw, 4 oz. .............................................................................105
baked, broiled, or microwaved, 4 oz. ....................................135

**Sugar,** beet or cane:
brown, 1 cup, not packed.................................................546
granulated, 1 cup............................................................773
granulated, 1 tbsp...........................................................46
granulated, 1 tsp.............................................................15
powdered or confectioner's, 1 cup, sifted .....................389
powdered or confectioner's, 1 tbsp., unsifted................31
**Sugar, maple,** 1 tsp.......................................................11
**Sugar apple,** fresh, 1 medium, 2⅞" diam. ...............146
**Sugar loaf squash** (*Frieda's*), ¾ cup, 3 oz.................30
**Sugar snap peas,** see "Peas, edible pod"
**Summer sausage:**
(*Johnsonville* Old World), 2 oz....................................190
(*Johnsonville* Original/Beef/Garlic), 2 oz. ..................180
(*Old Smokehouse*), 2 oz.............................................200
beef and pork, .8-oz. slice .............................................77
stick, all varieties (*Johnsonville* Summer Stix), 1-oz. stick.......120
**Sunfish,** pumpkinseed, meat only:
raw, 4 oz. .....................................................................109
baked, broiled, or microwaved, 4 oz. ...........................129
**Sunflower seed,** shelled, except as noted:
(*Arrowhead Mills*), ¼ cup...........................................180
(*Frito-Lay*), 1 oz..........................................................180
(*Planters*), ¼ cup........................................................200
in shell (*Planters*), 3.25-oz. pkg. ...............................300
in shell, roasted and salted (*Planters*), 3-oz. pkg........280
in shell, roasted and salted (*Planters*), ¾ cup.............160
dried, in shell, 1 cup (edible yield 1.6 oz.) ...................262
dry roasted, kernels, 1 oz..............................................165
oil roasted, kernels, 1 oz. .............................................174
**Sunflower seed butter,** 1 tbsp....................................93
**Sunflower seed flour,** partially defatted, 1 cup .........209
**Swamp cabbage,** fresh:
raw, chopped, 1 cup .......................................................11
boiled, drained, chopped, 1 cup .....................................20
**Sweet dumpling squash** (*Frieda's*), ¾ cup, 3 oz........30
**Sweet peas,** see "Peas, green"
**Sweet potato,** fresh:
raw, 5" long, 4.7 oz.......................................................137

**Sweet potato (*cont.*)**
raw, cubed, 1 cup .................................................................140
baked in skin, 1 large, 6.3 oz.............................................185
baked in skin, mashed, 1 cup.............................................206
boiled w/out skin, 1 medium, 5.3 oz. ..................................159
boiled w/out skin, mashed, 1 cup .......................................344
**Sweet potato, canned:**
whole (*Royal Prince/Trappey*), 3 pcs. ...............................200
cut (*Allens/Princella/Sugary Sam*), ⅔ cup..........................160
pieces, vacuum pack, 1 cup ...............................................182
mashed (*Princella/Sugary Sam*), ⅔ cup ............................120
mashed, vacuum pack, 1 cup..............................................232
in syrup, drained, 1 cup......................................................212
candied or orange pineapple (*Royal Prince*), ½ cup................210
**Sweet potato, frozen:**
baked, cubed, 1 cup ...........................................................176
candied (*Mrs. Paul's*), 5 oz..............................................140
candied w/apple (*Mrs. Paul's*), 1¼ cup .............................175
**Sweet potato leaf,** steamed, 1 cup...................................22
**Sweet roll,** see "Bun, sweet"
**Sweet and sour sauce,** 2 tbsp.:
(*Kikkoman*) ...........................................................................35
(*Kraft*) ..................................................................................60
(*La Choy* Duck Sauce) ..........................................................60
(*San-J*) .................................................................................50
w/pineapple (*Contadina*).......................................................40
**Sweetener,** artificial (*Sweet'n Low*), 1 pkt............................4
**Sweetbreads,** see "Pancreas" and "Thymus"
**Swiss chard,** fresh:
raw (*Frieda's*), 1 cup, 3 oz. ...............................................15
boiled, drained, chopped, 1 cup ..........................................35
**Swisswurst** (*Johnsonville*), 2.71-oz. link .......................240
**Swordfish,** meat only:
raw, 4 oz. ............................................................................137
baked, broiled, or microwaved, 4 oz. ..................................176
**Syrup,** see "Pancake syrup" and specific listings
**Szechuan sauce** (*San-J*), 1 tsp. .......................................5

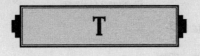

**FOOD AND MEASURE**          **CALORIES**

**Tabouli:**
(*Cedarlane* Salad), ½ cup ...........................................................180
(*Cedar's* Taboule), 2 tbsp. ...........................................................30
***Taco Bell,*** 1 serving:
breakfast items:
   burrito, country ...........................................................270
   burrito, double bacon and egg ...........................................480
   burrito, fiesta ...........................................................280
   burrito, grande ...........................................................420
   hash brown nuggets ...........................................................280
   quesadilla, bacon ...........................................................450
   quesadilla, cheese ...........................................................380
   quesadilla, sausage ...........................................................430
burrito, bean ...........................................................370
burrito, *Big Beef* ...........................................................400
burrito, *Big Beef Supreme* ...........................................................510
burrito, *Big Chicken Supreme* ...........................................................460
burrito, grilled chicken ...........................................................390
burrito, chili cheese ...........................................................330
burrito, 7 layer ...........................................................520
burrito, *Supreme* ...........................................................430
*Chalupa Baja,* beef ...........................................................420
*Chalupa Baja,* chicken or steak ...........................................................400
*Chalupa Santa Fe,* beef ...........................................................440
*Chalupa Santa Fe,* chicken ...........................................................420
*Chalupa Santa Fe,* steak ...........................................................430
*Chalupa Supreme,* beef ...........................................................380
*Chalupa Supreme,* chicken or steak ...........................................................360
*Gordita Baja,* beef ...........................................................360
*Gordita Baja,* chicken or steak ...........................................................340
*Gordita Santa Fe,* beef ...........................................................380
*Gordita Santa Fe,* chicken or steak ...........................................................370
*Gordita Supreme,* beef, chicken, or steak ...........................................................300

*Taco Bell* (*cont.*)

taco ..................................................................................170
taco, *Double Decker* ..............................................330
taco, *Double Decker Taco Supreme* ................380
taco, soft ..........................................................210
taco, soft, grilled chicken or grilled steak..............200
taco, soft, grilled steak *Supreme*........................240
*Taco Supreme*...................................................210
*Taco Supreme,* soft..............................................260
specialties:
   *Big Beef Meximelt* ........................................290
   Mexican pizza...............................................540
   Mexican pizza, beef ......................................530
   Mexican pizza, chicken..................................520
   quesadilla, cheese .......................................350
   quesadilla, chicken .......................................400
   taco salad, w/salsa .......................................850
   taco salad w/out shell, w/salsa .....................430
   tostada..........................................................250
nachos and sides:
   *Big Beef Nachos Supreme* .............................440
   nachos...........................................................320
   *Nachos BellGrande*........................................760
   *Nachos BellGrande,* chicken or steak.............740
   Pintos 'n Cheese ...........................................180
   rice, Mexican.................................................190
   twists, cinnamon............................................180
ice cream dessert, *Choco Toco* ...........................310
**Taco dinner mix:**
(*Taco Bell Home Originals*), 2 tacos*......................280
(*Ortega*), 2 shells, 1 tbsp. sauce, ⅛ pkt. seasoning................150
soft (*Chi-Chi's Kit*), 2 shells and seasoning................300
soft (*Ortega*), 2 tortillas, 1 tbsp. sauce, ⅕ pkt. seasoning........240
soft (*Taco Bell Home Originals*), 2 tacos*...............410
white or yellow (*Chi-Chi's* Kit), 2 shells, seasoning .................200
**Taco pocket,** frozen (*Michelina's*), 5.5-oz. pkg. .........350
**Taco sauce:**
(*Chi-Chi's*), 1 tbsp....................................................15
medium or mild (*Taco Bell Home Originals*), 2 tbsp....................15

**Taco seasoning mix:**
(*Chi-Chi's* Fiesta/*El Torito*), ⅕ pkg. ...............................25
(*Lawry's* Spices & Seasonings), 2 tsp. ......................15
(*Ortega*), 1 tbsp. ...............................................20
(*Taco Bell Home* Originals), 2 tsp. ............................20
chicken (*Lawry's* Spices & Seasonings), 2 tsp. ..............20
**Taco shell:**
(*Ortega*), 2 shells ..............................................120
(*Taco Bell Home Originals*), 3 shells ..........................150
tostada (*Ortega*), 2 shells ....................................130
white or yellow (*Chi-Chi's*), 2 shells .........................170
yellow (*Ortega*), 2 shells .....................................120
**Tahini:**
(*Arrowhead Mills*), 2 tbsp. ....................................190
paste, 1 tbsp. ..................................................95
**Tamale,** canned:
beef (*Hormel*), 7.5-oz. can ....................................200
beef (*Hormel* Jumbo), 2 pcs. ...................................190
beef, regular or hot-spicy (*Hormel*), 2 pcs. ..................140
chicken (*Hormel*), 2 pcs. ......................................130
**Tamale pie,** frozen, Mexican (*Amy's*), 8-oz. pie ............220
**Tamale pocket,** frozen, Mexican (*Amy's*), 4.5 oz. ...........250
**Tamari,** see "Soy sauce"
**Tamarillos** (*Frieda's*), 4.2 oz. ............................45
**Tamarind,** fresh, raw:
(*Frieda's*), 1.1 oz. ...........................................70
pulp, 1 cup .....................................................287
**Tangerine,** fresh, raw:
(*Dole*), 2 medium ..............................................70
1 large, 2½" diam. ..............................................43
sections, 1 cup .................................................86
**Tangerine, canned,** ½ cup, except as noted:
in juice, 1 cup .................................................92
in light syrup (*Del Monte*) ....................................80
in light syrup (*Del Monte Fruit Cup*), 4 oz. ..................70
in light syrup (*Dole*) .........................................80
in light syrup (*S&W*) ..........................................90
**Tangerine juice,** 8 fl. oz., except as noted:
fresh ...........................................................106

**Tangerine juice** (*cont.*)
frozen\*, sweetened................................................................111
**Tapioca,** dry:
(*Minute*), 1½ tsp.................................................................20
pearl, 1 cup.......................................................................544
**Tapioca pudding**, see "Pudding" and "Pudding and pie
   filling mix"
**Tarama,** see "Caviar"
**Taramosalata,** see "Caviar spread"
**Taro,** fresh:
raw (*Frieda's*), ⅔ cup..........................................................85
raw, sliced, 1 cup...............................................................117
cooked, sliced, 1 cup..........................................................187
**Taro, Tahitian,** fresh:
raw, sliced, 1 cup.................................................................55
cooked, sliced, 1 cup............................................................60
**Taro chips,** 1 oz.................................................................141
**Taro leaf:**
raw, 1 leaf, 11" by 6½", .4 oz..................................................4
raw, 1 cup...........................................................................12
steamed, 1 cup....................................................................35
**Taro shoots,** fresh:
raw, sliced, ½ cup..................................................................5
cooked, sliced, 1 cup............................................................20
**Tarragon, dried,** ground, 1 tsp.................................................5
**Tartar sauce,** 2 tbsp.:
(*Kraft*)................................................................................90
(*Kraft Free*)........................................................................25
lemon and herb flavor (*Kraft*).............................................150
**Tea** (see also "Tea, iced"), brewed:
8 fl. oz.\*...............................................................................2
all flavors, instant (*General Foods International*), 8 fl. oz.\*........70
herb, all types, 8 fl. oz.\*.........................................................2
**Tea, iced,** 8 fl. oz.:
(*Nestea Cool*).....................................................................80
(*Schweppes*).......................................................................90
all flavors (*Crystal Light*).......................................................5
lemon (*Nestea* Diet)..............................................................3
lemon, peach, or raspberry (*Nestea*)......................................80

sweet (*Nestea*)................................................................65
**Tea, iced, mix:**
plain (*Nestea* 100%/100% Decaf), 2 tsp........................0
plain (*Nestea* Sun Tea), 1 tsp. ....................................0
plain or flavored (*Crystal Light*) ...................................5
herb tea, lemon bliss or orange spice (*Nestea*), 1 tbsp. ............15
lemon (*Nestea/Nestea* Decaf/*Nestea* Sugar Free), 2 tsp................5
lemon (*Nestea Ice Teaser*), ⅛ tub ................................5
lemon, and sugar (*Nestea*), 2 tbsp.............................80
lemon, sweetened w/sugar, 3 rounded tsp. ...................23
lemonade (*Nestea*), 2 tbsp. ........................................80
**Tempeh,** ½ cup .........................................................160
**Teriyaki entree,** frozen, stir-fry (*Lean Cuisine Everyday Favorites*), 10-oz. pkg. ..........................................290
**Teriyaki sauce,** 1 tbsp., except as noted:
(*Annie Chun's/Annie Chun's* Hot & Spicy)....................25
(*House of Tsang* Korean) ...........................................30
(*Kikkoman* Baste & Glaze), 2 tbsp..............................50
(*Kikkoman* Marinade & Sauce/Marinade & Sauce Lite)..............15
(*Lawry's* Marinade) ....................................................25
(*San-J*) ......................................................................40
honey mirin (*Sun Luck*) ...............................................30
w/honey and pineapple (*Kikkoman* Baste & Glaze), 2 tbsp. ........80
roasted garlic (*Kikkoman* Marinade & Sauce)................25
steak (*Lawry's* Weekday Gourmet Marinade)..................25
**Thuringer cervelat,** see "Summer sausage"
**Thyme,** fresh, 1 tbsp..................................................1
**Thyme, dried,** ground, 1 tsp ........................................4
**Thymus,** 4 oz.:
beef, braised .............................................................362
veal, braised ..............................................................197
**Tikka sauce,** see "Curry sauce"
**Tilefish,** meat only:
raw, 4 oz. ...................................................................109
baked, broiled, or microwaved, 4 oz. ...........................167
**Toaster pastry,** 1 pc.:
apple, cherry, strawberry, or brown sugar cinnamon (*Toaster Strudel*)....................................................................190
apple cinnamon (*Pop-Tarts*).........................................200

**Toaster pastry (*cont.*)**

apple cinnamon, cheese, or strawberry (*Pop-Tarts Pastry
  Swirls*) ................................................................260
berry, wild, frosted (*Pop-Tarts*) ...............................210
blueberry (*Eggo*)...................................................120
brown sugar cinnamon, frosted (*Pop-Tarts* Low Fat) .............190
brown sugar cinnamon, plain or frosted (*Pop-Tarts*)...............210
berry or strawberry, frosted (*Pop-Tarts Snak-Stix*) ..................190
blueberry, plain or frosted (*Pop-Tarts*)......................................200
blueberry or raisin bran (*Thomas' Toast-R-Cakes*) ....................90
brown sugar cinnamon, frosted (*KoolStuf* Toastettes) .............190
cherry, frosted (*KoolStuf* Toastettes Burst) ...............................190
cherry, plain or frosted (*Pop-Tarts*).............................................200
chocolate chip or cinnamon (*Thomas' Toast-R-Cakes*) ...........100
chocolate fudge, frosted (*Pop-Tarts*)...........................................200
chocolate fudge, frosted (*Pop-Tarts* Low Fat) ...........................190
chocolate vanilla creme, frosted (*Pop-Tarts*)..............................200
cinnamon (*Eggo*) ................................................................130
cream cheese and strawberry (*Toaster Strudel*) ........................200
corn (*Thomas' Toast-R-Cakes*)........................................................100
fudge, frosted (*KoolStuf* Toastettes)................................................180
grape, frosted (*Pop-Tarts*).................................................................200
raspberry, frosted (*Pop-Tarts*) ........................................................210
s'mores, frosted (*KoolStuf Honey Maid*) .......................................90
s'mores, frosted (*Pop-Tarts*) ...........................................................200
strawberry (*Eggo*)...............................................................................130
strawberry, plain or frosted (*KoolStuf* Toastettes) ....................180
strawberry, plain or frosted (*Pop-Tarts*)......................................200
strawberry, plain or frosted (*Pop-Tarts* Low Fat) ......................190
watermelon, frosted (*Pop-Tarts*) ....................................................210
*Wild Magicburst,* frosted (*Pop-Tarts*).........................................200
*Wild Tropical Blast,* frosted (*Pop-Tarts*) ...................................210
**Toffee baking bits** (*Skor*), ½ oz. ................................................70
**Toffee topping** (*Hershey's Heath* Shell), 2 tbsp. .......................230
**Tofu:**
extra firm (*Nasoya* Organic), 3.2 oz. .............................................90
firm (*Nasoya* Organic), 3.2 oz. ........................................................80
5 spice (*Nasoya* Organic), 3 oz. .....................................................70
French country (*Nasoya* Organic), 3.17 oz.....................................70

silken (*Nasoya* Organic), 3.2 oz............................................50
silken, firm (*Mori-Nu* Lite), 3 oz. ...................................35
silken, soft (*Mori-Nu*), 3 oz. .........................................45
soft (*Nasoya* Organic), 3.2 oz.......................................60
dried, frozen (koyadofu), .6-oz. piece.........................82
fried, ½-oz. piece.........................................................35
salted and fermented (fuyu), .4-oz. block ..................13
**Tofu dish,** ½ cup, except as noted:
(*Cedarlane* Cottage Style Salad) ..............................190
(*Cedarlane* Egg Free Salad) ....................................180
(*Cedarlane* Ranchero Salad)....................................140
**Tomatillo,** fresh:
(*Frieda's*), ½ cup, 3 oz.................................................25
1 medium, 1.2 oz............................................................11
**Tomato,** ripe, fresh:
orange, 3.9 oz...............................................................18
red, raw, 2⅗" diam........................................................26
red, raw, baby (*Frieda's* Roma), ⅔ cup, 3 oz...............20
red, raw, cherry tomato, 1 cup......................................31
red, raw, chopped or diced, 1 cup................................38
red, boiled, 2 medium, 8.7 oz.......................................66
red, boiled, 1 cup..........................................................65
red, stewed, 1 cup........................................................80
red or yellow (*Frieda's* Tear Drop), ⅔ cup, 3 oz. .........20
yellow, 7.5 oz................................................................32
**Tomato, canned** (see also "Tomato sauce"), ½ cup, except as noted:
whole, peeled (*Contadina*).............................................25
whole, peeled, plain or w/basil (*Muir Glen* Organic).....30
whole, peeled, in juice (*Del Monte*)..............................25
chunky, chili style (*Del Monte*) ....................................30
chunky, pasta style (*Del Monte*) ..................................45
crushed, all styles (*Contadina*), ¼ cup.........................20
crushed, original or Italian (*Del Monte*) ........................45
crushed, w/basil (*Muir Glen* Organic), ¼ cup ...............25
crushed, w/garlic (*Del Monte*) ......................................50
diced:
    (*Contadina*)............................................................30
    (*Del Monte/Del Monte* No Salt)..............................25

**Tomato, canned (*cont.*)**
    all varieties (*Muir Glen* Organic) ............................................25
    w/basil, garlic, and oregano (*Del Monte*)..............................50
    w/roasted garlic or Italian herbs (*Contadina*) .........................45
    w/garlic or green pepper and onion (*Del Monte*) ..................40
    w/green chili peppers or jalapenos (*Del Monte*)....................30
    w/green chilies (*Chi-Chi's*), ¼ cup .......................................70
    w/onion (*Contadina*).............................................................40
ground, peeled (*Muir Glen* Organic), ¼ cup ............................10
paste or puree, see "Tomato paste" and "Tomato puree"
stewed (*Muir Glen* Organic) ....................................................30
stewed, all styles (*Contadina*)..................................................35
stewed, all styles, except Italian (*Del Monte*) ..........................35
stewed, Italian (*Del Monte*).....................................................30
wedges (*Del Monte*) ................................................................35
**Tomato, dried:**
1 pc., 32 pcs. per cup..................................................................5
packed in oil, drained, 1 pc., 36 pcs. per cup ..............................6
halves or chopped (*Frieda's*), ⅓ cup......................................100
sun-dried, in sunflower oil, in jars (*Rienzi*), 4 pcs., 1.4 oz.......130
vegetable blend (*Frieda's* Tomato Toss), ½ cup......................100
yellow, halves or chopped (*Frieda's*), ½ cup...........................220
**Tomato, green,** raw, 1 large, 6.4 oz........................................44
**Tomato, green, pickled,** halves (*Claussen*), 1 oz......................5
**Tomato, sun-dried,** see "Tomato, dried"
**Tomato juice,** bottled or canned:
(*Campbell's/Campbell's Healthy Request*), 8 fl. oz. ..................50
(*Del Monte*), 8 fl. oz................................................................50
(*Del Monte* Not from Concentrate), 8 fl. oz. .............................40
(*Muir Glen* Organic), 5.5 fl. oz.................................................40
(*Sacramento*), 8 fl. oz..............................................................40
**Tomato juice blend,** 8 fl. oz.:
beef (*Beefamato*) .....................................................................50
clam (*Clamato* Bloody Caesar) ................................................50
clam (*Clamato* Cocktail/Picante Cocktail)................................60
**Tomato paste,** canned, 2 tbsp.:
(*Contadina* 100%) ...................................................................30
(*Del Monte*).............................................................................30
(*Muir Glen* Organic).................................................................30

Italian, regular or w/roasted garlic (*Contadina*)............................35
**Tomato preserves** (*Smucker's*), 1 tbsp. ......................50
**Tomato puree, canned,** ¼ cup:
(*Contadina*) ......................................................................20
(*Muir Glen* Organic)............................................................20
**Tomato relish,** in jars, 1 tbsp:
(*Patak's*)...........................................................................10
green (*Braswell's*) .............................................................20
hot (*Braswell's*)..................................................................10
sun-dried (*Peloponnese*) ...................................................25
**Tomato sauce,** canned (see also "Pasta sauce" and "Tomato,
    canned"), ¼ cup, except as noted:
(*Contadina/Contadina* Italian Style) .................................15
(*Contadina* Extra Thick & Zesty).......................................20
(*Del Monte/Del Monte* No Salt) ........................................20
all styles (*Muir Glen* Organic)............................................20
w/garlic and onions (*Contadina*) .......................................20
w/herbs and cheese, ½ cup.................................................40
**Tongue,** beef, simmered, 4 oz.........................................321
**Tortellini, packaged,** dry, cheese, spinach, or tricolor cheese
    (*Real Torino*), 2.3 oz. .................................................250
**Tortellini, refrigerated** (see also "Tortelloni"):
beef and roasted garlic (*Di Giorno*), 1 cup...............................340
cheese (*Contadina Buitoni*), ¾ cup........................................250
cheese, mixed (*Contadina Buitoni*), ¾ cup.............................260
cheese, 3 (*Contadina Buitoni*), ¾ cup ...................................250
cheese, 3 (*Di Giorno*), ¾ cup ..............................................250
chicken, herb (*Contadina Buitoni*), ¾ cup .............................260
spinach cheese (*Contadina Buitoni*), ¾ cup ...........................260
**Tortellini entree, canned:**
cheese (*Chef Boyardee*), ½ of 15-oz. can ...............................230
meat (*Chef Boyardee*), ½ of 15-oz. can ..................................260
**Tortellini entree, frozen,** cheese and chicken (*Healthy Choice*
    Bowl), 8.7-oz. pkg. ......................................................250
**Tortelloni** (see also "Tortellini"), refrigerated, 1 cup:
cheese and roasted garlic (*Contadina Buitoni*) .........................270
chicken and prosciutto (*Contadina Buitoni*) .............................360
lemon chicken (*Di Giorno*) ...................................................270
mozzarella garlic (*Di Giorno*)................................................300

**Tortelloni (*cont.*)**
mozzarella and herb (*Contadina Buitoni*)................................320
mozzarella and pepperoni (*Contadina Buitoni*).....................350
mushroom and cheese (*Contadina Buitoni*)...........................290
pesto (*Di Giorno*)................................................................320
portobello mushroom (*Di Giorno*)........................................310
sausage, sweet, or sun-dried tomato (*Contadina Buitoni*).......320
**Tortilla,** 1 pc., except as noted:
corn, blue or yellow (*Cedarlane* Organic Lowfat), 2 pcs.,
    1.6 oz. ................................................................................100
flour (*Cedarlane* Organic Fat Free), 2 pcs., 1.6 oz...................120
whole wheat (*Cedarlane* Organic Fat Free), 2 pcs., 1.6 oz. ......120
**Tortilla chip,** see "Corn chip, puff, and similar snacks"
**Tostada shell,** see "Taco shell"
**Trail mix:**
(*Planters* Caramel Nut Crunch), 3 tbsp. ................................140
(*Planters* Flamin' Cajun Crunch), ⅓ cup ...............................130
(*Planters* Nuts, Seeds & Raisins), 3 tbsp..............................160
**Tree fern,** cooked, chopped, ½ cup.......................................28
**Triticale,** whole grain, 1 cup...............................................645
**Triticale flour,** whole grain, 1 cup.......................................439
**Trout,** meat only:
mixed species, raw, 4 oz. .....................................................168
mixed species, baked, broiled, or microwaved, 4 oz. ..............216
rainbow, farmed, raw, 4 oz....................................................157
rainbow, farmed, baked, broiled, or microwaved, 4 oz............192
rainbow, wild, raw, 4 oz.........................................................135
rainbow, wild, baked, broiled, or microwaved, 4 oz................170
**Trout, smoked,** fillet (*Ducktrap River*), 2 oz........................110
**Trout, smoked, canned,** golden fillets, in olive oil, drained
    (*Reese*), 3.75-oz. can.......................................................110
**Trout, smoked, pâté** (*Ducktrap River*), ¼ cup.......................130
**Tuna,** meat only:
bluefin, raw, 4 oz. ................................................................163
bluefin, baked, broiled, or microwaved, 4 oz. ........................208
skipjack, raw, 4 oz. ..............................................................117
skipjack, baked, broiled, or microwaved, 4 oz. ......................150
yellowfin, raw, 4 oz...............................................................123
yellowfin, baked, broiled, or microwaved, 4 oz.......................158

**Tuna, canned:**
fillet, drained (*Starkist* Select Prime Light), 2 oz...........................60
light, in oil, drained (*Bumble Bee*), 2 oz., approx. ¼ cup..........110
light, in oil, drained, chunk (*Starkist*), 2 oz................................110
light, in olive oil (*Progresso*), ¼ cup ........................................160
light, in water (*Bumble Bee*), 2 oz., approx. ¼ cup....................60
light, in water, chunk (*Starkist/Starkist* Low Fat/Sodium), 2 oz...60
white, in oil, drained, solid (*Bumble Bee*), 2 oz. .........................90
white, in oil, drained, solid (*Starkist*), 2 oz. ...............................90
white, in water:
    albacore, drained (*Bumble Bee*), 2 oz., approx. ¼ cup .........70
    chunk (*Starkist/Starkist* Low Fat/Sodium), 2 oz. ..................60
    solid (*Starkist*), 2 oz. ........................................................70
**Tuna burger,** frozen (*Ocean Beauty*), 3.2-oz. burger...................90
**Tuna entree,** frozen, 1 pkg.:
casserole (*Healthy Choice* Entree), 9 oz....................................240
casserole (*Stouffer's*), 10 oz....................................................380
and noodles, homestyle (*Marie Callender's*), 12 oz. .................600
**Tuna entree mix** (*Tuna Helper*), 1 cup\*, except as noted:
au gratin, creamy pasta, tetrazzini, or tuna melt ......................300
broccoli, cheesy or garden cheddar ...........................................290
broccoli, creamy or fettuccine Alfredo .......................................310
pasta, cheesy or tuna Romanoff.................................................280
pasta salad, ⅔ cup\* .................................................................370
tuna pot pie..............................................................................440
**Tuna salad,** canned or packaged:
(*Bumble Bee* Original), 3.5 oz....................................................190
w/crackers (*Bumble Bee* Fat Free), 3.5 oz.................................180
w/crackers (*Bumble Bee* Kit), 3.8 oz. .......................................250
w/crackers (*Bumble Bee* Original), 3.5 oz. ................................280
w/crackers (*Starkist* Kit), 1 pkg................................................190
w/out crackers (*Bumble Bee* Fat Free), 2.75 oz. .........................90
w/out crackers (*Bumble Bee* Original), 2.75 oz. .........................190
**Turban squash** (*Frieda's*), ¾ cup, 3 oz....................................30
**Turbot,** European, meat only:
raw, 4 oz. ................................................................................108
baked, broiled, or microwaved, 4 oz. ........................................138
**Turkey,** fresh, all classes, roasted, 4 oz., except as noted:
meat w/skin .............................................................................236

**Turkey (*cont.*)**

| | |
|---|---:|
| meat only | 193 |
| meat only, chopped or diced, 1 cup | 238 |
| skin only, 1 oz. | 125 |
| dark meat, w/skin | 251 |
| dark meat only | 212 |
| dark meat only, chopped or diced, 1 cup | 262 |
| light meat, w/skin | 223 |
| light meat only | 178 |
| light meat only, chopped or diced, 1 cup | 220 |
| back, meat w/skin | 276 |
| breast, meat w/skin | 214 |
| leg, meat w/skin | 236 |
| wing, meat w/skin, 6.6 oz. | 426 |
| wing, meat w/skin | 260 |

**Turkey, canned,** 2 oz., w/broth, except as noted:

| | |
|---|---:|
| (*Hormel* Chunk) | 70 |
| white (*Hormel* Chunk) | 60 |
| 5-oz. can | 232 |
| drained, 1 cup | 220 |

**Turkey, frozen or refrigerated:**

| | |
|---|---:|
| whole, hen, raw (*Empire* Kosher), 4 oz. | 120 |
| whole, young (*Norbest Family Tradition* 16–24 lb.), 4 oz. | 170 |
| whole, young (*Norbest Family Tradition* 8–16 lb.), 4 oz. | 190 |
| whole, basted, young (*Norbest* 16–24 lb.), 4 oz. | 160 |
| whole, basted, young (*Norbest* 8–16 lb.), 4 oz. | 170 |

whole, cooked, 3 oz.:

| | |
|---|---:|
| hen, dark (*Perdue/Perdue* Frozen) | 180 |
| hen, white (*Perdue/Perdue* Frozen) | 150 |
| tom, dark (*Perdue/Perdue* Frozen) | 160 |
| tom, white (*Perdue/Perdue* Frozen) | 140 |
| whole, hickory smoked, young (*Norbest*), 3 oz. | 145 |
| breast, raw, hen, half (*Empire* Kosher), 4 oz. | 160 |
| breast, basted (*Norbest*), 4 oz. | 160 |
| breast, boneless or boneless roast (*Norbest*), 4 oz. | 135 |

breast, cooked, 3 oz., except as noted:

| | |
|---|---:|
| whole or half, cooked (*Perdue*) | 150 |
| half, broth marinated, cooked (*Perdue*) | 130 |
| roast, w/sweet and sour sauce (*Empire* Kosher), 5 oz. | 160 |

boneless, skinless (*Perdue Fit 'N Easy* London Broil) .........110
cutlet, boneless, skinless (*Perdue Fit 'N Easy* Thin Sliced),
   2.4 oz. ...............................................................................90
fillet, boneless, skinless (*Perdue Fit 'N Easy*) ......................110
tenderloin, boneless, skinless (*Perdue Fit 'N Easy*) ............110
tenderloin, cracked black pepper (*Perdue*) .............................90
drumsticks (*Empire* Kosher), 4 oz. .........................................110
nuggets, cooked (*Louis Rich*), 4 pcs., 3.25 oz. ........................260
tenders, raw (*Empire* Kosher), 4 oz. .......................................120
thigh, raw (*Empire* Kosher), 4 oz. ...........................................160
wing, raw (*Empire* Kosher), 4 oz. ...........................................205
wing, cooked (*Perdue*) ............................................................160
wing drumette, cooked (*Perdue*), 3.3-oz. pc. ..........................180
**Turkey, ground:**
(*Norbest*), 4 oz. ......................................................................170
raw, all types and styles (*Perdue Fit 'N Easy*), 4 oz. ...............170
cooked, all types and styles (*Perdue Fit 'N Easy*), 3 oz. ..........160
**Turkey bacon** (*Louis Rich*), ½-oz. slice .......................................35
**Turkey bologna:**
(*Louis Rich* 50% Less Fat), 1-oz. slice......................................50
(*Louis Rich Variety-Pak*), 3 slices, 2.2 oz. .............................120
**Turkey dinner,** frozen, 1 pkg.:
breast, w/gravy, stuffing and mashed potatoes (*Swanson*
   *Traditional Favorites*), 11.75 oz. ...........................................330
breast, traditional (*Healthy Choice* Meal), 10.5 oz. ..................290
and gravy, w/stuffing (*Banquet Extra Helping*), 17 oz. ..............620
and gravy, w/stuffing (*Freezer Queen*), 9.25 oz. ........................230
roast, country inn (*Healthy Choice* Meal), 10 oz. ......................250
white meat w/gravy, stuffing and mashed potatoes (*Swanson*
   *Hungry-Man*), 16¾ oz. ..........................................................500
**Turkey entree, canned or packaged:**
and dressing (*Dinty Moore American Classics*), 1 bowl ..........290
stew (*Dinty Moore*), 1 cup .......................................................140
**Turkey entree, frozen,** 1 pkg., except as noted:
breast, grilled, w/rice pilaf (*Marie Callender's*), 11.75 oz. .........310
breast, honey roast (*Banquet*), 9 oz. .......................................270
breast, medallions, w/gravy (*Boston Market*), 8 oz. .................210
breast, medallions, w/mashed potato and gravy (*Boston
   Market*), 15.5 oz. ...................................................................470

**Turkey entree, frozen (*cont.*)**
breast, roast (*Healthy Choice* Entree), 8.5 oz............................220
breast, roast (*Stouffer's Hearty Portions*), 16 oz........................460
breast, roast (*Stouffer's* Homestyle), 9⅝ oz. ...........................310
breast, roast (*Lean Cuisine Café Classics*), 9.75 oz. .................270
breast, roast (*Lean Cuisine Hearty Portions*), 14 oz. .................320
croquettes, gravy and (*Freezer Queen* Family), 1 patty
   w/gravy..................................................................................140
divan (*Healthy Choice* Bowl), 9.5 oz..........................................250
gravy and, w/stuffing (*Michelina's*), 8 oz. ..................................260
gravy and, w/stuffing (*Morton*), 9 oz. .......................................240
w/gravy and mashed potato (*Boston Market*), 15½ oz...........470
w/gravy and mashed potato (*Marie Callender's* Family), 2 pcs.
   turkey w/gravy and ½ cup potato.....................................310
and gravy and stuffing (*Marie Callender's*), 14 oz....................500
and gravy, stuffing, and mashed potatoes (*Freezer Queen*),
   8.5 oz. ............................................................................210
homestyle (*Lean Cuisine Everyday Favorites*), 9⅜ oz. .............240
pie/pot pie:
   (*Banquet*), 7 oz. .................................................................370
   (*Empire* Kosher), 1 pie.........................................................470
   (*Marie Callender's*), 9.5 oz. .................................................690
   (*Stouffer's*), 10 oz. ..............................................................520
   (*Swanson*), 7 oz. .................................................................400
   white meat (*Swanson Hungry-Man*), 17 oz........................440
roasted (*Lean Cuisine Skillet Sensations*), ½ of 24-oz. pkg. ....220
sliced, gravy and:
   (*Banquet* Hot Sandwich Toppers), 4-oz. bag......................160
   (*Freezer Queen* Family), ⅙ pkg...........................................60
   (*Freezer Queen* Cook-in-Pouch), 5 oz................................70
   homestyle (*Banquet* Family), 2 slices w/gravy ...................140
tenderloins, glazed (*Lean Cuisine Cafe Classics*), 9 oz. ...........260
tetrazzini (*Stouffer's*), 10 oz.....................................................400
white meat (*Banquet* Mostly White Meat), 9.25 oz....................270
**Turkey giblets,** simmered, chopped or diced, 1 cup................242
**Turkey gravy,** in jars, ¼ cup:
(*Boston Market* Roasted) ..............................................................25
(*Franco-American*).........................................................................25
(*Franco-American* Fat Free) ..........................................................20

(*Franco-American* Slow Roasted/Slow Roasted Fat Free)...........30
**Turkey gravy mix,** roasted (*Knorr*), 1 tbsp................................25
**Turkey ham:**
(*Carl Buddig*), 2.5-oz. pkg. ......................................................100
(*Healthy Deli* 95% Fat Free), 2 oz.................................................70
(*Louis Rich Variety-Pak*), 3 slices, 2.2 oz. ...............................80
(*Norbest*), 3 oz. .............................................................................90
hickory smoked (*Perdue Deli*), 2 oz. ........................................60
honey roasted (*Sara Lee*) .............................................................70
**Turkey lunch meat** (see also "Turkey ham," etc.), breast, 2 oz.,
    except as noted:
(*Boar's Head* Golden/Golden Skinless)...................................60
(*Boar's Head* Premium Lower Sodium) ...................................60
(*Carl Buddig*), 2.5-oz. pkg. ......................................................110
(*Hebrew National* 97% Fat Free), 5 slices, 2 oz. .......................50
(*Hormel Light and Lean* 97), 1-oz. slice....................................30
Black Forest (*Healthy Deli* 99% Fat Free Gourmet)....................60
browned (*Healthy Choice*) .............................................................50
browned (*Norbest* Gold Label Deli) .............................................60
Cajun or honey (*Perdue Carving*) ...............................................50
cracked pepper (*Sara Lee*), 3 slices, 2 oz. ...............................60
flame seared (*Healthy Deli* 98% Fat Free) .................................60
glazed, oven cooked (*Healthy Deli* 98% Fat Free Gourmet)........60
hickory smoked (*Louis Rich Variety-Pak* Fat Free), 4 slices,
    2 oz..........................................................................................45
hickory smoked, pan roasted (*Perdue Carving Classics*)............70
honey, oven cooked (*Healthy Deli* 98% Fat Free Gourmet) ........60
honey roasted (*Carl Buddig*), 2.5-oz. pkg. ...............................110
honey roasted (*Carl Buddig*), 9 slices, 2 oz. .............................85
honey roasted (*Sara Lee*) .............................................................60
honey roasted (*Sara Lee* Deli), 2 slices, 1.6 oz. .........................50
honey roasted and smoked (*Healthy Choice*)..............................60
honey roasted and smoked (*Healthy Choice Deli Thin Savory
    Selections*), 6 slices, 1.9 oz. ....................................................70
honey smoked or mesquite smoked (*Perdue Carving*)..............50
Italian style, oven cooked (*Healthy Deli* 98% Fat Free) ..............70
maple (*Boar's Head Maple Glazed Honey Coat*) .........................70
mesquite smoke, oven roasted (*Healthy Deli* 99% Fat Free) ......60
mesquite smoked (*Louis Rich Carving Board*), 3 slices, 1.9 oz. 50

**Turkey lunch meat (*cont.*)**
oven cooked (*Healthy Choice Deli Thin Deli Traditions*), 6 slice,
  1.9 oz............................................................................60
oven cooked (*Healthy Deli* 99% Fat Free Gourmet) ...................60
oven roasted (*Healthy Choice*), 1-oz. slice ...................................30
oven roasted (*Healthy Deli* 99% Fat Free) ....................................60
oven roasted (*Louis Rich Carving Board*), 6 slices, 2.1 oz. .......60
oven roasted (*Louis Rich* Fat Free) ...............................................50
oven roasted (*Louis Rich Free*), 1-oz. slice .................................20
oven roasted (*Norbest* Bronze Label Deli)....................................60
oven roasted (*Norbest* Gold Label Deli/Silver Label Deli) ...........55
oven roasted (*Perdue Carving*).....................................................70
oven roasted (*Perdue* Deli).............................................................50
oven roasted (*Perdue HealthSense*) .............................................60
oven roasted (*Sara Lee*) ................................................................60
oven roasted (*Sara Lee* Deli), 2 slices, 1.6 oz. ...........................45
oven roasted, rotisserie flavored (*Sara Lee*), ...............................70
oven roasted or smoked (*Carl Buddig*), 2.5-oz. pkg. .................110
oven roasted or smoked (*Carl Buddig*), 9 slices, 2 oz. ................80
oven roasted or smoked (*Russer*) ..................................................50
pan roasted (*Perdue Carving Classics*) .........................................70
pepper (*Healthy Deli* Tutta Bella) .................................................60
pepper, cracked, pan roasted (*Perdue Carving Classics*)............50
pepper, cracked (*Sara Lee*) ...........................................................60
peppered (*Sara Lee*) .......................................................................50
roast (*Boar's Head Ovengold*) .......................................................60
roasted (*Boar's Head Salsalito*) ....................................................60
roasted (*Healthy Choice* 10 oz.), 1-oz. slice ................................50
roasted (*Healthy Choice Hearty Deli Flavor*), 3 slices, 2 oz........60
roasted and smoked (*Healthy Choice* 10 oz.), 1-oz. slice ..........35
rotisserie seasoned or smoked (*Healthy Choice Deli Thin Deli*
  *Traditions*), 6 slices, 1.9 oz. .................................................60
salsa (*Healthy Choice*) ...................................................................60
skinless (*Perdue Carving Classics* Pan Roasted) ........................60
smoked, white (*Norbest*) ................................................................70
smoked (*Carl Buddig* Premium Lean), 2.5-oz. pkg......................60
smoked (*Healthy Choice*), 1-oz. slice ...........................................30
smoked (*Oscar Mayer Free*), 4 slices, 1.8 oz. .............................40
smoked, brick oven style (*Healthy Deli* 99% Fat Free)................60

smoked, hardwood (*Sara Lee*) ...............................................60
smoked, hardwood (*Sara Lee* Deli), 2 slices, 1.6 oz. ..................45
smoked, hickory (*Boar's Head*) ............................................70
smoked, hickory (*Norbest* Gold Label Deli) .............................60
smoked, honey mesquite (*Norbest* Gold Label Deli)..................50
smoked, mesquite (*Healthy Choice Deli Thin Savory Selections*),
   6 slices, 1.9 oz. ..............................................................70
smoked, mesquite (*Hormel Light and Lean* 97), 1-oz. slice .......30
smoked, mesquite (*Sara Lee*).................................................60
smoked, mequite or pepper (*Boar's Head*)...............................60
smoked, skinless (*Healthy Choice*)..........................................50
Southwest grill (*Healthy Choice*) ............................................60
**Turkey lunch meat,** canned, oven roasted (*Spam*), 2 oz............70
**Turkey patties,** breaded, battered, fried, 1-oz. patty...................79
**Turkey pastrami,** 2 oz.:
(*Boar's Head*) .....................................................................60
(*Healthy Deli* 95% Fat Free)................................................70
(*Norbest*) ...........................................................................70
hickory smoked (*Perdue* Deli) ..............................................70
**Turkey pepperoni,** sliced (*Hormel Pillow*), 17 slices, 1.1 oz......80
**Turkey pocket,** frozen, 4.5-oz. pc.:
broccoli and cheese (*Lean Pockets*).....................................230
and ham, w/cheddar (*Lean Pockets*)....................................290
and ham, w/cheese (*Hot Pockets*)........................................310
and ham, w/Swiss (*Croissant Pockets*).................................320
**Turkey roll,** light and dark meat, 2 oz.....................................85
**Turkey salami** (*Louis Rich Variety-Pak*), 3 slices, 2.2 oz........100
**Turkey sticks,** breaded, battered, fried, 2.25-oz. stick..............179
**Turmeric, dried,** ground, 1 tsp. ..............................................8
**Turnip,** fresh or stored:
raw, 1 large, 6.5 oz. ............................................................49
raw, cubed, 1 cup ...............................................................35
boiled, drained, mashed, 1 cup ...........................................48
**Turnip, frozen:**
unprepared, mashed, ⅓ of 10-oz. pkg. .................................15
boiled, drained, 1 cup .........................................................36
**Turnip greens,** fresh:
raw, chopped, 1 cup ............................................................15
boiled, drained, chopped, 1 cup ...........................................29

**Turnip greens, canned:**
(*Allens/Sunshine*) .........................................................................25
chopped, w/diced turnip (*Allens/Sunshine*) ...............................30
**Turnip greens, frozen,** chopped, 1 cup:
(*Birds Eye*) ....................................................................................30
boiled, drained, w/turnips.............................................................28
w/diced root (*Birds Eye*).............................................................25
**Turnover,** frozen, apple or raspberry (*Pepperidge Farm*),
    1 pc. ........................................................................................290
**Twists pasta entree,** canned, w/meat sauce (*Franco*-American
    Superiore Hearty), 1 cup.......................................................250

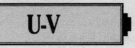

## U-V

**FOOD AND MEASURE**                                      **CALORIES**

**Uzbek melon** (*Frieda's*), 1 cup, 1.4 oz. ...................................35
**Vanilla extract,** 1 tbsp. ...................................................37
**"Vanilla extract," imitation:**
1 tbsp..........................................................................31
nonalcoholic, 1 tbsp. ........................................................7
**Veal,** meat only, 4 oz., except as noted:
cubed, leg and shoulder, braised, lean only ...........................213
ground, broiled .............................................................195
leg, braised or pan fried, lean w/fat...................................239
leg, braised, lean only....................................................230
leg, pan fried, lean only .................................................208
leg, roasted, lean w/fat ..................................................181
leg, breaded, pan fried, lean and fat ..................................250
leg, breaded, pan fried, lean only .....................................234
loin, roasted, lean w/fat .................................................246
loin, roasted, lean only ..................................................199
loin chop, braised, lean w/fat ..........................................322
loin chop, braised, lean w/fat, 2.8 oz. (6.9 oz. raw w/bone) .....227
loin chop, braised, lean only............................................256
loin chop, braised, lean only, 2.4 oz. (6.9 oz. raw w/bone) ......156
rib, braised, lean w/fat ..................................................285
rib, braised, lean only ...................................................247
rib, roasted, lean w/fat ..................................................259
rib, roasted, lean only ...................................................201
shoulder, whole, braised, lean w/fat...................................259
shoulder, whole, braised, lean only ...................................226
shoulder, whole, roasted, lean w/fat..................................209
shoulder, whole, roasted, lean only ...................................193
shoulder, arm, braised, lean w/fat .....................................268
shoulder, arm, braised, lean only ......................................228
shoulder, arm, roasted, lean w/fat .....................................208
shoulder, arm, roasted, lean only ......................................186
shoulder, blade, braised, lean w/fat....................................255

**Veal** (*cont.*)

shoulder, blade, braised, lean only ...............................225
shoulder, blade, roasted, lean w/fat...........................211
shoulder, blade, roasted, lean only ...........................194
sirloin, braised, lean w/fat .........................................286
sirloin, braised, lean only...........................................231
sirloin, roasted, lean w/fat .........................................229
sirloin, roasted, lean only ..........................................191

**Veal dinner,** parmigiana, frozen, 1 pkg.:

(*Freezer Queen*), 9 oz. .............................................330
(*Swanson*), 11¼ oz. .................................................390
(*Swanson Hungry-Man*), 18¼ oz. .............................630

**Veal entree,** parmigiana, frozen, 1 pkg., except as noted:

(*Banquet*), 8.75 oz. ..................................................330
(*Freezer Queen*), 1 patty ........................................170
(*Stouffer's Hearty Portions*), 17.5 oz.......................630
(*Stouffer's* Homestyle), 11⅝ oz. ..............................410

**Vegetable dish, canned or in jars:**

curry, mild (*Patek's* Aloo Mattar Sabzi), 1½ cups.................240
curry, mild (*Patek's* Tikka Masala), 1½ cups ......................190
salad (*Hanover*), ⅓ cup ................................................80
and sauce, hot and spicy (*House of Tsang* Szechuan),
  .½ cup...............................................................70
and sauce, sweet and sour (*House of Tsang* Hong Kong),
  ½ cup.................................................................160
and sauce, teriyaki (*House of Tsang* Tokyo), ½ cup .................100

**Vegetable dish, frozen:**

Alfredo (*Green Giant*), ¾ cup ......................................80
and pasta, see "Pasta dish, frozen"

**Vegetable entree,** frozen (see also specific listings), 1 pkg.:

and chicken pasta bake (*Stouffer's*), 12 oz. ............................380
country, and beef (*Lean Cuisine Cafe Classics*), 9 oz. .............210
parmigiana (*Freezer Queen* Cook-in-Pouch), 5 oz. ...................190
parmigiana, w/tomato sauce (*Morton*), 8.75 oz......................290
pie/pot pie:

  (*Cedarlane* Less Fat), 7.4 oz. .....................................390
  (*Cedarlane* Sante Fe/Mediterranean), 7.4 oz.......................490
  (*Amy's*), 7.5 oz. .................................................420
  (*Amy's* Country), 7.5 oz. .........................................370

(*Amy's* Nondairy), 7.5 oz. ....................................................320
cheese (*Banquet*), 7 oz. ....................................................340
w/beef (*Morton*), 7 oz. ....................................................340
w/chicken (*Morton*), 7 oz. ....................................................320
w/turkey (*Morton*), 7 oz. ....................................................310
stir-fry, w/rice (*Michelina's*), 8 oz. .....................................240
wrap, couscous (*Cedarlane* Low Fat), 6 oz. ....................220
wrap, pizza (*Cedarlane* Low Fat), 6 oz. ..........................220
wrap, rice and teriyaki (*Cedarlane* Low Fat), 6 oz. ......280

**Vegetable entree mix,** fresh, 1 cup*:
lo mein stir-fry (*Mann's*) ....................................................330
teriyaki stir-fry (*Mann's*) ....................................................340

**Vegetable entree mix,** frozen:
Alfredo tortellini (*Freshlike Meal Starter*), 1 cup* .........280
cashew stir-fry (*Freshlike Meal Starter*), 1 cup* ............230
cheesy cheese (*Freshlike Meal Starter*), 1 cup* ............270
lo mein, Oriental (*Birds Eye Easy Recipe Creations*),
   2¼ cups ......................................................................230
Parmesan, creamy (*Freshlike Meal Starter*), 1 cup* .....300
Parmesan, garlic, roasted (*Birds Eye Easy Recipe Creations*),
   2¼ cups ......................................................................240
primavera, basil herb (*Birds Eye Easy Recipe Creations*),
   2¼ cups ......................................................................260
sweet and sour w/pineapple tidbits (*Birds Eye Easy Recipe
   Creations*), 1⅔ cups ..................................................200
sweet/sour blend (*Freshlike Meal Starter*), 1 cup* .........270
Szechwan, spicy (*Freshlike Meal Starter*), 1 cup* ..........270
Szechwan w/cashews (*Birds Eye Easy Recipe Creations*),
   2¼ cups ......................................................................180
teriyaki blend (*Freshlike Meal Starter*), 1 cup* ..............230
tortellini Parmigiana (*Birds Eye Easy Recipe Creations*),
   2¼ cups ......................................................................240

**Vegetable juice,** canned:
(*V8/V8* Picante/Spicy), 8 fl. oz. ..........................................50
(*V8* Low Sodium), 8 fl. oz. ..................................................60
all varieties (Muir Glen), 5.5 fl. oz. ......................................50
tomato and chili (*Snap-E-Tom*), 10 fl. oz. ........................60
tomato and chili (*Snap-E-Tom*), 6 fl. oz. ..........................40

**Vegetable oyster,** see "Salsify"
**Vegetable pie,** see "Vegetable entree"
**Vegetable pocket,** frozen, 1 pc.:
"cheese," nondairy (*Amy's* Soy Cheeze), 4.5 oz. ....................270
pie (*Amy's*), 5 oz. ...........................................................300
Mediterranean or roasted (*Amy's*), 4.5 oz. ...............................220
**Vegetable,** see specific listings
**Vegetables, mixed,** fresh, Asian stir-fry (*Frieda's*), 3 oz. ...........15
**Vegetables, mixed, canned,** ½ cup:
(*Del Monte*) ...................................................................40
(*Green Giant*) .................................................................60
**Vegetables, mixed, frozen:**
(*Birds Eye*), ⅓ cup ..........................................................50
(*Freshlike*), ⅔ cup ...........................................................60
(*Seabrook Farms*), ⅔ cup ...................................................70
boiled, drained, ½ cup ......................................................54
California (*Freshlike*), 1 cup ...............................................30
country (*Freshlike*), ⅔ cup .................................................45
gumbo blend (*Birds Eye*), ¾ cup ..........................................40
Oriental (*Birds Eye*), ½ cup ................................................60
Oriental stir-fry (*Freshlike*), 1 cup ........................................30
midwestern (*Freshlike*), ¾ cup ............................................25
seasoning (*Birds Eye*), ¾ cup .............................................20
soup (*Birds Eye/Freshlike*), ⅔ cup .......................................45
stew (*Birds Eye*), ¾ cup ....................................................40
stew (*Freshlike*), ⅔ cup .....................................................45
stir-fry (*Birds Eye*), ½ cup ..................................................60
winter (*Freshlike*), 1 cup ...................................................25
**Vegetables, mixed, pickled** (*Krinos* Giardinara), ¼ cup ..............0
**Vegetarian burger,** see "Burger, vegetarian"
**Vegetarian dinner,** frozen, 1 pkg.:
"salisbury steak" (*Amy's* Country Dinner), 11 oz. ......................380
veggie loaf (*Amy's*), 10 oz. ................................................260
**Vegetarian entree,** frozen (see also specific listings), 1 pkg.:
shepherd's pie (*Amy's*), 8 oz. .............................................160
stew (*Yves* Veggie Country Stew), 10.6 oz. .............................160
**Venison,** roasted, 4 oz. ...................................................179
**Vermicelli entree, mix,** roasted garlic and olive
oil (*Pasta Roni*), approx. 1 cup* .........................................360

**Vienna sausage,** see "Sausage, canned"
**Vindaloo sauce,** see "Curry sauce"
**Vinegar:**
balsamic (*Regina*), 1 tbsp...................................................5
cider, 1 cup ................................................................34
cider, 1 tbsp. ...............................................................2
rice (*Nakano*), 1 tbsp. ....................................................1
rice, seasoned (*Nakano*), 1 tbsp....................................0
rice, seasoned, balsamic blend (*Nakano*), 1 tbsp. ..........15
white, distilled (*Indian Summer*), 1 tbsp. .........................0
wine, red or white, plain or flavored (*Regina*), 1 tbsp..........0

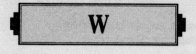

## W

**FOOD AND MEASURE**                                     **CALORIES**

**Waffle,** frozen, 2 pcs., except as noted:
(*Aunt Jemima* Homestyle)........................................................200
(*Aunt Jemima* Low Fat)...........................................................170
(*Eggo* Homestyle)....................................................................190
(*Eggo* Homestyle Low Fat).....................................................160
(*Eggo* Mini's Homestyle).........................................................260
(*Eggo* Nutri-Grain)..................................................................170
(*Eggo* Nutri-Grain Low Fat)....................................................140
(*Eggo* Special K).....................................................................120
(*Hungry Jack* Homestyle)........................................................180
apple cinnamon, blueberry, or chocolate chip (*Eggo*) .............200
banana bread or buttermilk (*Eggo*) ........................................190
blueberry (*Aunt Jemima*)........................................................210
blueberry (*Eggo* Nutri-Grain Low Fat) ....................................150
blueberry (*Hungry Jack*)........................................................210
buttermilk (*Aunt Jemima*)........................................................200
buttermilk (*Hungry Jack*)........................................................190
multi-bran (*Eggo* Nutri-Grain) ................................................160
nut and honey (*Eggo*)..............................................................220
oat, golden (*Eggo*)..................................................................140
sticks (*Aunt Jemima* Homestyle), 3 pcs.................................310
sticks, chocolate chip (*Aunt Jemima*), 3 pcs. ........................330
sticks, cinnamon sugar (*Aunt Jemima*), 3 pcs........................320
strawberry (*Eggo*), 2 pcs........................................................200
**Waffle mix,** see "Pancake mix"
**Walnut,** dried, shelled:
(*Planters*), ⅓ cup....................................................................210
black, 1 oz................................................................................172
black, chopped, ¼ cup .............................................................190
English, 1 oz. ...........................................................................185
English, chopped, ¼ cup ..........................................................196
**Walnut topping** (*Smucker's* Spoonable Toppings), 2 tbsp.......170
**Wasabi root,** fresh, raw, sliced, 1 cup.....................................142

**Wasabi sauce,** in jars (*Sushi Chef*), 1 tbsp. ..............................90
**Water chestnuts,** Chinese, fresh:
(*Frieda's*), 1 tbsp., 1.1 oz................................................30
4 whole, 1.3 oz. .............................................................35
sliced, ½ cup ................................................................60
**Water chestnuts,** Chinese, canned:
4 whole, 1 oz. ...............................................................14
sliced, ½ cup ................................................................35
**Watercress,** fresh, raw:
(*Frieda's*), 1 cup, 3 oz...................................................10
chopped, 1 cup ...............................................................4
**Watermelon,** fresh:
1" slice, 10" diam. .......................................................152
balls or diced, 1 cup .....................................................49
yellow seedless (*Frieda's*), ½ cup ...................................25
**Watermelon-cherry drink mix,** 8 fl. oz.*:
(*Kool-Aid*)..................................................................100
(*Kool-Aid* Sugar Sweetened) ...........................................60
**Watermelon drink** (*Kool-Aid Splash*), 8 fl. oz...................110
**Watermelon seed kernels,** dried:
¼ cup.........................................................................150
1 oz. .........................................................................158
**Wax bean,** fresh, see "Green bean"
**Wax bean, canned** (*Del Monte*), ½ cup .............................20
**Wax gourd,** fresh, boiled, drained, cubed, 1 cup..................23
**Welsh rarebit,** frozen (*Stouffer's*), ½ cup ......................120
*Wendy's,* 1 serving:
sandwiches:
   bacon cheeseburger, jr. ...........................................380
   *Big Bacon Classic*..................................................580
   cheeseburger, jr. or kid's meal .................................320
   cheeseburger, jr., deluxe .........................................360
   chicken, breaded ...................................................440
   chicken, grilled .....................................................310
   chicken, spicy.......................................................410
   chicken club .........................................................470
   hamburger, single, plain...........................................360
   hamburger, single, w/everything.................................420
   hamburger, jr. or kid's meal .....................................270

**Wendy's** (*cont.*)

sandwich components and condiments:

| | |
|---|---|
| American cheese | 70 |
| American cheese, jr. | 45 |
| bacon, 1 pc. | 20 |
| bun, kaiser | 190 |
| bun, sandwich | 160 |
| chicken fillet, breaded | 230 |
| chicken fillet, grilled | 110 |
| chicken fillet, spicy | 210 |
| hamburger patty, 4 oz. | 200 |
| hamburger patty, 2 oz. | 100 |
| ketchup, 1 tsp. | 10 |
| lettuce, 1 leaf | 15 |
| mayonnaise, 1½ tsp. | 30 |
| mustard, ½ tsp. | 0 |
| mustard, honey, reduced calorie, 1 tsp. | 25 |
| onion, 4 rings | 5 |
| pickle, 4 slices | 0 |
| tomato, 1 slice | 5 |

*Fresh Stuffed Pitas,* w/dressing:

| | |
|---|---|
| chicken Caesar | 490 |
| Classic Greek | 440 |
| garden ranch chicken | 480 |
| garden veggie | 400 |
| pita dressing, Caesar vinaigrette, 1 tbsp. | 70 |
| pita dressing, garden ranch sauce, 1 tbsp. | 50 |
| chicken nuggets, 5 pcs. | 230 |
| chicken nuggets, kid's, 4 pcs. | 190 |

chicken nuggets sauce, 1-oz. pkt.:

| | |
|---|---|
| barbecue | 45 |
| honey | 90 |
| honey mustard | 130 |
| sweet and sour | 50 |

chili:

| | |
|---|---|
| large, 12 oz. | 310 |
| small, 8 oz. | 210 |
| cheddar cheese, shredded, 2 tbsp. | 70 |
| saltine crackers, 2 pcs. | 25 |

baked potato:
    plain...................................................................................310
    bacon and cheese .............................................................530
    broccoli and cheese .........................................................470
    cheese ..............................................................................570
    chili and cheese................................................................630
    sour cream and chives......................................................380
    sour cream or whipped margarine, 1 pkt. ............................60
fries, *Biggie*.............................................................................470
fries, *Great Biggie* ..................................................................570
fries, medium..........................................................................390
fries, small..............................................................................270
salads-to-go, fresh, w/out dressing:
    Caesar side salad or deluxe garden .................................110
    grilled chicken ..................................................................200
    side salad ...........................................................................60
    soft breadstick..................................................................130
    taco chips .........................................................................210
    taco salad .........................................................................380
dressing, 2 tbsp., except as noted:
    blue cheese ......................................................................180
    French ..............................................................................120
    French, fat free ...................................................................35
    Italian Caesar....................................................................150
    ranch, *Hidden Valley* .......................................................100
    ranch, *Hidden Valley,* reduced fat/calorie...........................60
    salad oil, 1 tbsp..................................................................120
    Thousand Island..................................................................90
    wine vinegar, 1 tbsp. .............................................................0
desserts:
    chocolate chip cookie........................................................270
    *Frosty,* large.....................................................................540
    *Frosty,* medium ................................................................440
    *Frosty,* small....................................................................330
**Wheat, whole grain,** 1 cup, except as noted:
durum .....................................................................................651
hard red, spring......................................................................632
hard red, winter (*Arrowhead Mills*), ¼ cup .............................160
hard white...............................................................................657

**Wheat, whole grain (*cont.*)**

soft red winter ........................................................................556

soft white ................................................................................571

**Wheat, parboiled,** see "Bulgur"

**Wheat, sprouted,** 1 cup ........................................................214

**Wheat bran** (see also "Cereal, ready-to-eat"):

(*Arrowhead Mills*), ¼ cup ......................................................35

crude, 1 cup ...........................................................................125

raw (*Hodgson Mill* Untoasted), ¼ cup ....................................30

**Wheat flakes,** rolled (*Arrowhead Mills*), ⅓ cup .....................110

**Wheat flour** (see also "Semolina flour"), ¼ cup, except as noted:

(*La Piña*) .................................................................................100

(*Wondra*) .................................................................................100

all varieties (*Gold Medal/Red Brand*) ....................................100

all varieties, except whole wheat (*Robin Hood*) .....................100

all purpose, bleached (*Pillsbury*) ...........................................100

bread (*Hodgson Mill*) .............................................................100

bread (*Pillsbury*) ....................................................................100

cake (*Softasilk* Velvet) ...........................................................100

cake, white (*Swans Down*) .....................................................100

(*Hodgson Mill* 50/50), scant ¼ cup ........................................100

pastry (*Arrowhead Mills*) ........................................................110

seasoned (*Hodgson Mill Kentucky Kernel*) ..............................90

self-rising, white, all purpose, 1 cup .......................................443

self-rising, white, tortilla mix, 1 cup .......................................450

white, unbleached (*Arrowhead Mills*), ⅓ cup ..........................160

white, unbleached (*Hodgson Mill*), scant ¼ cup .....................100

white, unbleached (*Hodgson Mill* Organic Natural) .................100

white, unbleached (*Pillsbury* Best) ........................................100

whole grain, 1 cup ..................................................................407

whole wheat (*Hodgson Mill*) ..................................................100

whole wheat (*Robin Hood*) ......................................................90

whole wheat, graham (*Hodgson Mill/Hodgson Mill* Organic),
scant ¼ cup .......................................................................100

whole wheat, stone ground (*Arrowhead Mills*) ........................130

**Wheat germ:**

raw (*Arrowhead Mills*), 3 tbsp. ................................................50

raw (*Hodgson Mill* Untoasted), 2 tbsp. ....................................55

toasted (*Kretschmer* Original), 2 tbsp. ....................................50

toasted, honey crunch (*Kretschmer*), 1⅔ tbsp. ..........................50
**Wheat gluten:**
(*Arrowhead Mills* Vital), 3 tbsp. ......................................35
(*Hodgson Mill* Vital), 1 tbsp. ...........................................30
**Wheels and cheese entree,** frozen (*Michelina's*), 8 oz. ...........300
**Whelk,** meat only:
raw, 4 oz. ...........................................................155
boiled, poached, or steamed, 4 oz. ...........................................312
**Whipped topping,** see "Cream topping"
**Whiskey sour mix,** bottled (*Mr & Mrs T*), 4 fl. oz. ..................100
**White chocolate baking chips,** see "Baking chocolate"
**White chocolate topping,** see "Chocolate topping"
**White bean,** mature:
dry, 1 cup ..........................................................673
boiled, 1 cup ......................................................245
small, dry, 1 cup ................................................722
small, boiled, 1 cup ..........................................254
**White bean, canned,** lightly seasoned (*S&W*), ½ cup ............80
**White sauce mix** (*Knorr* Classic), 2 tsp. or ¼ cup* .................25
**Whitefish,** meat only:
raw, 4 oz. ..........................................................153
baked, broiled, or microwaved, 4 oz. .........................................195
smoked, 4 oz. ....................................................122
**Whiting,** meat only:
raw, 4 oz. ..........................................................102
baked, broiled, or microwaved, 4 oz. .........................................130
**Wiener,** see "Frankfurter"
**Wild rice:**
dry (*Lundberg* Organic), ¼ cup ...............................160
dry, ¼ cup .........................................................143
cooked, 1 cup ....................................................166
**Wild rice blend,** see "Rice"
**Wild rice dish,** see "Rice dish"
**Wine:**
dessert, 3.5-fl.-oz. glass .......................................158
dessert, 1 fl. oz. ................................................45
dessert, dry, 3.5-fl.-oz. glass ................................130
dessert, dry, 1 fl. oz. ...........................................37
table, red, 3.5-fl.-oz. glass ...................................74

**Wine (*cont.*)**
table, red, 1 fl. oz. ...............................................................21
table, rosé, 3.5-fl.oz. glass.................................................73
table, rosé, 1 fl. oz. ............................................................21
table, white, 3.5-fl.-oz. glass.............................................70
table, white, 1 fl. oz. ..........................................................20
**Wine, cooking:**
burgundy (*Regina*), 2 tbsp. .............................................25
rice (*Sun Luck* Mirin), 1 tbsp. .........................................20
rice (*Sushi Chef*), 1 tbsp. ................................................50
sauterne (*Regina*), 2 tbsp. ..............................................20
sherry (*Regina*), 2 tbsp.....................................................35
**Winged bean,** fresh:
raw, 1 pod, .6 oz. ................................................................8
raw, sliced, 1 cup...............................................................22
boiled, drained, 1 cup .......................................................24
**Winged bean, mature:**
dry, 1 cup.........................................................................744
boiled, 1 cup ....................................................................253
**Winter melon** (*Frieda's*), 3 oz. .......................................0
**Winter radish,** see "Radish, black"
**Wolf fish,** Atlantic, meat only:
raw, 4 oz. .........................................................................109
baked, broiled, or microwaved, 4 oz. .............................140
**Wonton wrapper:**
(*Frieda's*), 4 pcs., 1 oz. ....................................................80
(*Nasoya*), 8 pcs., 2.1 oz....................................................160
**Worcestershire sauce,** 1 tsp.:
(*Crosse & Blackwell*)............................................................5
(*Heinz*)..................................................................................0
(*Lea & Perrins*) .....................................................................5
**Wrap,** unfilled, 1 pc.:
plain, jalapeno, or southwestern (*Aladdin Bread*), 2 oz...........190
garlic pesto (*Cedar's*), 2.5 oz. .......................................190
garlic pesto or whole wheat (*Aladdin Bread*), 2 oz....................180
Southwestern or tomato and basil (*Cedar's*), 2.5 oz..................185
spinach (*Cedar's*), 2.5 oz................................................180

# Y-Z

**FOOD AND MEASURE**                                    **CALORIES**

**Yam,** fresh:
raw, cubed, 1 cup ....................................................................177
baked or boiled, cubed, 1 cup ...............................................158
**Yam, canned or frozen,** see "Sweet potato"
**Yam, mountain, Hawaiian,** fresh:
raw, 14.8 lb. ...........................................................................281
raw, cubed, ½ cup ....................................................................46
steamed, cubed, 1 cup ............................................................119
**Yam, name** (*Frieda's*), ¾ cup, 3 oz. .....................................100
**Yam bean tuber,** fresh:
raw, sliced, ½ cup ....................................................................46
boiled, drained, 4 oz. ...............................................................43
**Yard-long bean,** fresh:
(*Frieda's*), ¾ cup, 3 oz. ..........................................................40
raw, sliced, 1 cup .....................................................................43
boiled, drained, chopped, 1 cup ..............................................49
**Yard-long bean, mature:**
raw, 1 cup ...............................................................................580
boiled, 1 cup ...........................................................................202
**Yautier root,** fresh, raw, sliced, 1 cup ...................................132
**Yeast:**
dry (*Hodgson Mill*), 5/16 oz. ...................................................30
fast rise (*Hodgson Mill*), 5/16 oz. ...........................................25
**Yellow bean,** fresh:
raw, 1 cup .................................................................................34
boiled, drained, 1 cup ..............................................................44
**Yellow bean, mature:**
raw, 1 cup ...............................................................................676
boiled, 1 cup ...........................................................................255
**Yellow squash,** see "Crookneck squash"
**Yellowtail,** meat only:
raw, 4 oz. ...............................................................................166
baked, broiled, or microwaved, 4 oz. .....................................212

**Yogurt,** 8 oz., except as noted:
plain:
    (*Colombo* Classic)......................................................130
    (*Colombo* Fat Free 32 oz.) ....................................100
    (*Dannon* Lowfat) ....................................................150
    (*Dannon* Natural).....................................................170
    (*Dannon* Nonfat) .....................................................130
    (*Stonyfield Farm* All Natural Nonfat)....................100
    (*Stonyfield Farm* Organic Lowfat)........................110
    (*Stonyfield Farm* Organic Whole Milk).................180
all fruit flavors:
    (*Breyers* Blended/Smooth & Creamy), 4.4 oz. ...130
    (*Breyers* Light) .......................................................120
    (*Colombo* Light)......................................................120
    (*Dannon* Blended Nonfat), 4 oz.............................100
    (*Dannon Light* Nonfat) ...........................................120
    (*Dannon Light Snap 'n Stack* Nonfat), 4 oz. .........60
    (*Dannon Snap 'n Stack* Fruit on the Bottom), 4 oz...110
    (*Jello-O* Lowfat), 4.4 oz. .......................................130
    (*Light n' Lively* Lowfat), 4.4 oz. ............................130
    (*Light n' Lively Free*), 4.4 oz..................................70
    (*Yoplait* Custard Style/Light), 6 oz. ......................190
    (*Yoplait* 99% Fat Free), 6 oz.................................170
    (*Yoplait* 99% Fat Free), 4 oz.................................110
    except banana/strawberry, lemon and vanilla (*Colombo*
      Classic).................................................................220
    except cookies 'n cream (*Dannon Crunch*)............170
apple cinnamon (*Dannon* Fruit on the Bottom).........210
apple cobbler (*Breyers* Smooth & Creamy) ..............230
banana/strawberry (*Colombo* Classic) ......................230
berries, mixed (*Dannon* Fruit on the Bottom) ...........210
berry, mixed, or blueberry (*Breyers* Lowfat) .............230
blueberry (*Dannon* Fruit on the Bottom)...................220
blueberry French vanilla (*Dannon* Double Delights), 6 oz........180
blueberries 'n cream (*Breyers* Smooth & Creamy)....240
boysenberry (*Dannon* Fruit on the Bottom) ..............210
cherry (*Dannon* Fruit on the Bottom).......................220
cherry, black (*Breyers* Lowfat) ................................240
cherry, black, parfait (*Breyers* Smooth & Creamy)...240

cherry cheesecake (*Dannon* Double Delights), 6 oz. ...............180
chocolate cheesecake (*Dannon* Double Delights), 6 oz. ..........200
coconut cream pie (*Yoplait*), 6 oz. .............................................190
coffee (*Dannon*) ...........................................................................220
cookies 'n cream (*Dannon Crunch* Lowfat) ................................150
cranberry raspberry (*Dannon*) ....................................................220
lemon (*Colombo* Classic) .............................................................180
lemon (*Dannon*) ............................................................................220
lemon (*Yoplait*), 6 oz. ...................................................................180
lemon meringue pie (*Dannon* Double Delights), 6 oz. ..............180
orange vanilla cream (*Breyers* Smooth & Creamy) .................230
peach (*Breyers* Lowfat) ...............................................................240
peach (*Dannon* Fruit on the Bottom) ...........................................210
peach, tropical (*Dannon* Fruit on the Bottom) ...........................250
peaches 'n cream (*Breyers* Smooth & Creamy) .......................230
piña colada (*Yoplait*), 6 oz. .........................................................170
pineapple (*Breyers* Lowfat) .........................................................240
raspberries 'n cream (*Breyers* Smooth & Creamy) ..................230
raspberry Bavarian cream (*Dannon* Double Delights), 6 oz......170
raspberry or strawberry (*Breyers* Lowfat) ................................230
raspberry or strawberry (*Dannon* Fruit on the Bottom) ............210
strawberry (*Breyers* Smooth & Creamy Classic) .....................230
strawberry (*Colombo* Low Fat 32 oz.) ........................................190
strawberry (*Dannon Sprinkl'ins* Lowfat), 4.1 oz. ......................130
strawberry banana (*Breyers* Lowfat) .........................................240
strawberry banana split (*Breyers* Smooth & Creamy) .............240
strawberry cheesecake (*Dannon* Double Delights), 6 oz. .........170
vanilla (*Breyers* Lowfat) ..............................................................220
vanilla (*Colombo* Classic) ...........................................................180
vanilla (*Colombo* Fat Free 32 oz.) ..............................................160
vanilla (*Dannon*) ...........................................................................230
vanilla (*Dannon Sprinkl'ins* Lowfat), 4.1 oz. .............................120
vanilla (*Stonyfield Farm* Organic Whole Milk) ..........................230
vanilla (*Stonyfield Farm* Organic Lowfat) .................................170
vanilla, French (*Colombo* Low Fat 32 oz.) .................................180
vanilla, French, strawberry or raspberry (*Dannon* Fruit on the
   Bottom) .......................................................................................240
**Yogurt, frozen,** ½ cup:
*Bananafana* (*Edy's/Dreyer's*) ....................................................120

**Yogurt, frozen** *(cont.)*
(*Ben & Jerry's Cherry Garcia*) ................................................170
(*Ben & Jerry's Chocolate Cherry Garcia*)................................190
(*Ben & Jerry's Chunky Monkey*) ...........................................200
(*Ben & Jerry's Ooey Gooey Cake*) ........................................190
black cherry vanilla swirl (*Edy's/Dreyer's* Fat Free) ..................90
caramel praline crunch (*Edy's/Dreyer's* Fat Free) ...................100
chocolate (*Breyers* All Natural)..............................................130
chocolate (*Häagen-Dazs* Fat Free) ........................................140
chocolate (*Stonyfield Farm* Organic Nonfat) ..........................100
chocolate fudge (*Edy's* Fat Free) ...........................................100
chocolate fudge brownie (*Ben & Jerry's*)................................190
chocolate chip cookie dough (*Ben & Jerry's*) ........................200
chocolate *Heath Bar Crunch* (*Ben & Jerry's*) ......................210
chocolate mint chip (*Stonyfield Farm* Organic Lowfat).............130
crème caramel (*Stonyfield Farm* Organic Lowfat)....................120
coffee (*Häagen-Dazs* Fat Free)..............................................140
coffee (*Stonyfield Farm* Decaf Organic Nonfat)........................90
coffee fudge sundae (*Edy's* Fat Free) ....................................100
cookies 'n cream (*Edy's/Dreyer's*) ..........................................110
dulce de leche (*Häagen-Dazs* Lowfat) ...................................190
(*Edy's/Dreyer's* Mumbo Jumbo) .............................................120
(*Edy's/Dreyer's* Hokey Pokey) ...............................................140
mocha almond fudge (*Stonyfield Farm* Organic Lowfat) ..........130
raspberry (*Stonyfield Farm* Organic Nonfat) ...........................100
strawberry (*Breyers* All Natural).............................................120
strawberry (*Häagen-Dazs* Nonfat) .........................................140
tin roof sundae (*Edy's/Dreyer's* Ultimate)...............................130
toffee crunch (*Edy's/Dreyer's Heath*) ......................................120
vanilla (*Dreyer's*)..................................................................100
vanilla (*Edy's*)......................................................................130
vanilla (*Edy's/Dreyer's* Fat Free).............................................90
vanilla (*Häagen-Dazs* Fat Free) .............................................140
vanilla (*Stonyfield Farm* Organic Nonfat) .................................90
vanilla or vanilla/chocolate/strawberry (*Breyers* All Natural) ....120
vanilla chocolate swirl (*Edy's/Dreyer's* Fat Free).......................90
vanilla raspberry swirl (*Häagen-Dazs* Fat Free) ......................130
**Yogurt bar,** frozen (*Ben & Jerry's Cherry Garcia*), 1 bar..........250
**Yokan,** from mature adzuki beans, .5-oz. slice ............................36

**Yu choy sum** (*Frieda's*), 1 cup, 3 oz. ..........................................20
**Yuca root** (*Frieda's*), ½ cup, 3 oz. ..........................................100
**Ziti,** see "Pasta"
**Zucchini,** fresh:
raw, w/skin, sliced, 1 cup ..............................................................16
raw, w/skin, chopped, 1 cup..........................................................17
raw, baby, 1 large, .6 oz. ..................................................................3
raw, baby (*Frieda's*), ⅔ cup, 3 oz. ..............................................20
raw, baby, 1 medium, .4 oz. ............................................................2
boiled, drained, w/skin, sliced, 1 cup .............................................29
boiled, drained, w/skin, mashed, ½ cup .........................................19
**Zucchini,** canned:
Italian style, 1 cup..........................................................................66
w/tomato sauce, Italian style (*Del Monte*), ½ cup .....................30
**Zucchini,** frozen:
w/skin, unprepared, 10-oz. pkg.......................................................48
w/skin, boiled, drained, 1 cup .........................................................38

# Corinne T. Netzer

## SHE KNOWS WHAT'S GOOD FOR YOU!

___ 22563-9  THE COMPLETE BOOK OF FOOD COUNTS
5th Edition / $7.50

___ 23455-7  THE CORINNE T. NETZER CALORIE COUNTER FOR THE YEAR
2002 / $6.99

___ 22609-0  BIG BOOK OF MIRACLE CURES / $6.99

___ 21109-3  THE BRAND NAME CALORIE COUNTER / $5.99

___ 23682-7  THE CORINNE T. NETZER CARBOHYDRATE COUNTER
7th Edition / $6.50

___ 20739-8  THE CHOLESTEROL CONTENT OF FOOD
Revised and Updated / $5.50

___ 22055-6  THE CORINNE T. NETZER FAT GRAM COUNTER
Revised and Updated / $5.99

___ 22335-0  THE COMPLETE BOOK OF VITAMIN AND
MINERAL COUNTS / $6.50

___ 50410-4  THE CORINNE T. NETZER DIETER'S DIARY / $9.95

___ 50821-5  THE DIETER'S CALORIE COUNTER Third Edition / $11.95

NF3 9/01